GASTROINTESTINAL EMERGENCIES

GASTROINTESTINAL EMERGENCIES

edited by

Ian T. Gilmore

MA, MD, FRCP,

Consultant Physician, Royal Liverpool University Hospital

and

Robert Shields

DL, MD, DSc, FRCS(Edin), FRCS(Eng), FACS, FCS(SA)

Professor and Head of Department of Surgery, University of Liverpool and
Royal Liverpool University Hospital

W B Saunders Company
Harcourt Brace Jovanovich, Publishers
London   Philadelphia   Toronto
Sydney   Tokyo

W. B. Saunders Company   24–28 Oval Road
London NW1 7DX, England

West Washington Square
Philadelphia, PA 19105, USA

1 Goldthorne Avenue
Toronto, Ontario M8Z 5T9, Canada

ABP Australia Ltd
44–50 Waterloo Road
North Ryde, NSW 2113
Australia

Harcourt Brace Jovanovich Japan Inc.
Ichibancho Central Building, 22-1 Ichibancho
Choyoda-ku, Tokyo 102, Japan

First published 1992

This book is printed on acid free paper

A catalogue record for this book is available from the British Library

ISBN 0–7020–1558–X

Typeset by Mathematical Composition Setters Ltd., Salisbury, Wiltshire, UK, and printed in Great Britain by The University Press, Cambridge.

CONTENTS

CONTRIBUTORS

A. ALLAN MD, FRCS, Consultant Surgeon, Good Hope Hospital, Birmingham, B75 7RR, UK.

J. ALEXANDER-WILLIAMS MD, FRCS, Professor of Gastrointestinal Surgery, The General Hospital, Birmingham, B4 6NH, UK.

DION R. BELL MB, ChB, FRCP, FFPHM, DTM and H, Lately Reader in Tropical Medicine, Liverpool School of Tropical Medicine and Honorary Consultant Physician, Royal Liverpool University Hospital, Liverpool, UK.

DAVID C. CARTER MD, FRCS(Ed), FRCS(Glasg), Regius Professor of Clinical Surgery, University of Edinburgh, Honorary Consultant Surgeon, The Royal Infirmary of Edinburgh, Scotland, UK.

R. A. COBB MS, FRCS, Senior Surgical Registrar, John Radcliffe Hospital, Oxford, OX3 9DU, UK.

A. CUSCHIERI, MD, ChM. FRCS(Eng), FRCS(Edin), Professor of Surgery, Ninewells Hospital and Medical School, Dundee, DD1 9SY, Scotland, UK.

DAVID PAUL DRAKE MA, MB, BChir, FRCS, DCH, The Hospitals for Sick Children, London, Institute of Child Health, Guildford Street, London, WC1, UK.

JOHN L. DUNCAN ChM, FRCS (Ed.), Consultant Surgeon, Raigmore Hospital, Inverness, Scotland.

P. W. DYKES MD, FRCP, FRACP, Consultant Physician, The General Hospital, Steelhouse Lane, Birmingham, B4 6NH, UK.

DAVID J. GERTNER BSc, MB, MRCP, Senior Registrar, The Royal London Hospital, Whitechapel, London, E1 1BB. Former Research Fellow, St Mark's Hospital.

I. T. GILMORE MA, MD, FRCP, Consultant Physician, Royal Liverpool University Hospital, Prescot Street, Liverpool, L7 8XP, UK.

M. R. B. KEIGHLEY FRCS, Barling Professor of Surgery, Queen Elizabeth Hospital, Queen Elizabeth Medical Centre, Edgbaston, Birmingham, B15 2TH, UK.

A. N. KINGSNORTH MS, FRCS, Senior Lecturer in Surgery, University of Liverpool, PO Box 147, Liverpool, L69 3BX and Consultant Surgeon, Broadgreen Hospital, Thomas Drive, Liverpool, L14 3LB.

M. J. S. LANGMAN MD, FRCP, Professor of Medicine, University of Birmingham Medical School, Queen Elizabeth Hospital, Birmingham, B15 2TH, UK.

M. LAVELLE-JONES FRCS, Department of Surgery, Ninewells Hospital and Medical School, Dundee, DD1 9SY, Scotland, UK.

JOHN E. LENNARD-JONES MD, FRCP, Consultant Gastroenterologist, St Mark's Hospital, London, EC1V 2PS, Emeritus Professor of Gastroenterology, University of London, UK.

ADRIAN MARSTON MA, DM, MCh, FRCS, MD, Consultant Surgeon, The Middlesex and University College Hospital, Mortimer Street, London W1A 8AA, UK.

ANTHONY I. MORRIS BSc(Hons), MSc, MD, FRCP, Consultant Physician, Royal Liverpool University Hospital, Prescot Street, Liverpool, L7 8XP, Clinical Lecturer, University of Liverpool.

JOHN G. O'GRADY MD, MRCPI, Senior Lecturer, Institute of Liver Studies, King's College Hospital, London, SE5, UK.

I. R. SANDERSON MRCP, Academic Department of Paediatric Gastroenterology, Queen Elizabeth Hospital for Children, Hackney Road, London, E2 8PS, UK.

ROBERT SHIELDS Kt, DL, MD, DSc, FRCS, FACS, FCS(SA), Head of Department, Department of Surgery, The University of Liverpool, PO Box 147, Liverpool L69 3BX, UK and Honorary Consultant Surgeon, Royal Liverpool University Hospital and Broadgreen Hospital, Liverpool.

J. H. SNYMAN MB, ChB, MMed(Chir), South African Medical Research Council Research Fellow, Department of Surgery, Universitase Hospital, Bloemfontain 9300, South Africa.

CHRISTOPHER J. STODDARD MD, FRCS, Consultant Surgeon, Royal Hallamshire Hospital, Glossop Road, Sheffield, S10 2JF, UK.

B. A. TAYLOR MA, MCh, FRCS, Senior Lecturer in Surgery, University of Liverpool, PO Box 147, Liverpool, L69 3BX, and Honorary Consultant Surgeon, Royal Liverpool Hospital, Prescot Street, Liverpool, L7 8XP and Broadgreen Hospital, Thomas Drive, Liverpool L14 3LB, UK.

W. E. G. THOMAS BSc, MBBS, FRCS, MS, Consultant Surgeon, Royal Hallamshire Hospital, Glossop Road, Sheffield S10 2JF, UK.

J. A. WALKER-SMITH MD(Sydney), FRCP(Ed. & Lon), FRACP, Academic Department of Paediatric Gastroenterology, Queen Elizabeth Hospital for Children, Hackney Road, London, E2 8PS, UK.

R. P. WALT MD, MRCP, Senior Lecturer in Medicine, University of Birmingham Medical School, Queen Elizabeth Hospital, Birmingham, B15 2TH, UK.

ROGER WILLIAMS MD, FRCP, FRCS, FRCPE, FRACP, Director and Consultant Physician, Institute of Liver Studies, King's College Hospital, London SE5 9RS, UK.

R. C. N. WILLIAMSON MA, MD, MChir, FRCS, Professor and Director of Surgery, Royal Postgraduate Medical School, Hammersmith Hospital, London, W12 0NN, UK.

FOREWORD

The practice of modern gastroenterology requires not only expertise in the out-patient department and endoscopy suite but also the ability to react swiftly and appropriately to urgent and life-threatening illnesses precipitating admission to hospital. In practice, this often requires close co-operation between physician and surgeon, and we have felt it appropriate to maintain these close ties throughout this book. It is not intended as a pocketbook for the resident on his way to a gastrointestinal emergency but as a distillate of current thinking on the overall management strategy, in a timeframe of days or sometimes weeks. Authors have been chosen for their practical experience in dealing with the specific conditions covered.

Acute gastrointestinal haemorrhage remains one of the most frequent and demanding emergencies, and so there is no apology for devoting the first five chapters to it. Non-operative intervention is in vogue, but many clinicians are uncertain about its use except in specialized centres or occasional patients. It is hoped that a balanced view emerges through the different contributions on these and other topics. The chapters are also linked by each having a concluding section on outstanding problems and future prospects.

We would like to thank the contributors for the high standard of their chapters, the publishers for their co-operation and Miss Dawn Armitage for secretarial assistance.

I

UPPER GASTROINTESTINAL HAEMORRHAGE—EPIDEMIOLOGY

M. J. S. Langman and R. P. Walt

THE PROBLEM

Acute upper gastrointestinal bleeding occurs in approximately one in 2000 of the population each year and therefore causes about 30 000 admissions in the United Kingdom. About half the cases are associated with peptic ulceration and death rates vary between 5% and 10%, particularly with age. Mortality rates have remained persistently high, probably because ulcer bleeding is becoming increasingly a problem of the elderly. Similar trends probably apply elsewhere.

Incidence

Overall frequency data indicate that between 40 and 150 individuals per 100 000 population are admitted to hospital with haematemesis and melaena in Western communities (Table 1). Such overall data are however of little value. The causes of bleeding are heterogeneous, and their impact has differed with time and according to age.

Causes

Table 2 shows the frequency of detection of the various causes of bleeding in a number of representative series, demonstrating the general frequency of duodenal

TABLE I

Frequency of upper gastrointestinal bleeding in European series

	Reference	Crude rates per 100 000 population
Oxford, England	Schiller et al (1970)	47
Aberdeen, Scotland	Johnston et al (1973)	116
Rural Sweden	Herner et al (1965)	144

TABLE 2
Percentage distribution by diagnostic categories of cases of acute upper gastrointestinal bleeding

	UK		Australia	USA	
	Oxford 1963–1967[a]	Nottingham 1975–1979[b]	Newcastle 1964–1974[c]	Texas 1976–1977[d]	Texas 1981[e]
Duodenal ulcer	30.1	23.2	29.6	26.3	22.0
Gastric ulcer	14.1	25.5	19.5	21.1	18.0
Gastric cancer	2.6	3.0	0.9	2.1	2.0
Acute gastric lesions		6.7 ⎫	15.7	2.1	6.0
Oesophagitis and ulcer	Not ⎱	12.2 ⎭		—	—
Mallory–Weiss syndrome	stated ⎰		4.0	23.2	16.0
Oesophageal varices	3.1	1.9	4.6	20.0	20.0
Other known diagnoses	31.0	—	10.2	2.2	—
Diagnosis unclear	19.2	27.4	Not stated	3.1	16.0
	688	526	568	95	100

[a] Schiller et al (1970); [b] Dronfield et al (1982); [c] Duggan (1986); [d] Graham (1980); [e] Peterson et al (1981).

and gastric ulceration. Cross comparison is difficult. Acute lesions are classified separately by some but ignored by others, who probably include them as gastric and duodenal ulcers. They generally do not present difficult problems of management. In addition, the chances of detecting acute lesions will fall rapidly if endoscopy is delayed, but if lesions are so evanescent it seems doubtful if it would have been worth detecting them in the first place. Also, the type of institution in which the study takes place may greatly influence the pattern of admission and hence of diagnosis. Thus hospitals for the indigent in the United States are likely to see bleeding oesophageal varices more often than private institutions; similarly there is a high admission rate to hospitals in continental Europe because national alcohol consumption is still relatively high.

Deaths

Ulcer disease is a common and important cause of death, usually the result of complications. Table 3 shows that of some 6000 deaths in England and Wales in 1986 slightly more were associated with bleeding than with perforation. Gastric ulcer deaths were more common in women than men whilst duodenal ulcer deaths tended to be more often in men with bleeding, and more often in women with perforation.

Overall totals are comparatively unrevealing. Age-specific data (Table 4) show that death rates with bleeding rise between 50- and 100-fold with increasing age, both for gastric and duodenal ulcers and in men and women.

Death rates from acute upper gastrointestinal bleeding have fallen considerably between the 1920s and the end of the Second World War but have fallen little if at all since (Table 5). The improvement during the initial 20 years probably represents the benefit coming from blood transfusion. Apparent lack of

TABLE 3
Deaths in England and Wales from peptic ulcer in 1986 (OPCS, 1988)

Site	Total		Bleeding	Perforation	Both
Stomach	M	1122	467	244	—
	F	1385	547	387	
Duodenum	M	1803	649	639	16
	F	1527	438	713	25
Peptic unspecified	M	523	165	94	—
	F	603	207	137	

TABLE 4
Deaths per 100 000 population in England and Wales from bleeding gastric and duodenal ulcer (OPCS, 1988)

	Age (years)				
	0–49	50–59	60–69	70–79	80+
Gastric					
Men	0.06	1.2	4.6	11.8	27.7
Women	0.03	0.8	2.4	7.0	24.8
Duodenal					
Men	0.1	2.0	5.9	17.8	34.8
Women	0.04	0.4	2.3	6.0	18.9

TABLE 5
Death rates from upper gastrointestinal bleeding and proportions of patients aged 60 and over

		No. of patients	% aged 60 and over	% dying
Birmingham[a]	1926–1931	123	6	22
London[b]	1921–1930	137	10	21
Oxford[c]	1938–1947	305	28	19
London[d]	1940–1947	687	33	10
Aberdeen[e]	1941–1948	476	29	14
Oxford[f]	1953–1957	674		10
	1958–1962	787	47	8
	1963–1967	688		9
	Overall	2149	47	9
Birmingham[g]	1971–1973	300	48	10
North-east Scotland[h]	1967–1968	817	49	14
Newcastle (NSW)[i]	1964–1969	568	33	8
Nottingham[j]	1975–1977	526	Unknown	11

[a] Bulmer (1932); [b] Burger and Hartfall (1934); [c] Lewin and Truelove (1949); [d] Jones (1947); [e] Needham and McConachie (1950); [f] Schiller et al (1970); [g] Allan and Dykes (1976); [h] Johnston et al (1973); [i] Duggan (1986); [j] Dronfield et al (1982).

improvement since seems likely to be associated in great part with rising patient age. Comparison with data from elsewhere is hampered by a paucity of figures covering a reasonable time span and also by the variable contribution of liver disease. However comparable trends seem to be evident in Australia (Kang and Piper, 1980; Rofe et al, 1985).

PEPTIC ULCER HAEMORRHAGE

Table 6 shows data from a single large group of ulcer patients. It confirms the generally held beliefs that duodenal bleeding is more common than gastric ulcer haemorrhage, that duodenal ulcers tend to be more common in men, and that patients with gastric ulcer may be more likely to die than duodenal ulcer patients. However this difference may only reflect the higher average age of gastric ulcer patients since in those dying the ages of gastric and duodenal ulcer patients were virtually the same.

Mortality rates in the Nottingham series are somewhat higher than those recorded elsewhere but it is difficult to know whether this indicates a real difference and hence by implication inferior management, or poorer general condition due to other diseases, or, as seems likely, greater age. Thus Duggan (1986) recorded a mortality rate of 3.6% in duodenal ulcer patients and 8.9% in those with gastric ulcer, but the average age of the patients with bleeding would seem to have been 50 years.

Prognostic indices

Those who are elderly presumably withstand rebleeding poorly or may be more likely to die if operated upon. Useful prognostic indicators have been sought, but apart from endoscopic predictive stigmata, little of note has emerged. Swain et al (1986) noted that 54 of 93 patients (58%) with visible vessels suffered rebleeding compared with two of 36 (6%) with other stigmata and none of 107 without stigmata. This trend is in broad conformity with earlier suggestions (Foster et al, 1978).

TABLE 6
Peptic ulcer bleeding Nottingham 1975–1980
(Vellacott et al, 1982)

	Ulcer site	
	Gastric	Duodenal
No.	398	510
% male	49.5	79.2
Mean age (years)	67	61
% dying	13.3	9.6
Mean age in those dying	73	74

Predisposing factors

Drug-induced ulcer

Aspirin intake has long been accepted as causing acute upper gastrointestinal bleeding although the frequency of the sequence has been contested. Broadly similar trends have now been noted for non-aspirin non-steroidal anti-inflammatory drugs.

The literature concerned with drug-induced ulcer has been cogently criticized by Kurata et al (1982), who drew attention to poor design, lack of proper controls and small studies. However the weight of evidence overwhelmingly indicates that drug-induced damage poses a significant clinical problem.

Aspirin Much of the published evidence is now 20 or more years old and suffers from the defects of poor design and also from the inability of the available endoscopes to examine the duodenum. Many diagnoses were therefore made radiologically, with inherent uncertainty about their value particularly if suggesting duodenal ulcer on the basis of cap deformity. Secondly, the exemplar of the aspirin lesion was believed to be an acute gastric erosion although it is now clear that these form a minor proportion of diagnosed disease. Table 7 shows data obtained in some of these, and in more recent studies. Raised relative risks are uniformly apparent although the level of risk varies considerably. The findings of these retrospective case control studies can be contrasted with the outcome of trials of cardiovascular prophylaxis (Table 8) where risks appear to be negligible. The reason for the divergence is unclear, but may partly depend upon patient selection.

Our own recently acquired data suggest (Faulkner et al, 1988) that risks are elevated by between two- and fourfold for both gastric and duodenal ulcer. Relative risks are difficult to put into perspective unless we can measure underlying absolute risk. However if half of all haematemesis and melaena is due to gastric and duodenal ulcer, and the overall number of cases of bleeding is 30 000 in a 60 million population, then there must be approximately 15 000 cases of ulcer bleeding or one in every 4000 people each year. If aspirin doubles the risk, then in a taker the risk should be of the order of one episode for every 2000 takers. Another way of examining the problem is to calculate attributable risk by standard

TABLE 7

Retrospective case control data on the risk of aspirin-associated haematemesis and melaena

	Relative risk	95% confidence interval
Kelly (1956)	11.6	3.3–50.3
Alvarez and Summerskill (1958)	5.8	2.9–11.8
Allibone and Flint (1958)	1.1	0.6–11.8
Muir and Cossar (1959)	6.1	3.0–12.3
Parry and Wood (1967)	4.6	2.8– 7.6
Coggon et al (1982)	4.8	2.4–10.7

TABLE 8

Results of cardiovascular surveillance studies concerning aspirin-associated gastrointestinal bleeding

	Relative risk	95% confidence interval
Elwood et al (1974)	1.0	0.3–3.8
Aspirin Myocardial Infarction Study Research Group (1980)	1.7	1.3–2.1
Canadian Cooperative Study Group (1978)	—	0.2–2.3
The Coronary Drug Project Research Group (1976)	1.1–1.9	—
Fields et al (1977)	1.3	0.6–2.7

TABLE 9

Non-steroidal anti-inflammatory drugs included in lists of the ten drugs most frequently reported to cause adverse drug reactions in 1982 (Griffin, 1986)

Australia	Indomethacin, naproxen, sulindac
Denmark	Benoxaprofen, fenbufen, ibuprofen
Finland	Piroxicam tolmetin
France	Acetylsalicylic acid
Germany	Benoxaprofen, diclofenac, piroxicam
Ireland	Indomethacin, piroxicam
Italy	Diclofenac, diflunisal, zomepirac
Japan	Indomethacin, mefanamic acid, piroxicam sulindac
New Zealand	Naproxen, sulindac
Sweden	Piroxicam
United Kingdom	Benoxaprofen, fenbufen, piroxicam, zomepirac

epidemiological methods; it would seem to be approximately 0.10, indicating that about 1 in every 10 ulcer bleeds (at least in the population aged 60 and over who were studied) were caused by aspirin, or about 1000 episodes annually in the 10 000 ulcer patients aged 60 and over. Whether the same risk applies to younger patients is unclear because the requisite case control studies have not been done.

Non-aspirin non-steroidal anti-inflammatory drugs The introduction of each new non-aspirin non-steroidal anti-inflammatory drug (non-aspirin NSAID) has been quickly followed by reports of adverse effects, most of them gastrointestinal (Table 9). Spontaneous reports are biased samples of a total group of unknown size, and in which association cannot necessarily be taken to indicate causation. The true size of the problem can only be determined by methodical retrospective or prospective study (Langman, 1989).

Three retrospective case control comparisons have been reported in the United Kingdom, but one of these was concerned solely with ulcer perforation (Collier and Pain, 1985). The second examined antecedent drug intake in patients with life-threatening complications, haemorrhage or perforation, who underwent surgery or died. In the third (Somerville et al, 1986), we examined antecedent drug intake of all types in all patients admitted with bleeding gastric and duodenal ulcers over

TABLE 10
Relative risks of ulcer and its complications

Non-aspirin NSAIDs				95% confidence interval
Ulcer occurrence				
Gastric	Australia	5.0	(Duggan et al, 1986)	1.4–26.9
	Australia	4.7	(McIntosh et al, 1985)	1.3–16.6
Duodenal	Australia	1.1	(Duggan et al, 1986)	0.4– 3.7
Ulcer complications				
Bleeding	UK	3.8	(Somerville et al, 1986)	2.2– 6.4
	USA	1.5	(Carson et al, 1987)	1.1– 4.9
Perforation	USA	1.6	(Jick et al, 1987)	0.7– 3.7
Death	USA	4.7	(Griffin et al, 1988)	3.1– 7.2

a 2-year period, matching those over 60 with controls, both hospital in-patient and community. Relative risks were raised by approximately three- to fourfold.

Suggestions have been made that NSAID-induced damage is a particular problem of the elderly or of the very elderly, and that drug exposure is associated with a particular risk of dying. The data in Table 10 show that relative risks vary according to the study carried out, but that the risks for ulcer complications and for death are rather similar. This supports the concept that the NSAID taker may not be at special risk of death over and above that associated with NSAID-associated occurrence of that complication (Henry et al, 1987). The United States data (Jick et al 1987, Carson et al 1987, Griffin et al 1988) are of interest because the methodology employed was that of surveillance in NSAID script recipients and controls. A fourth study of script recipients in the UK has given a result in broad conformity (Beardon et al, 1989).

Whether the elderly or extreme elderly are at particular risk is unclear since case control data collected from younger individuals are not available. However the burden of disease is likely to be greatest in older people simply because they are the most likely to take NSAIDs.

Calculations suggest that about 20% of all bleeding ulcer in those over 60, or about 2000 cases a year, are non-aspirin NSAID induced (Somerville et al, 1986), so that approximately a third of the total set of ulcer bleeds in those aged 60 and over is likely to be aspirin or non-aspirin NSAID-induced. It is unclear whether the lesions responsible are new or pre-existing. Many of the patients, however, have been completely symptom free before admission, so that avoidance of NSAIDs by those with pre-existing ulcer or dyspepsia may be an ineffective method of preventing severe NSAID-associated damage.

Corticosteroids Though having a strong reputation for causing peptic ulcer complications, the evidence in favour is essentially anecdotal outside meta-analysis combining data from all clinical trials (Messer et al, 1983). Risks appear to be modest, except in association with high dose treatment, and the burden of disease is probably small given, at least by NSAID standards, the small usage of corticosteroids.

Alcohol

Though it is frequently claimed that alcohol intake predisposes to upper gastrointestional bleeding, supportive evidence is poor beyond the obvious association between alcoholic cirrhosis and variceal bleeding. Coggon et al (1982) found a small excess of heavy alcohol consumers, 56 out of 346, in those with bleeding (16%) compared with 33 out of 346 (10%) in matched controls. The claim often made that alcohol and aspirin act synergistically to cause bleeding is also unsupported by epidemiological data.

Genetic factors

The early finding that blood group O was associated with peptic ulceration was followed by evidence that complications, certainly bleeding (Langman and Doll, 1965) and possibly perforation of ulcer, especially duodenal ulcer, were particularly associated. The basis is unclear; a marginal depression of plasma factor VIII levels has been detected in individuals of group O (Preston and Barr, 1964), but whether this accounts for the association of blood group with bleeding is unclear.

Seasonality

Varied patterns have been described. These have been of more frequent bleeding in spring and autumn, or in the winter. The cause of the variation described is uncertain. It may simply mirror the seasonal exacerbation of ulcer (Langman, 1964).

NON-ULCER BLEEDING

Apart from varying frequency, comparisons are hindered because clinicians vary in the classifications they apply. The liver disease group may be easier to define but the type responsible and severity seem likely to be important prognostic factors. Thus alcoholic and chronic viral disease are likely to differ in outcome. De Dombal et al (1986), in a multinational study which included 44 centres in 21 countries collecting data from over 4000 patients, found that age, a history of liver disease, continued bleeding and indications of initially profuse haemorrhage (haemoglobin below 10 g/dl and a systolic blood presence below 90 mmHg) correlated best with rebleeding, none of which seems unexpected.

Predisposing factors

Variceal haemorrhage is the most important cause of non-ulcer bleeding, but the predisposing causes are poorly understood. Factors invoked have included deteriorating liver function, particularly large varices, concomitant oesophageal acid–peptic attack, the presence of ascites and fluctuating portal pressure. Evidence has tended to conflict, thus normal lower oesophageal sphincter pressures have been reported (Eckhardt et al, 1976), according poorly with the concept that associated reflux is important. Elsewhere, Lebrec et al (1980) concluded that in alcoholic cirrhosis portal pressure had no predictive value, whereas the size of varices did.

CONCLUSIONS AND THE WAY FORWARD

Death rates from haematemesis and melaena have changed little in the last 40 years despite improvements in resuscitating methods and in diagnostic techniques. The lack of change in death rates almost certainly reflects the greater age of patients with ulcer bleeding, who form the majority of those dying in recent years, compared with up to the time of the Second World War. Variceal bleeding remains uncommon, except in populations with high rates of alcohol consumption or where special factors, such as endemic schistostomiasis, prevail, and outcome tends to reflect the severity of underlying liver disease. Predisposing factors are poorly understood, but use of non-steroidal anti-inflammatory drugs by the elderly appears to account for a quarter to a third of all ulcer bleeding. The advanced age of the generality of patients indicates that simpler non-operative methods of treatment have much to commend them.

REFERENCES

Allan RN & Dykes PW (1976) A study of the factors influencing mortality rates from gastrointestinal haemorrhage. *Quarterly Journal of Medicine* **45**: 533–550.
Allibone A & Flint FJ (1958) Bronchitis aspirin smoking and other factors in the aetiology of peptic ulcer. *Lancet* **2**: 179–182.
Alvarez AS & Summerskill WHJ (1958) Gastrointestinal haemorrhage and salicylates. *Lancet* **1**: 920–928.
Armstrong CP & Blower AL (1987) Non steroidal anti-inflammatory drugs and life-threatening complications of peptic ulceration. *Gut* **28**: 527–532.
Aspirin Myocardial Infarction Study Research Group (1980) A randomized controlled trial of aspirin in persons recovered from myocardial infarction. *Journal of the American Medical Association* **243**: 661–669.
Beardon PHG, Brown SV & McDevitt DG (1989) Gastrointestinal events in patients prescribed non steroidal anti-inflammatory drugs: a controlled study using record linkage in Tayside. *Quarterly Journal of Medicine* **71**: 497–505.
Bulmer E (1932) Mortality from haematemesis. *Lancet* **2**: 720–722.
Burger F & Hartfall SJ (1934) Haematemesis in peptic ulcer. *Guy's Hospital Report* **84**: 197–209.
Canadian Cooperative Study Group (1978) A randomized trial of aspirin and sulfinpyrazone in threatened stroke. *New England Journal of Medicine* **299**: 53–58.
Carson JL, Strom BL, Soper KA, West SL & Morse ML (1987) The association of non steroidal anti-inflammatory drugs with upper gastrointestinal bleeding. *Archives of Internal Medicine* **147**: 85–88.
Coggon D, Langman MJS & Spiegelhalter DJ (1982) Aspirin, paracetamol, haematemesis and melaena. *Gut* **23**: 340–344.

Collier DS & Pain JA (1985) Non steroidal anti-inflammatory drugs and peptic ulcer perforation. *Gut* **26**: 359–363.

de Dombal FT, Clarke JR, Clamp SE, Malizia G, Kotwal MR & Morgan AG (1986) Prognostic factors in upper GI bleeding. *Endoscopy* **18**: 6–10.

Dronfield MW, Langman MJS, Atkinson M, Balfour TW, Bell GD, Vellacott KD, Amar SS & Knapp DR (1982) Outcome of endoscopy and barium radiography for acute upper gastrointestinal bleeding: controlled trial in 1037 patients. *British Medical Journal* **284**: 545–548.

Duggan JM (1986) Haematemesis patients should be managed in special units. *Medical Journal of Australia* **144**: 247–250.

Duggan JM, Dobson AJ, Johnson H & Fahey P (1986) Peptic ulcer and non steroidal anti-inflammatory agents. *Gut* **27**: 929–933.

Eckhardt VF, Grace ND & Kantrowitz PA (1976) Does lower esophageal sphincter pressure incompetency contribute to esophageal variceal bleeding? *Gastroenterology* **71**: 185–189.

Elwood PC, Cochrane AL, Burr ML, Williams G & Welsley E (1974) A randomized controlled trial of acetyl salicylic acid in the secondary prevention of mortality from myocardial infarction. *British Medical Journal* **1**: 436–440.

Faulkner G, Prichard P, Somerville K & Langman MJS (1988) Aspirin and bleeding peptic ulcers in the elderly. *British Medical Journal* **297**: 1311–1313.

Fields WS, Lemak NA, Frankowski RF & Hardy RJ (1977) Controlled trial of aspirin in cerebral ischemia. AITIA study. *Stroke* **8**: 301–315.

Foster DN, Miloszewski KJA & Losowsky MS (1978) Stigmata of recent haemorrhage in diagnosis and prognosis of upper gastrointestinal bleeding. *British Medical Journal* **1**: 1173–1177.

Graham DY (1980) Limited value of early endoscopy in management of acute upper gastrointestinal bleeding. Prospective controlled trial. *American Journal of Surgery* **140**: 284–290.

Griffin JP (1986) Survey of the spontaneous adverse drug reaction reporting schemes in fifteen countries. *British Journal of Clinical Pharmacology* **22 (supplement)**: 835–1005.

Griffin MR, Ray WA & Schaffner W (1988) Non steroidal anti-inflammatory drug use and death from peptic ulcer in elderly persons. *Annals of Internal Medicine* **109**: 359–363.

Henry DA, Johnston A, Dobson A & Duggan JM (1987) Fatal peptic ulcer complications and the use of non steroidal anti-inflammatory drugs, aspirin and corticosteroids. *British Medical Journal* **295**: 1227–1228.

Herner B, Kallgand B & Lauritsen A (1965) Haematemesis and melaena from a limited reception area during a five year period. *Acta Medica Scandinavica* **177**: 483–492.

Jick SS, Perera DR, Walker AM & Jick H (1987) Non steroidal anti-inflammatory drugs and hospital admission for perforated peptic ulcer. *Lancet* **ii**, 380–382.

Johnston SJ, Jones PF, Kyle J et al (1973) Epidemiology and cause of gastrointestinal haemorrhage in North East Scotland. *British Medical Journal* **3**: 655–660.

Jones FA (1947) Haematemesis and melaena with special reference to bleeding peptic ulcer. *British Medical Journal* **2**: 441–446.

Kang JY & Piper DW (1980) Improvement in mortality rates in bleeding peptic ulcer disease. *Medical Journal of Australia* **1**: 213–215.

Kelly J (1956) Salicylate ingestion, a frequent cause of gastric hemorrhage. *American Journal of Medical Science* **232**: 119–127.

Kurata JH, Elashoff JD & Grossman MI (1982) Inadequacy of the literature on the relationship between drugs, ulcers and gastrointestinal bleeding. *Gastroenterology* **82**: 373–382.

Langman MJS (1964) The seasonal incidence of bleeding from the upper gastrointestinal tract. *Gut* **5**: 142–144.

Langman MJS (1989) Epidemiologic evidence on the association between peptic ulceration and anti-inflammatory drug use. *Gastroenterology* **96**: 640–646.

Langman MJS & Doll R (1965) ABO blood groups and secretor status in relation to clinical characteristics of peptic ulcer. *Gut* **6**: 270–273.

Lebrec D, De Fleury P, Rueff B, Nahum H & Benhamon JP (1980) Portal hypertension, size of esophageal varices, and risk of gastrointestal bleeding in alcoholic cirrhosis. *Gastroenterology* **79**: 1139–1144.

Lewin DC & Truelove SC (1949) Haematemesis with special reference to chronic peptic ulcer. *British Medical Journal* **1**: 383–386.

McIntosh JH, Byth K & Piper DW (1985) Environmental factors in aetiology of chronic gastric ulcer. A case-control study of exposure variables before the first symptoms. *Gut* **26**: 789–798.

Messer J, Reitman D, Sacks HS, Smith H & Chalmers TC (1983) Association of adrenocortico steroid therapy and peptic ulcer disease. *New England Journal of Medicine* **309**: 21–29.

Muir A & Cossar IA (1959) Aspirin and gastric haemorrhage. *Lancet* **1**: 539–541.

Needham, CD & McConachie JA (1950) Haematemesis and melaena. *British Medical Journal* **2**: 133–138.

Office of Population Censuses and Surveys (1988) *Mortality Statistics. Cause.* HMSO, London.

Parry DJ & Wood PHN (1967) Relationship between aspirin taking and gastroduodenal haemorrhage. *Gut* **8**: 301–307.

Peterson WL, Barnett CC, Smith HJ, Allen MH & Corbett DB (1981) Routine early endoscopy in upper gastrointestinal tract bleeding. *New England Journal of Medicine* **304**: 925–929.

Preston AE & Barr A (1964) The plasma concentration of factor VIII in the normal population. *British Journal of Haematology* **10**: 238–245.

Rofe SB, Duggan JM, Smith ER & Thursby CJ (1985) Conservative treatment of gastrointestinal haemorrhage. *Gut* **26**: 481–484.

Schiller KFR, Truelove SC & Williams DG (1970) Haematemesis and melaena, with special reference to factors influencing outcome. *British Medical Journal* **2**: 7–14.

Somerville K, Faulkner G & Langman MJS (1986) Non steroidal anti-inflammatory drugs and bleeding peptic ulcer. *Lancet* **1**: 462–464.

Swain CP, Storey DW, Bown SG, Heath J, Mills TN, Salmon PR, Northfield TC, Kirkham J & O'Sullivan PO (1986) Nature of the bleeding vessel in recurrent bleeding gastric ulcers. *Gastroenterology* **90**: 595–608.

The Coronary Drug Research Project Group (1976) Aspirin in coronary heart disease. *Journal of Chronic Disease* **29**: 625–642.

Vellacott KD, Dronfield MW, Atkinson M & Langman MJS (1982) Comparison of surgical and medical management of bleeding peptic ulcers. *British Medical Journal* **284**: 548–551.

2

UPPER GASTROINTESTINAL HAEMORRHAGE—ENDOSCOPIC APPROACHES TO DIAGNOSIS AND TREATMENT

A. I. Morris

INTRODUCTION

Acute upper gastrointestinal bleeding is one of the commonest medical emergencies accounting for over 25 000 admissions to hospitals in the UK each year with an annual admission rate of approximately 100 per 100 000 population. Thus a district general hospital serving a population of 250 000 would expect to see 250 cases a year, almost 4 patients a week. The introduction of fibre optic endoscopy in the early 1970s, although improving the diagnostic accuracy, did not alter the mortality from this condition. Indeed the overall mortality has remained almost constant over the last 50 years at around 10% (Allan and Dykes, 1976; Cutler and Mendeloff, 1981). This disappointing lack of improvement in the face of better diagnosis, resuscitation, anaesthesia and surgery has spurred many gastroenterological physicians and surgeons to look for non-operative ways of reducing the mortality and morbidity from acute gastrointestinal bleeding.

It is thought that one of the main reasons for this continued high mortality is the progressively increasing age of the population (Hunt et al, 1979; Morris et al, 1984). However, closer inspection of the literature has revealed two findings of interest. Firstly Piper and Stiel (1986) in their comprehensive review of the natural history and mortality trends of acute upper gastrointestinal haemorrhage found evidence from three studies that the mortality rate was less than 2% if only bleeding from peptic ulceration was considered. These authors make the point that the three studies from London (La Brooy et al, 1979), Birmingham (Hoare et al, 1979) and Sydney (Kang and Piper, 1980) all originate from units with a long-standing special interest in the management of acute upper gastrointestinal haemorrhage. Secondly Kang and Piper (1980) looked at the age-related mortality rates for patients with acute upper gastrointestinal haemorrhage not due to variceal, cancer or stress-related ulcer, and found that there was 'a marked reduction in the mortality of those over 60 years' from 1939 to 1977. Clearly progress has and can be made in this demanding area, but such changes are masked by the low mortality seen in younger age groups. In addition the progressively increasing age of the population means that in many units the average age of patients admitted with such problems is well over 70.

CAUSES OF ACUTE GASTROINTESTINAL BLEEDING

With the introduction of widespread fibre optic endoscopy services it became clear that many minor mucosal lesions had been missed when the diagnosis of the cause of bleeding had relied on clinical and radiological means. In one report from the UK the causes of upper gastrointestinal bleeding were found to be gastric ulceration in 25.3%, duodenal ulceration 25.1%, gastric/duodenal erosions 22%, oesophagitis in 12.1%, Mallory–Weiss tear and oesophageal varices both 3.7% and gastric carcinoma 0.9% (Holman et al, 1990). The remaining 7% included other rare causes of gastrointestinal bleeding and patients with no identifiable source. In many series varices and Mallory–Weiss tears each contribute about 10% to the total.

The rare causes of upper gastrointestinal bleeding are given in Table 1. The reasons why in a small but definite proportion of cases no identifiable source for bleeding is found are also of some interest—the lesion was missed, the site was not considered and examined or the lesion had healed (Table 2).

The proportion of cases with variceal bleeding is greater in countries where alcohol consumption is higher and where hepatitis B virus infection is common.

In recent years upper gastrointestinal bleeding has been associated with the

TABLE I

Causes of upper gastrointestinal bleeding

Common (10–30%)
Duodenal and gastric ulceration
Oesophagitis
Gastritis
Duodenitis
Varices
Mallory–Weiss tear

Less common (1–5%)
Carcinomas
Bleeding diathesis
Leiomyomas
Aortic aneurysm fistula

Rare (less than 1%)
Dieulafoy lesion
Angiomas
Hereditary haemorrhagic telangiectasia
Pseudoxanthoma elasticum
Ehlers–Danlos syndrome
Haemobilia
Pancreatic bleeding
Foreign body

TABLE 2
Acute upper gastrointestinal bleeding
with no cause found (10%)

Lesion missed
  Site obscured (blood, clot, etc)
  Gastric fundus not fully
  examined
  Inexperienced operator
  Lesion healed

Intermittent bleeding
  Delay in investigating
  Lesion healed

Site not considered/reached
  Nasopharynx
  Second part duodenum or
  beyond
  Biliary tract
  Pancreas

ingestion of non-steroidal anti-inflammatory drugs (NSAIDs) taken for arthritic and locomotor disorders. In patients bleeding from peptic ulceration almost 35% had ingested NSAIDs in the week prior to presentation, the majority (84%) being over the age of 60 (Holman et al, 1990).

PRESENTATION

Patients usually present with haematemesis, melaena, or both. Occasionally patients may present with dizziness prior to the bleeding becoming overt. This is often followed by the passage of melaena as the only sign of bleeding. In patients with arteriosclerosis a brisk bleed, with resulting hypotension, may precipitate myocardial ischaemia or even a stroke.

INITIAL MANAGEMENT AND RESUSCITATION

The initial management depends on the clinical state of the patient. The main priority is to resuscitate the patient and preserve oxygenation of vital organs. The patient should be examined to ascertain if there are: (a) signs of hypovolaemia or shock; (b) clues to the aetiology of the haemorrhage (Table 3).

Particular attention should be paid to signs of sympathetic overactivity, such as sweating and pallor, as well as to blood pressure and pulse rate. Thirst may be a prominent symptom in a hypovolaemic patient. If doubt exists about hypovolaemia, central venous pressure (CVP) monitoring or the insertion of a Swann–Ganz catheter may be necessary. Evidence of hypovolaemia, demands immediate resuscitation.

TABLE 3
Physical signs as clues to the aetiology of upper gastrointestinal bleeding

Clinical features	Possible gastrointestinal abnormality
Signs of portal hypertension	Varices
Telangiectasia (lips, tongue)	Gastroduodenal telangiectasia
Signs of bleeding diathesis	Mucosal bleeding or varices
Arthritis	Peptic ulceration or gastritis
Weight loss	Carcinoma, gastric ulcer
Epigastric mass	Carcinoma
Abnormal skin (elasticity/scarring)	Pseudoxanthoma elasticum/Ehlers–Danlos syndrome

The hypovolaemic patient

For those patients who are clearly hypovolaemic with low blood pressure, tachycardia and/or signs of sympathetic overactivity the first priority is to obtain venous access using a wide-bore cannula. In such patients central venous pressure monitoring is of considerable help, but a central line should be inserted only by an experienced doctor after the initial peripheral venous cannulation. Central venous pressure monitoring should also be considered for all patients requiring large volumes of blood, for those patients with cardiac, renal or respiratory problems, and in the elderly. Even if these patients are not shocked, they tolerate transfusion less well and are at risk of developing heart failure from fluid overload. The patient should be nursed flat or slightly head down and have oxygen administered. Blood for cross-matching and haemoglobin extinction should be taken immediately and, if required, platelet count, prothrombin time, liver function tests and urea and electrolytes. Apart from the clotting factors the other tests are not usually urgent.

If it is thought that the patient might have chronic liver disease or be in a high risk category (homosexuals or i.v. drug abusers), their hepatitis B and possibly HIV status should be checked.

While blood is being cross-matched either crystalloids or a dextran plasma expander should be infused, bearing in mind that these have no oxygen carrying capacity. As soon as blood is available this should be given quickly to raise the CVP to normal. In the most severely ill patient it may be necessary to transfuse universal donor blood. If it is apparent within a short period of time that the vital signs are not improving despite adequate blood replacement a surgeon should be called for consultation immediately. Also those patients who continue to bleed with large fresh haematemesis in whom their vital signs improve with resuscitation should be seen by the surgeons and a decision made about taking them to the operating room. Providing there is no absolute contraindacation to operation, these two groups of patients, the unresuscitable and those continuing to bleed heavily, should be taken straight to the operating room, anaesthetized and a cuffed endotracheal tube inserted to protect their airway. It is then usually prudent to perform an on-table endoscopy to identify the source of bleeding. It is particularly important to exclude varices, for if these are found then they should either be injected or, if there is nobody of sufficient skill and training, a balloon tamponade tube should be inserted (Chapter 4). It is particularly helpful to the surgeon about to undertake the laparotomy to identify the non-variceal source, but may not be feasible because of free blood within the lumen. Providing the patient's condition is not too critical, gastric lavage with ice cold water can be of some value in both reducing the bleeding and enabling the endoscopist to define the source. With or without an endoscopic diagnosis the patient should then proceed to laparotomy as a life-saving procedure.

In those patients unsuitable for such emergency operation because of coincident cardiac, respiratory or other systemic disease and in those who refuse operation there are two options, either therapeutic endoscopy or interventional radiology, both of which will be discussed later. Pharmacological management in such ill patients rarely has a part to play. Intravenous vasopressin or more recently somatostatin or its analogue may be tried, however in bleeding ulcers somatostatin has little effect (Christiansen et al, 1989).

Nasogastric intubation with gastric lavage using ice cold water to which nordrenaline may be added, is sometimes used, particularly in the USA, as a means of reducing mucosal blood flow and haemorrhage. This may give time to both resuscitate the patient and enable other therapeutic options to be considered.

However, the majority of hypovolaemic patients respond well to resuscitation and do not require emergency measures to stop bleeding. Between 80% and 90% of patients admitted with upper gastrointestinal haemorrhage stop bleeding spontaneously. Once the patient is fit to move from the Accident and Emergency Department he or she should be transferred to an appropriate ward with expertise in the management of gastrointestinal bleeding. There is now accumulating evidence that the mortality can be reduced to less than 5% if such patients are managed by a joint team of gastroenterologist and gastrointestinal surgeon. This joint approach is facilitated by having a designated ward area for gastrointestinal bleeding patients, where not only the doctors but also the nursing staff can become expert in the management of these patients. Careful monitoring is essential and remains the responsibility of the doctor. Once the patient has been successfully resuscitated it is sensible to arrange for an early endoscopy (within hours) to identify the source of the blood loss. There is evidence to suggest that delay in performing endoscopy reduces the diagnostic yield (Forrest and Finlayson, 1974).

The non-hypovolaemic patient

These patients can be divided into two categories, those with a trivial bleed of altered blood or specks of fresh blood, and those requiring transfusion who on admission are not hypovolaemic.

The principal indications for transfusion other than hypovolaemia are observed loss of large amount of blood or initial haemoglobin of less than 10 g/dl.

Non-hypovolaemic patients who do not require transfusion should have an indwelling intravenous cannula inserted and be admitted for observation. All patients bleeding from the upper gastrointestinal tract should be fasted until they have a diagnostic endoscopy. For those patients who do not require transfusion the endoscopy can be performed on the next available elective list.

If no lesion is seen at the endoscopy and the patient has had a trivial bleed,

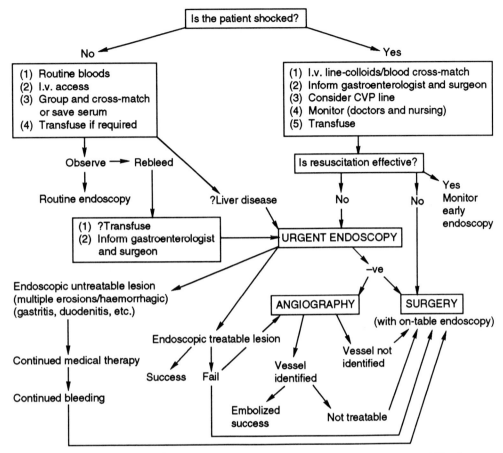

FIGURE 1   Flow diagram of suggested management of acute upper gastrointestinal bleeding

in most cases the patient can be discharged. Many are young, and the bleed is associated with an alcoholic binge. In older patients with definite but small haematemesis and negative endoscopy the patient should be discharged but kept under review.

If bleeding recurs then endoscopy should be repeated. Should this be again negative and there were no technical problems to impede adequate visualization further investigation of the patient may be indicated (Figure 1).

PROGNOSIS

Because of the mortality associated with acute upper gastrointestinal bleeding much effort has gone into the investigation of risk factors that will predict which individual patient is likely to suffer most from bleeding. Most of these studies have focused on those patients bleeding from peptic ulceration as this accounts for 60–70% of all upper gastrointestinal bleeds.

Increasing risk of mortality has been shown (Balint et al, 1977) to be associated

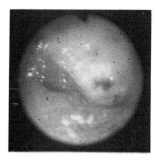

FIGURE 2 Endoscopic appearance of a visible vessel in the base of a peptic ulcer

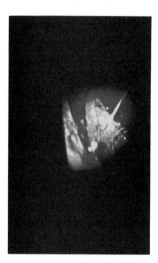

FIGURE 3 Endoscopic appearance of a spurting vessel in the base of a peptic ulcer

with: (a) chronic rather than actute ulceration; (b) gastric rather than duodenal ulceration; (c) age over 60; (d) continued or recurrent bleeding; (e) ulcer pain persisting after admission; (f) presence of other serious concomitant disease.

Many gastroenterologists would believe that age, continued or recurrent bleeding or presence of concomitant disease would be risk factors also for patients bleeding from causes other than peptic ulcer, although there is no proof for this.

On endoscopy there are some important visual clues as to which patient is likely to rebleed from his or her ulcer. Rebleeding increases the mortality rate almost tenfold (Avery Jones, 1956; Macleod and Mills, 1982) and thus these endoscopic signs have important predictive value. They are major stigmata of recent haemorrhage, namely: (a) a visible vessel in the base of an ulcer (Figure 2); (b) a spurting or oozing blood vessel (Figure 3); (c) a fresh adherent blood clot. The presence of any of these stigmata carries a greater than 50% chance of clinical rebleeding (Foster et al, 1978; Storey et al, 1981), and the recognition of this has led to rapid increase in endoscopic methods aimed at both stopping active haemorrhage and preventing recurrent bleeding.

ENDOSCOPIC THERAPY FOR UPPER GASTROINTESTINAL BLEEDING

The development of the modern fibre optic or video endoscope has enabled endoscopists to attempt to directly attack the site of bleeding. Any modern endoscope can be used but in general the larger the biopsy channel the better. Luminal contents including blood are aspirated through this channel to allow visualization of the mucosal surface and narrow channels such as those found in the very slim paediatric endoscopes are very easily blocked by blood clot. Even standard channel instruments (2.8 mm internal diameter) are liable to this problem, and most specialized units prefer to use large diameter biopsy channel instruments (3.4 mm or greater internal diameter) both to help reduce channel blockage and to improve aspiration of intraluminal blood.

The introduction of a therapeutic device down the biopsy channel will severely limit the suction available to the endoscopist. A nasogastric tube passed down alongside the endoscope will aid in aspirating luminal contents. This can be accompanied by gastric lavage to enhance visualization of the mucosal surface. Another approach is to use a twin channel endoscope (Figure 4), allowing one channel for therapy and the other for suction.

The disadvantage of larger or twin channel endoscopes is that their diameter makes them less flexible, making inspection of the duodenal bulb more difficult. Patients who are bleeding are at particular risk of hypoxia, hypotension and aspiration. Emergency endoscopies must be performed by an experienced doctor to maximize the diagnostic yield and to allow endoscopic therapy to be used if appropriate. Trained endoscopy assistants or nursing staff should be available to care for the patient and look after the equipment. The use of pulse oximeters greatly helps in the monitoring of such patients. Many endoscopists prefer to

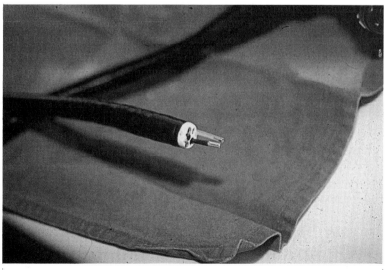

FIGURE 4 A twin-channel therapeutic fibre optic endoscope

undertake endoscopy in a dedicated endoscopy suite where the equipment is available and familiar. Out of normal working hours however, many hospitals use the operating room. Although this has the advantage of having more staff available to assist, they are not always specifically trained in the techniques and the use of theatre time may be limited by other cases. If therapeutic endoscopy is to be undertaken, this may dictate where the procedure is performed, as some laser equipment is fixed in site by plumbing and wiring.

TYPES OF ENDOSCOPIC THERAPY THAT ARE AVAILABLE

Much ingenuity has been shown in endoscopically controlling bleeding and preventing rebleeding. There are basically four techniques (Table 4): (a) topical; (b) injectable; (c) thermal; (d) mechanical. Each technique has its devotees and critics. There is no single technique that is universally accepted, and although there are now many published studies few are adequately controlled randomized trials with enough statistical power to convince all. In addition there are very few trials comparing one haemostatic technique with another.

Topical therapy

The aim is to seal the bleeding point by forming a plug of either blood or some other substance.

Tissue adhesives

Only a few studies have been reported in man, the main problem being the delivery systems. It has been reported that the catheter may become stuck either within the endoscope or to the mucosa. After an initial encouraging study with control of bleeding in five out of six patients (Martin et al, 1977) a subsequent controlled trial in 52 patients failed to show benefit from this technique (Peura et al, 1982). Because of problems with the delivery systems this technique has never become popular.

Collagen

Klein et al (1982) have used microcrystalline collagen to stop bleeding by inducing clotting as well as forming a gel over the site of bleeding. It would seem unlikely that this would stop arterial spurting but it may have a role in oozing lesions. This technique is not widely used, again because of delivery problems and the lack of strong supporting data.

Clotting factors

As with collagen there is very little evidence that the topical application of either thrombin or fibrinogen has any significant role in upper gastrointestinal bleeding.

TABLE 4

Specific therapies for acute upper gastrointestinal bleeding

Oesophageal varices
  Vasopressin
  Sengstaken tube
  Injection sclerotherapy

Ulcers
  Ulcer healing drugs
  Electrocoagulation ⎫
  Thermocoagulation ⎪ If visible
  Photocoagulation   ⎬ vessel
  Injection therapy ⎭

Arteriographic embolization

Vascular abnormalities
  Electrocoagulation
  Thermocoagulation
  Photocoagulation
  Injection therapy

Ferromagnetic tamponade

The novel idea of using a viscous slurry of iron powder, thrombin and a suspending agent held against the site of bleeding by a strong magnetic force has been tried in both animals and humans. According to the authors initial haemostasis was achieved in most patients but when the external magnetic field was turned off rebleeding occurred in about half. This is another technique that has not been actively pursued.

Although of interest none of these techniques has proven to be practical on a large scale although they all have the attraction that no additional expensive equipment is needed.

Thermal techniques

These methods are designed to produce local heat at the point of bleeding to coagulate proteins and cause their contraction. It is this shrinkage of tissue to narrow the vascular lumen that is the chief haemostatic mechanism, with secondary thrombosis within the vessel. In addition, direct pressure at the site further helps in preventing bleeding by sealing the vessel. All these methods are applicable only if the bleeding point or lesion can be reached by the relevant probe. Some lesions high on the lesser curve, in the fundus or in the duodenal bulb cannot be reached by a standard forward viewing endoscope, and better access may be achieved by use of an oblique or side viewing one. With all the current techniques it has been estimated that 75% of those patients with major stigmata of recent haemorrhage have accessible lesions (Bown, 1985).

Diathermy techniques

There are several techniques available using either monopolar, bipolar or liquid spray electrodes. Diathermy equipment is relatively cheap in comparison with other endoscopic methods for delivering local heat.

Monopolar electrode The first technique used a monopolar electrode and a distant patient plate. The disadvantage is that there is little control of the depth of tissue injury and perforation is a possibility. In addition, the electrode tends to stick to the coagulum and when it is removed there is the possibility of pulling off the coagulum, inducing further bleeding (Laurence and Cotton, 1987). To avoid this the addition of an irrigating port at the end of the probe theoretically allows a film of water to prevent such sticking. Monopolar electrodes have been shown to be effective in the production of both initial and permanent haemostasis and in two controlled trials (Papp, 1982; Moreto et al, 1987) reduction in rebleeding rate has been confirmed. In the earlier study the need for operation was also reduced. Similar results have been achieved with a liquid monopolar electrode (Freitas et al, 1985).

Bi- or multipolar electrode As a bipolar electrode would be difficult to orientate endoscopically, a multipolar electrode consisting of three linked pairs of bipolar electrodes has been produced (Bicap, ACMI, USA; Figure 5). This electrode is connected to the control unit (Figure 6) and has an integral water pump to spray water through the end of the probe in an attempt to prevent sticking. Two controlled trials have failed to show significant benefit (Goudie et al, 1984; Kernohan et al, 1984); one has shown a reduction in rebleeding (O'Brien et al, 1986); a fourth has demonstrated a reduction in bleeding, need for operation, length of stay, transfusion requirements and total cost (Laine, 1987). Why such discrepancies exist is uncertain, but expertise and probe size are likely to be factors.

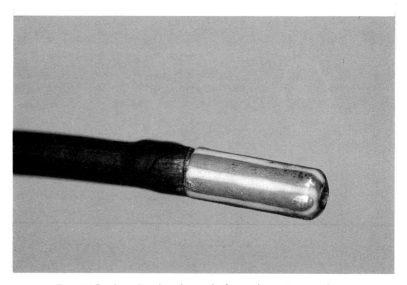

FIGURE 5 A multipolar electrode for endoscopic coagulation

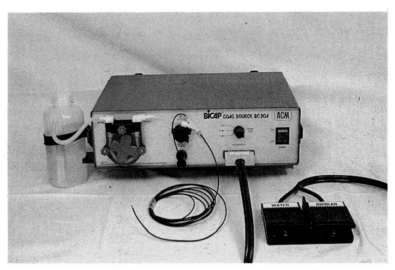

FIGURE 6 Control unit for multipolar electrocoagulation

In none of the studies involving diathermy techniques has a reduction in mortality been demonstrated.

Heater probe

Designed by Auth in the USA this equipment consists of a heating coil in a ceramic tip coated with aluminium and covered by a non-stick coating of Teflon. The coil is heated to 250°C and the amount of energy administered controlled by a microcomputer (Figure 7). Two sizes of probe are available but the larger requires the use of a large channel endoscope and the system is moderately expensive. This equipment also has a water pump to prevent sticking and to wash away blood and secretions (Figure 8). Only one controlled trial has shown it to be effective in both producing initial haemostasis and preventing rebleeding (Fullarton et al, 1989). Again, no study has shown a reduction in mortality by this method.

Laser photocoagulation

Laser therapy in the upper gastrointestinal tract has been used since the late 1970s, initially for the treatment of bleeding. Two types have been used, the argon laser and the Nd YAG laser. Initial studies employed the poorly penetrating blue-green argon laser and three controlled studies have been reported (Swain et al, 1981; Vallon et al, 1981; Jensen et al, 1984). The first showed benefit in terms of need for operation and mortality only when patients with inaccessible ulcers were excluded. The second trial excluded inaccessible ulcers from entry and showed benefit for both of these endpoints. The third study was too small for statistical analysis.

The introduction of the more powerful infra-red Nd YAG laser (Figure 9) renewed interest in this field. On account of its greater tissue penetration, this

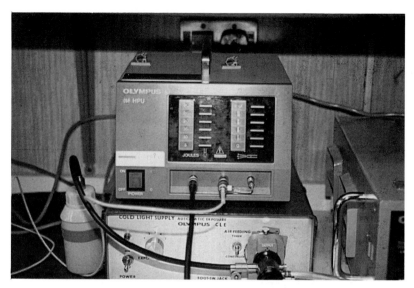

FIGURE 7   Control unit for endoscopic heater probe

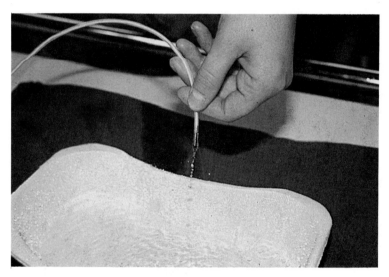

FIGURE 8   Heater probe with water jet

laser is more likely to be effective against larger vessels and to produce full-thickness damage and therefore perforation. As the beam is infra-red and thus invisible, an aiming beam is added by a secondary helium–neon laser. The laser beam is transmitted, as with the argon laser, down a single quartz fibre encased in polythene overtube. A coaxial stream of gas or saline is used to cool the tip and keep it free of secretions. Figure 10 shows a laser fibre with the helium–neon aiming beam clearly visible. Most operators aim to produce a circle of laser burns around the bleeding point before aiming at the centre of the blood vessel. Only occasionally does laser treatment initiate bleeding which can usually be stemmed

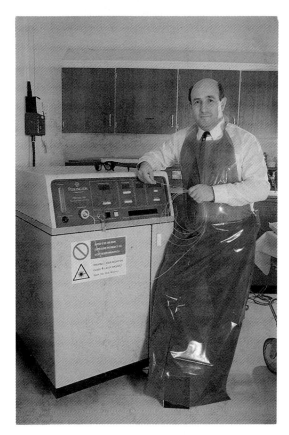

FIGURE 9 Infra-red Nd YAG laser

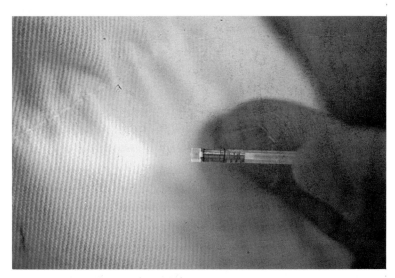

FIGURE 10 Sapphire tip with aiming beam

by further application of the laser provided the operator is quick enough. By using the laser at a distance of about 1 cm from the lesion there is no chance of the coagulum being touched or stuck on to the end of the laser fibre. This is one of the main advantages of laser therapy over the contact methods, and this type of laser use is described as being non-contact. More recently, by fitting laser light-transmitting artificial sapphires to the tip of the fibre (Figure 11) it has been possible to seal blood vessels, and there are some protagonists of this contact mode of laser use. Although animal studies have suggested better heat sealing of blood vessels by this means there have been no clinical trials reported employing this method.

Of the clinical trials that have been published using the Nd YAG laser only four out of the eight have been suitable for proper analysis as the others have either been poorly designed or flawed in other ways. Swain et al (1986) demonstrated a reduction in rebleeding rate, need for operation and mortality, while Rutgeerts et al (1982) were able to demonstrate a reduction only in rebleeding. The smallest study from Glasgow (Macleod et al, 1983) showed a significant reduction in the need for operation as the only significant benefit. The final and only negative study was that of Krejs et al published in 1987. In this study 281 patients were excluded because they were too unstable for laser therapy, the laser was malfunctioning or the lesion was inaccessible. The authors had thus selected a low risk group of patients, with only two having active arterial bleeding. In addition there were multiple operators and this must call into question their expertise.

On balance there appears to be little doubt that laser therapy stops initial bleeding and is the only thermal method of haemostasis yet to be reported to reduce mortality, even if this is in only two studies. It is probably at least as efficient as the other methods at stopping rebleeding.

This beneficial effect of laser therapy may not seem justification enough to spend around £40 000. However, the St James's group in London have costed laser therapy and believe that this technique is cost effective. This is particularly the case because it will be used much more for the palliation of malignancy than the treatment of bleeding in most units.

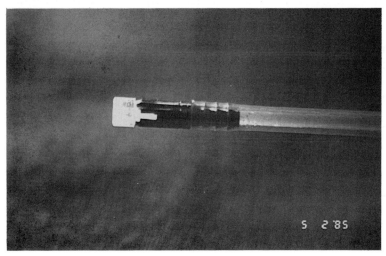

FIGURE 11   Nd YAG laser sapphire tip

Injection therapy

It is now well established that injection therapy is effective in treating oesophageal varices, haemorrhoids and varicose veins. It was thus inevitable that injection therapy would be tried in the treatment of non-variceal upper gastrointestinal haemorrhage. One of the main advantages of this type of therapy is that there is no significant capital cost, except for the provision of a sheathed flexible endoscopic injection needle, many of which are now disposable. A vasoconstrictor (1 : 10 000 adrenaline) or a sclerosant (ethanol or polidocanol) can be injected.

Injections are usually made in 0.5 ml or smaller aliquots with total volumes of up to 10 ml being administered in some studies. Adrenaline produces its haemostatic effect predominantly by vasoconstriction with added platelet aggregation. The sclerosants produce their effects by direct vascular thrombosis with secondary surrounding fibrosis. Chung et al in Hong Kong (1988) have demonstrated that adrenaline significantly reduced the volume of blood transfused, the length of hospital stay and the need for other treatment, while Asaki et al (1984) and Sugawa et al (1986) have both shown ethanol effectively to stop bleeding and, in the large Asaki study, to reduce the need for surgery.

There is one controlled trial of polidocanol (Panes et al, 1987) which showed a reduction in the need for transfusion, surgery and the length of stay, but the trial was flawed as each treated patient was injected with adrenalin prior to the polidocanol.

None of these studies has shown a significant reduction in mortality.

Comparative studies and combined therapeutic modes

There have been remarkably few comparative studies and details of these can be found in the extensive reviews by Fleischer (1986) and Steele (1989). Goff (1986) and Rutgeerts et al (1987) both failed to show any difference between the Nd YAG laser and the multipolar BICAP electrode. Northfield et al (1987) have shown the laser to be more effective than the heater probe in reducing mortality and rebleeding. Jensen et al (1988) failed to show a difference between the BICAP and the heater probe in stopping bleeding, but only the heater probe significantly reduced rebleeding and the need for surgery.

It is the author's view that the laser is probably more effective than the heater probe and that the heater probe is more effective than the BICAP. If the studies on injection therapy are confirmed this method would offer an effective low cost option, although Lin et al (1990) have shown that the heater probe is more effective than pure alcohol injection.

There are several reports of combining therapies, some of which seem to offer some benefit. In particular combining adrenaline injection prior to laser therapy appears to improve results possibly just by stopping the bleeding to enable the endoscopist to better aim the laser, or possibly by reducing the removal of heat by the blood flowing through the vessel (Rutgeerts et al, 1984).

OTHER METHODS OF PHYSICAL HAEMOSTASIS

Over the years attempts have been made to stop bleeding by the application of a variety of endoscopically placed devices. Haemostatic clips have been inserted with some difficulty, mostly in Japan, while Swain and colleagues in London are in the process of producing an endoscopic sewing machine. This group has also produced a rubber-banding machine to remove small ulcers, similar to the principle of banding of haemorrhoids. Endoscopically placed duodenal tamponade balloons have also been used on some occasions. There appears to be no limit to the ingenuity of endoscopists in trying to stop bleeding and save lives.

THE RELATIVE ROLES OF ENDOSCOPIC THERAPY AND OPERATION

While emergency operation is life saving, it carries a higher mortality and morbidity than elective operation, and patient selection, the timing of operation and the place of a preoperative trial of therapeutic endoscopy are matters of considerable debate.

The massively bleeding patient who can not be resuscitated and the patient who continues to bleed after, or as a result of, therapeutic endoscopy clearly require urgent operation. However, most endoscopists believe that an attempt at therapeutic endoscopy should be undertaken at the time of the diagnostic endoscopy if major stigmata of recent haemorrhage are seen and the chances of rebleeding are therefore high. An alternative view is that such patients should have operation without delay (Morris et al, 1984; Brearley et al, 1987). These authors, working in a specialized gastrointestinal bleeding unit, have shown that if such high risk patients are operated on early the mortality is less than in those in whom operation is delayed. However, not many units can achieve such low mortality rates for emergency operation. There is need for a comparison of the two approaches, each in expert hands.

Clearly joint management of high risk patients offers the best solution so that urgent operation is not unduly delayed by prolonged attempts at therapeutic endoscopy, while too precipitate surgery with its high mortality is not undertaken when less traumatic options are available.

CONCLUSIONS AND THE WAY FORWARD

There is enough evidence to suggest that all patients with upper gastrointestinal bleeding should be admitted under a team of interested physicians and surgeons to a special unit within the hospital. There should be clearly laid down policies on the management of these patients and their management should be under the supervision of a senior member of staff. Preferably joint ward rounds should take place, and on ongoing audit of the unit's activity will be essential to assess trends.

A full range of therapeutic endoscopic techniques is unlikely to be available to all units, but each should have a range available. It is essential that those performing these procedures should be adequately trained under the direct supervision of trained senior staff. The choice of what techniques should be used will depend at least in part on funding and facilities. Close ties with an interventional radiologist are of considerable help particularly in the occasional difficult case of obscure bleeding.

REFERENCES

Allan R & Dykes P (1976) A study of the factors influencing mortality rates from gastrointestinal haemorrhage. *Quarterly Journal of Medicine* **45**: 533–550.

Asaki S (1984) Endoscopic hemostasis by local absolute alcohol injection for upper gastrointestinal tract bleeding—a multicentre study. In Okabe H, Honda T & Oshiba S (eds) *Endoscopic Surgery*, pp 105–116. New York: Elsevier.

Avery Jones F (1956) Hematemesis and melena with special reference to causation and to the factors influencing the mortality from bleeding peptic ulcers. *Gastroenterology* **30**: 166–169.

Balint JA, Sarfel IJ & Fried MB (1977) *Gastrointestinal Bleeding. Diagnosis and Management*, pp 63–78. New York: J. Wiley.

Bown SG (1985) Controlled studies of laser therapy for haemorrhage from peptic ulcers. *Acta Endoscopica* **15**: 1–12.

Brearley S, Hawker PC, Morris DL, Dykes PW & Keighley MRB (1987) Selection of patients for surgery following peptic ulcer haemorrhage. *British Journal of Surgery* **74**: 893–896.

Christiansen J, Ottenjann R, & Von Arx F (1989) Placebo-controlled trial with the somatostatin analogue SMS 201-995 in peptic ulcer. *Gastroenterology* **97**: 568–574.

Chung SCS, Leung JWC, Steele RJC, Crofts TJ & Li AKC (1988) Endoscopic adrenaline injection for actively bleeding ulcers: a randomised trial. *British Medical Journal* **296**: 1631–1633.

Cutler JA & Mendeloff AI (1981) Upper gastrointestinal bleeding, nature and magnitude of the problem in the U.S. *Gastrointestinal Endoscopy* **26 (Supplement)**: 90–96.

Fleischer D (1986) Endoscopic therapy of upper gastrointestinal bleeding in humans. *Gastroenterology* **90**: 217–234.

Forrest JAH & Finlayson NDC (1974) The investigation of acute upper gastrointestinal haemorrhage. *British Journal of Hospital Medicine* **12**: 160–165.

Foster DN, Miloszewski KJA & Losowsky MS (1978) Stigma of recent haemorrhage in diagnosis and prognosis of upper gastrointestinal bleeding. *British Medical Journal* **1**: 1173–1177.

Freitas D, Donato, A & Monteiro JG (1985) Controlled trial of liquid monopolar electrocoagulation in bleeding peptic ulcers. *American Journal of Gastroenterology* **80**: 853–857.

Fullarton GM, Birnie GG, Macdonald A & Murray WR (1989) Controlled trial of heater probe treatment in bleeding peptic ulcers. *British Journal of Surgery* **76**: 541–544.

Goff JS (1986) Bipolar electrocoagulation versus Nd YAG laser photocoagulation for upper gastrointestinal bleeding lesions. *Digestive Disease Science* **31**: 906–910.

Goudie BM, Mitchell KG, Birnie GG & MacKay C (1984) Controlled trial of endoscopic bipolar electrocoagulation in the treatment of bleeding peptic ulcers. *Gut* **25**: A1185.

Hoare AM, Bradby GVH & Hawkes CT (1979) Cimetidine in bleeding peptic ulcer. *Lancet* **1**: 671–673.

Holman RAE, Davis M, Gough KR, Gartell P, Britton DC & Smith RB (1990) Value of a centralised approach in the management of haematemesis and melaena: experience in a district general hospital. *Gut* **31**: 504–508.

Hunt PS, Hansky J & Korman MG (1979) Mortality in patients with haematemesis and melaena: a prospective study. *British Medical Journal* **1**: 1238–1240.

Jensen DM, Machicado GA, Tapia JI & Elashoff J (1984) Controlled trial of endoscopic argon laser for severe ulcer hemorrhage. *Gastroenterology* **86**: 1125–1127.

Jensen, DM, Machicado GA, Kovacs TOG et al (1988) Controlled, randomised study of heater probe and BICAP for hemostasis of severe ulcer bleeding. *Gastroenterology* **94**: A208.

Kang JY & Piper DW (1980) Improvement in mortality rates in bleeding peptic ulcer. *Medical Journal of Australia* **1**: 213–215.

Kernohan RM, Anderson JR, McKelvey STD & Kennedy TL (1984) A controlled trial of bipolar electrocoagulation in patients with upper gastrointestinal bleeding. *British Journal of Surgery* **74**: 889–891.

Klein FA, Drueck C, Breuer RI et al (1982) Control of upper gastrointestinal bleeding with a microcrystalline collagen hemostat. *Digestive Disease Science* **27**: 981–985.

Krejs GJ, Little KH, Westergaard H, Hamilton JK, Spady DK & Polter DE (1987) Laser photocoagulation for the treatment of acute peptic ulcer bleeding. *New England Journal of Medicine* **316**: 1618–1621.

La Brooy SJ, Misiewicz JJ, Edwards J, Smith SJ, Haggie SJ, Libman L et al (1979) Controlled trial of cimetidine in upper gastrointestinal haemorrhage. *Gut* **20**: 892–895.

Laine L (1987) Multipolar electrocoagulation in the treatment of active upper gastrointestinal tract hemorrhage. *New England Journal of Medicine* **316**: 1613–1617.

Laurence BH & Cotton PB (1987) Bleeding gastroduodenal ulcers; non operative treatment. *World Journal of Surgery* **11**: 294–303.

Lin HJ, Lee FY, Kang WM, Tsai YT, Lee SD & Lee CH (1990) Heat probe thermocoagulation and pure alcohol injection in massive peptic ulcer haemorrhage: a prospective, randomised controlled trial. *Gut* **31**: 753–757.

Macleod IA & Mills PR (1982) Factors identifying the probability of further haemorrhage after acute upper gastrointestinal haemorrhage. *British Journal of Surgery* **69**: 256–258.

Macleod IA, Mills PR, Mackenzie JF, Joffe SN, Russell RI & Carter DC (1983) Neodymium yttrium aluminium garnet laser photocoagulation for major haemorrhage from peptic ulcer and single vessels: a single blind controlled study. *British Medical Journal* **286**: 345–348.

Martin TR, Onstad GR & Silvis SE (1977) Endoscopic control for massive UGI bleeding with a tissue adhesive (MBR 4197). *Gastrointestinal Endoscopy* **24**: 74.

Moreto M, Zaballa M, Ibanez S, Setien F & Figa M (1987) Efficacy of monopolar electrocoagulation in the treatment of bleeding gastric ulcer. *Endoscopy* **19**: 54–56.

Morris DL, Hawker PC, Brearley S, Simms M, Dykes PW & Keighley MRB (1984) Optimal timing of operation for bleeding peptic ulcer: prospective randomised trial. *British Medical Journal* **288**: 1277–1280.

Northfield TC, Matthewson K, Swain CP, Bland M, Kirkham JS & Bown SG (1987) Randomised comparison of Nd YAG laser, heater probe and no endoscopic therapy for bleeding peptic ulcer. *Gut* **28**: A1342.

O'Brien JD, Day SJ & Burnham WR (1986) Controlled trial of small bipolar probe in bleeding peptic ulcers. *Lancet* **1**: 464–467.

Panes J, Viver J, Forne M, Garcia-Olivares E, Marco C & Garau J (1987) Controlled trial of endoscopic sclerosis in bleeding peptic ulcers. *Lancet* **2**: 1292–1294.

Papp JP (1982) Endoscopic electrocoagulation in the management of upper gastrointestinal bleeding. *Surgical Clinics of North America* **62**: 797–806.

Peura DA, Johnson LF, Burkhalter EL et al (1982) Use of trifluroisopropyl cyanoacrylic polymer (MBR 4197) in patients with bleeding peptic ulcers of the stomach and duodenum: a randomised controlled study. *Journal of Clinical Gastroenterology* 4: 325–328.

Piper DW & Stiel D (1986) Natural history and mortality trends of acute upper gastrointestinal haemorrhage. In Hunt PS (ed.) *Clinical Surgery International. Volume 11. Gastrointestinal Haemorrhage*, chap. 1, pp 1–12. London: Churchill Livingstone.

Rutgeerts P, Vantrappen G, Broeckhaert L et al (1982) Controlled trial of YAG laser treatment of upper digestive hemorrhage. *Gastroenterology* 83: 410–416.

Rutgeerts P, Vantrappen G, Broeckhaert L et al (1984) A new and effective technique of YAG laser photocoagulation for severe upper gastrointestinal bleeding. *Endoscopy* 16: 115–117.

Rutgeerts P, Vantrappen G, Van Hootegem P et al (1987) Neodymium YAG laser photocoagulation versus multipolar electrocoagulation for the treatment of severely bleeding peptic ulcers: a randomised comparison. *Gastrointestinal Endoscopy* 33: 199–202.

Steele RJC (1989) Endoscopic haemostasis for non-variceal upper gastrointestinal haemorrhage. *British Journal of Surgery* 76: 219–225.

Storey DW, Bown SG, Swain CP et al (1981) Endoscopic prediction of recurrent bleeding in peptic ulcers. *New England Journal of Medicine* 305: 915–916.

Sugawa C, Fujita Y, Ikeda T & Walt AJ (1986) Endoscopic haemostasis of bleeding of the upper gastrointestinal tract by local injection of 98% dehydrated ethanol. *Surgery, Gynecology and Obstetrics* 162: 159–163.

Swain CP, Bown SG, Storey DW, Kirkham JS, Northfield TC & Salmon PR (1981) Controlled trial of argon laser photocoagulation in bleeding peptic ulcer. *Lancet* 2: 1313–1316.

Swain CP, Kirkham JS, Salmon PR, Bown SG & Northfield TC (1986) Controlled trial of Nd YAG laser photocoagulation in bleeding peptic ulcers. *Lancet* 1: 1113–1116.

Vallon AG, Cotton PB, Laurence BH, Miro JRA & Oses JCS (1981) Randomised trial of endoscopic argon laser photocoagulation in bleeding peptic ulcer. *Gut* 22: 228–233.

3

UPPER GASTROINTESTINAL HAEMORRHAGE—OVERVIEW OF TREATMENT

J. H. Snyman, P. W. Dykes and M. R. B. Keighley

INTRODUCTION

It has been calculated that in 1983 peptic ulceration caused over 4000 deaths in England and Wales (Taylor, 1985); as the most important complication, haemorrhage caused about 80% of these deaths. Mortality can be greatly reduced by careful attention to management detail. Further reduction requires safer and more effective means of arresting severe bleeding and to prevent its recurrence. Some progress has been made during the last decade in pharmacological and endoscopic ways to control the bleeding, but for many patients with life-threatening upper gastrointestinal bleeding, conventional surgical control of the bleeding vessel remains the only definitive therapy. Accurate selection of the patient who really needs surgery, choice of the ideal time and definition of the most appropriate operation are the most important decisions to be taken; they often need to be taken jointly by the physician and surgeon.

CLINICAL ASSESSMENT

The first responsibility of the clinician is to assess the severity of blood loss and resuscitate the patient. Patients may have a history that suggests severe loss of blood, for instance confusion, lightheadedness, tiredness, sweating and collapse. Important signs at examination are tachycardia, hypotension and cold, clammy extremities. Due to incomplete cardiovascular compensation, patients may have postural circulatory changes, with an increase in pulse rate of more than 20 beats per minute or a decrease in blood pressure of more than 20 mmHg when sitting up. A patient taking β-blocking drugs may not develop a tachycardia despite substantial blood loss.

A rapid careful history and physical examination may provide clues to the source of bleeding (Table 1). Unfortunately conventional clinical assessment does not always lead to the correct pathological diagnosis, even with the help of

TABLE I
1001 admissions with upper gastrointestinal bleeding at the General
Hospital, Birmingham, 1980–1986 (Snyman and Keighley, 1989)

Diagnosis	Admissions	Deaths	Mortality rate	% of mortality
Varices	67	32	48%	40
Carcinomata	41	16	39%	20
Duodenal ulcers	359	15	4%	18
Gastric ulcers	188	11	6%	14
Peptic ulcers	547	26	5%	32
Oesophagitis	85	0	0%	0
Mallory–Weiss	47	1	2%	1
Others	119	4	3%	5
No diagnosis	95	2	2%	2
Total	1001	81	8%	100

sophisticated computer programs (Thon et al, 1988). None the less, enquiry should be made about previous illnesses and previous operations as well as recent abdominal pain. Details should also be obtained of recent drug administration, particularly aspirin and other non-steroid anti-inflammatory drugs. These have been shown to have a substantial association with gastric haemorrhage particularly from superficial erosions (Langman et al, 1983). Smoking and drinking habits are also relevant. Various medications such as iron and bismuth can blacken the motions, mimicking melaena whilst haemoptysis or vomiting of swallowed blood can mimic haematemesis.

All patients should initially be managed with rapid resuscitation and steps taken to establish an early definitive diagnosis. It is very important quickly to exclude previous aortic surgery and portal hypertension, as the initial management of aortoduodenal fistula and bleeding varices substantially differs from that of bleeding peptic ulceration. Hyperactive bowel sounds may be a sign of continuing bleeding. As it is a rare finding with lower gastrointestinal bleeding, it also helps to distinguish between upper and lower gastrointestinal bleeding.

It is critically important to carefully assess the patient for underlying diseases, especially of the cardiovascular and respiratory systems, as these are major determinants of morbidity and mortality and have a profound effect on patient management (Allan and Dykes, 1976; Hunt, 1984). Patients with duodenal ulcers have a high incidence of atherosclerosis (Duggan, 1986) and should be carefully evaluated for coronary, cerebral and peripheral vascular disease.

Included in the clinical examination should be a search for Dupuytren's contracture, spider naevi, telangiectasia and haemangiomata on the skin and mucous membranes. Rare connective tissue disorders are indicated by hyperelasticity of the skin and hyperextensibility of joints (Callender, 1981). Impaired liver function indicates a bad prognosis and necessitates careful consideration of the most appropriate treatment plan. Though a variceal bleed is the most likely diagnosis in patients with clinical signs of portal hypertension, some patients may be bleeding from another lesion, particularly gastric erosions or peptic ulcers (Dave et al, 1983), and emergency endoscopy is mandatory for accurate diagnosis.

All diseases associated with a bleeding tendency should be excluded. A platelet count, prothrombin time and partial thromboplastin time are important early investigations.

Determination of haemoglobin and haematocrit, although a routine, is an inaccurate initial assessment of recent blood loss. Values may be normal despite a recent major haemorrhage until haemodilution has taken place. The plasma urea and creatinine levels are useful to distinguish between upper and lower gastrointestinal bleeding (Snook et al, 1986) as a raised urea with a relatively normal creatinine are usually found in upper gastrointestinal bleeding. Urea levels that remain elevated despite adequate resuscitation may be due to either continued upper gastrointestinal bleeding or impaired renal function.

RESUSCITATION

Resuscitation is critical to successful management of patients with severe gastrointestinal bleeding. Restoration of the circulating blood volume with intravenous crystalloid and colloid and subsequently by blood transfusion should be started as soon as possible after admission in all haemodynamically unstable patients. Haemodynamic stability is usually easily established but if not, continuous bleeding must be suspected and specific measures taken to arrest it. The haemoglobin level itself is usually corrected if less than 10 g%, and chronic blood loss will be suggested by a hypochromic and microcytic blood picture. It has been claimed that standard resuscitative transfusion is associated with an increased risk of rebleeding (Blair et al, 1986), but the evidence for this is inconclusive. Excessive transfusion should, however, be avoided as this may indeed be associated with rebleeding, thromboembolic complications and an increased risk of the transmission of infective disease.

CONTINUED OBSERVATION

Careful observation of the sick patient is the easiest and most important way to improve mortality rates. Reported mortality rates for bleeding peptic ulceration of around 10% (Madden and Griffith, 1986), are much too high and are largely due to errors in resuscitation and in the timing and nature of surgical intervention. This is bound to be worse when ill patients are scattered through a thinly staffed hospital. Although admission to intensive care is seldom necessary, a designated high dependency gastrointestinal unit is of enormous value. Hunt et al (1979a) aptly stated when commenting on improved mortality figures: 'Possibly the most important factor has been the formation of a unit with a combined medical and surgical approach in which patients are cared for by the same personnel familiar with all aspects of upper GI haemorrhage'. Only about 10% of patients are initially admitted to the intensive care unit including most of those with variceal bleeding. Continued or recurrent bleeding is diagnosed by careful monitoring of pulse rate and blood pressure (with postural changes), urine output, hyperactive bowel sounds and continued melaena stools as well as recurrent haematemesis. Frequent visits by medical and nursing personnel are essential to prevent delay in the diagnosis of rebleeding. Central venous pressure measurements are only used in patients admitted to the intensive care unit and seldom give information unobtainable more simply. Nasogastric tubes are not used to diagnose recurrent bleeding as they provide inaccurate information and are themselves irritant to the gastric mucosa.

SPECIFIC DIAGNOSIS

All patients who present with an upper gastrointestinal bleed require an upper gastrointestinal endoscopy to establish an accurate diagnosis. It is safest and of most help to perform this on a haemodynamically stable patient during working hours but still within 12 hours of admission, when appropriate skilled staff are available. Out of hours endoscopy should be done on stable patients with a presumed variceal bleed, patients believed to be at high risk for rebleeding and on those who fulfil the criteria for surgical intervention. In 10% of patients no endoscopic lesion can be demonstrated and here the four most likely possibilities are healed gastritis (perhaps due to irritant drugs), a duodenal ulcer in the blind angle of a forward viewing endoscope, a Mallory–Weiss tear and Dieulafoy syndrome.

Other investigations such as barium meal, radionuclide isotope studies and angiography are required in less than 1% of patients and are always second line procedures. These studies should be done if a small bowel cause of bleeding is suspected.

RISK FACTORS RESULTING IN DEATH

Rebleeding

Rebleeding is the most important single factor that adversely affects prognosis and increases the risk of death by up to 12 times (Jones, 1956).

Age

Very few deaths are recorded in patients less than 60 years of age (Morris et al, 1984). It is largely the increasing age of patients that is responsible for the unchanged mortality from bleeding peptic ulcers over the last 40 years, despite advances in medical management, anaesthesia and surgery (Figure 1). As age advances above 60 years, so does the incidence of associated cardiac, cerebral and general arteriosclerotic disease, and with them goes a rising mortality.

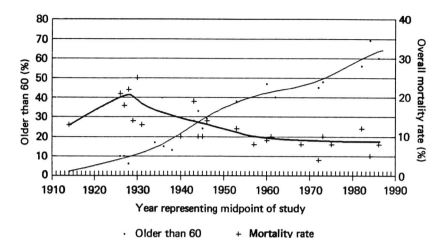

FIGURE I   Percentage of patients over 60 years of age and overall mortality rate for gastrointestinal
bleeding (adapted from Allan and Dykes, 1976)

Endoscopic stigmata

Endoscopic stigmata such as active bleeding, a visible vessel or adherent clot
known to be associated with an increased risk of rebleeding are also associated
with an increased mortality (Brearley et al, 1985).

In-patients

There is a very high mortality associated with upper gastrointestinal bleeds in
patients already hospitalized for another reason such as cardiorespiratory disease,
malignancy, cerebrovascular disease, liver disease or chronic renal failure. This
mortality rate is dependent on the severity of the underlying disease which
necessitated admission in the first place.

Source of bleeding

Different sources of bleeding have different mortalities. Peptic ulcer bleeding
carries a 5% mortality risk, much lower than that of variceal bleeding (50%) and
bleeding gastric (65%; Madden and Griffith, 1986) or oesophageal carcinoma.
However, as they are responsible for 50% of gastrointestinal bleed admissions,
peptic ulcers are responsible for most deaths, along with oesophageal varices
(Table 1).

Non-steroidal anti-inflammatory drugs

It is possible that non-steroidal anti-inflammatory drug (NSAID) intake is a risk
factor for both death and rebleeding. Armstrong and Blower (1987) studied 235

patients with a life-theatening complication of peptic ulceration, who either died or required emergency surgery. One hundred and three of these patients had a bleeding peptic ulcer. They found a very high incidence of NSAID intake in these patients (60%) compared to the hospital controls (10%). They also noted that nearly 80% of ulcer-related deaths occurred in patients using an anti-inflammatory agent. Another alarming finding was that in almost 60% of the patients the first sign of an ulcer was a life-threatening complication.

Miscellaneous

The presence of shock on admission (Clason et al, 1986; Hunt, 1987), transfusion of more than 5 units of blood (Himal et al, 1974), chronic rather than acute ulcer (Allan and Dykes, 1976) and gastric rather than duodenal ulcer (Allan and Dykes, 1976) have all been shown to be associated with an increased mortality. Mortality is also higher in patients going to surgery without a known diagnosis (Himal et al, 1974) thus supporting a policy of early endoscopy.

RISK FACTORS FOR REBLEEDING

It is logical to concentrate on risk factors for rebleeding (Table 2) as it is probably in this area that therapeutic intervention can have the greatest effect on reducing mortality. There are many definitions of rebleeding, many of them impractical as they do not use simple clinical indices. It is also important to define whether further haemorrhage means true recurrent bleeding, continued bleeding since admission or intermittent bleeding. We define an in-hospital recurrent haemorrhage as haematemesis or melaena associated with haemodynamic evidence of bleeding, and persistent bleeding as the need to transfuse 8 (patient older than 60) or 12 (patient less than 60) units of blood over a 48-hour period to keep the haemoglobin at a level of about 10 g/dl. Early and accurate diagnosis of rebleeding is essential—*early* to prevent the insult of severe shock and *accurate* to prevent

TABLE 2
Major risk factors for further bleeding from peptic ulcers

Reference	Risk factors	Risk of further bleeding
Bornman et al (1985)	Shock	48%
	Stigmata	24%
Clason et al (1986)	Age	
	Hb < 8 g/dl	71.4%
	Haematemesis	
	Stigmata	
Brearley et al (1987)	Major stigmata	53%
Hunt (1987)	Shock	70%
	Hb < 7 g/dl	30%

unnecessary operations or delayed treatment leading to a high mortality (Morris et al, 1984). Only haemodynamically significant rebleeding is a proper indication for surgery. In a patient with haemodynamic changes alone without evidence for fresh bleeding, other causes for shock, such as myocardial infarction or overwhelming infection, should carefully be excluded before rebleeding is diagnosed. An inadequate response in haemoglobin to a blood transfusion should also raise the suspicion of continued bleeding.

In a comprehensive statistical analysis Clason et al (1986) found four factors significantly associated with further haemorrhage: age over 60 years, haemoglobin less than 8 g/dl, a haematemesis as precipitating cause for admission and endoscopic stigmata of recent bleeding in a peptic ulcer. The association of clinical shock with endoscopic stigmata has been shown by Bornman et al (1985) as well as Clason et al (1986) to be a stronger predictor of rebleeding than either shock or stigmata alone. This has however been disputed by Hunt (1987) who judged shock on admission to be the single most important predictor of rebleeding, whilst other findings significantly associated with rebleeding were endoscopic stigmata, haemoglobin less than 7 g/dl, anaemia and gastric ulcer. Findings associated with a low incidence of rebleeding were the absence of endoscopic stigmata and a prepyloric ulcer. Age was not helpful in predicting rebleeding in this study.

Brearley et al (1987) identified several variables significantly associated with further haemorrhage from peptic ulcers, namely age older than 60, current medication, shock on admission, initial haemoglobin less than 10 g/dl, gastric ulcer and major endoscopic stigmata. Major endoscopic stigmata refer to fresh bleeding from the ulcer, fresh or altered blood clot or black slough adherent to the ulcer or a visible vessel protruding from the ulcer. Such patients have a 51–62% rebleeding rate compared with 5–10% for patients without these stigmata (Foster et al, 1978; Brearley et al, 1985).

We conclude that the more risk factors for rebleeding present, the more likely is the patient to suffer a recurrent haemorrhage (Table 2).

CONSERVATIVE MANAGEMENT

About 70–80% of peptic ulcers spontaneously stop bleeding and do not rebleed. Only 1–2% of patients will require immediate operation to control exsanguinating haemorrhage whilst about 25% of patients will require urgent surgery for recurrent or continued bleeding, usually within 72 hours of admission.

Local measures

There are no satisfactory studies which adequately examine the effectiveness of local measures such as intragastric lavage with ice water, saline or noradrenaline. The best that can be said about lavage is that it might be useful in preparing the upper gastrointestinal tract for endoscopic evaluation.

Pharmacological therapy

Control of gastrointestinal haemorrhage pharmacologically might be considered from the standpoint of factors operating in the gut lumen, factors relating to the circulation in the gut wall and the coagulability of blood. It is the first and fundamentally least probable of these factors that has paradoxically received the most attention. This has been attempted in two major ways: alteration of gastric acidity and inhibition of proteolysis.

Factors operating in the gut lumen

Antacids Antacids have been used for many years, the rationale being to prevent digestion of the clot by acid pepsin. Even with very high doses however (60 ml of magnesium aluminium hydroxide every 15 min) considerable individual variation occurs and many patients will still have an acid gastric content. Sodium bicarbonate is easier to administer but systemic alkalosis may follow. Milk drip therapy has also been used (Asby et al, 1963) either alone or as an adjunct to antacids, but no clinical benefit has been demonstrated.

Drugs inhibiting acid production The introduction of cimetidine provided a powerful tool for further examination of the antacid question and many trials have now been completed. In a review of the several randomized trials, Collins and Langman (1985) point to the inadequacies of trial design and the small numbers involved. They carried out an interesting statistical analysis, looking at three indices of hazard. There appeared to be overall risk ratios in treated versus control groups of 0.9 for persistent or recurrent bleeding, 0.8 for the need for surgery and 0.7 for mortality. Only for mortality did the 95% confidence interval for the odds ratio lie below 1.0, but when the analysis was done for gastric ulcers alone, the indices all reached the levels of significance. A further large multicentre study is in progress. The ultimate test for the effect of aid inhibition will be the results from the new drug omeprazole. Such studies are under way and should best answer the general question of whether rebleeding is affected by intragastric acidity.

Antiproteolytic drugs Attempts to inhibit proteolytic digestion of the clot have begun with an examination of tranexamic acid. Early studies were encouraging and suggested that oral and intravenous administration reduced transfusion requirements, rebleeding rates, frequency of surgery and mortality (Biggs et al, 1976; Engqvist et al, 1979). More recent studies have continued to show a benefit and from Sweden comes a convincing report of 3 days intravenous followed by 3 days of oral therapy (Staël von Holstein et al, 1987). There was a significant reduction in transfusion requirements and the need for surgery. A recent analysis of 1267 patients entered into six randomized trials indicated that treatment with tranexamic acid was associated with a 20–30% reduction in rebleeding, a 30–40% reduction in operation rate and a 40% reduction in mortality (Henry and O'Connell, 1989).

Studies in Birmingham have shown that proteolytic activity appeared to relate more to concentrations of tryspin than pepsin or serum protease. A study was, therefore, set up to study the effect of intragastric administration of the antitryptic drug aprotinin on rebleeding rates. This study is still in progress.

Factors relating to the circulation in the gut wall

Somatostatin and vasopressin have both been used in attempts to affect mucosal blood flow. Most studies have included very small numbers (Magnussen et al, 1985; Söderlund, 1987) and there are as yet no convincing benefits. Peptic ulcer bleeding occurs from large tortuous arterioles immobile in a mass of scar and inflammatory tissue. Hormonal control of blood flow seems more possible in the mucosa of the patient with multiple erosions.

Factors affecting the coagulability of blood

Non-steroidal anti-inflammatory drugs (NSAIDs) are well proven to have an effective antiplatelet effect by the inhibition of platelet aggregation. With aspirin this effect on platelet function is poorly reversible, while all other NSAIDs will only inhibit aggregation when they are present in the bloodstream. From the practical point of view this means that platelet function will return to normal approximately three half-lives after an NSAID is ceased and 4 days after aspirin is ceased (Brook, 1988).

Blair et al (1986) showed that a major upper gastrointestinal bleeding episode is accompanied by a hypercoagulable state, which gradually returns to normal in 3–4 days. This hypercoagulable state is partly reversed by the early administration of blood. They suggested that blood transfusion should where possible be delayed and only administered early if the haemoglobin is less than 8 g/dl or if the patient is shocked.

One of the several factors contributing to rebleeding may be fibrinolytic activity in the gastroduodenal wall. The first study on fibrinolysis in the stomach and duodenum was published by Cox et al in 1967. They found fibrinolytic activity in gastric venous blood but none in arterial blood flowing to the stomach. Furthermore, fibrinolytic activity was detected in the gastric venous blood of 11 of 13 patients with gastroduodenal ulcers, compared with 5 of 13 in the controls. Helgstrand (1983) demonstrated fibrinolytic activity in gastroscopic biopsy material comprising the mucosal lining and the lamina muscularis. A significantly higher level of activity was noted in the mucosa of patients with a history of haemorrhagic episodes than in those with no history of bleeding. Based on these observations tranexamic acid, previously discussed, may prevent rebleeding by inhibition of plasmin production in the gastric wall.

OUTCOME

Surprisingly little is known about the late outcome of patients treated surgically or conservatively for an upper gastrointestinal bleed. Hunt et al (1979b) described follow-up in 152 of 266 (57%) patients treated conservatively with bleeding duodenal ulceration. Over a mean period of 2.9 years 16 patients (10%) rebled, of whom 10 could again be treated conservatively. One patient died of a massive bleed at a different hospital. Twenty-five patients (18%) subsequently underwent emergency or elective surgery for duodenal ulcer complications.

Following admission for bleeding duodenal ulcer disease, Murray et al (1988) randomized their patients to receive either ranitidine or placebo for 2 years. Maintenance ranitidine therapy significantly reduced the incidence and symptoms of recurrent duodenal ulceration but unfortunately it did not prevent late rebleeding.

Murray et al (1986) have raised the question as to whether ulcer healing occurs as rapidly after gastrointestinal bleeding as in non-bleeding patients. They randomized 40 patients bleeding from duodenal ulceration to treatment with ranitidine or placebo and showed healing rates precisely in line with previous data in non-bleeding patients. In addition the placebo group was shown to smoke only half as much as those receiving ranitidine and yet still only achieve a healing rate of 25% at 1 month. It seems that histamine H_2 receptor antagonists (H2RAs) have a stronger influence on healing than alteration of lifestyle.

In a report on the late outcome of the non-operative treatment of bleeding gastric ulcers (Smart and Langman, 1986), 3% (4 out of 152) of the patients died due to late complications of gastric ulceration while another 16% suffered late rebleeding. The risk had however disappeared 6 years after the initial haemorrhage. Duggan (1986) has confirmed that this hazard applies much more to gastric than to duodenal ulcer patients. There is clearly a strong case for careful follow-up of all gastric ulcer patients. Curiously, duodenal ulcer bleeding was associated with an increased risk of late complications from cardiovascular disease.

ENDOSCOPIC THERAPY (Chapter 2)

All patients with arterial bleeding from ulcers as well as high risk patients with visible vessels (Lawrence and Cotton, 1987) should be considered for endoscopic therapy. Low risk patients with a visible vessel, adherent clot or slow oozing can be managed expectantly and treated endoscopically if rebleeding occurs.

INDICATIONS FOR SURGERY AND TIMING OF SURGERY

Emergency surgery is required to stem life-threatening haemorrhage, often in very unfit, ill-prepared elderly patients, and should be distinguished from early elective surgery. The aim of emergency surgical intervention is removal of the problem of continuing haemorrhage and its associated risk to life. Cure of the ulcer and prevention of recurrent ulceration are of secondary importance.

It is of the utmost importance to select those patients requiring early surgery, to optimize their preoperative treatment and to define the appropriate time for this intervention. Many deaths in upper gastrointestinal bleeding are not due to exsanguination but to thromboembolic phenomena consequent upon rapid changes in circulatory haemodynamics, leading to myocardial infarction, cerebrovascular accidents and pulmonary embolism (Allan and Dykes, 1976). It is therefore important to intervene before serious rebleeding with impaired tissue perfusion of vital organs occurs and to maintain circulatory stability. Mortality is substantially increased in older patients who require an initial transfusion of 4 or more units of blood to restore cardiovascular stability, because of poor cardiac reserve and a reduced ability to cope with rapid changes in blood volume (Devitt et al, 1966). Transfusion requirements of 4 units of blood indicate the need for urgent surgical intervention in patients over the age of 60 years (Morris et al, 1984). Younger patients can tolerate greater instability of the circulation; hence it is safe here to delay operative intervention, thus reducing the incidence of unnecessary emergency operations. Ideally, operations should be performed before rebleeding occurs in patients older than 60 years. The difficulty here lies in predicting which patients will rebleed. Thus about 50% of patients with a visible vessel in an ulcer base may be expected to bleed again (Storey et al, 1981). A blanket policy to operate on all elderly patients with a visible vessel would thus result in about 50% being operated upon unnecessarily. Thus although a visible vessel indicates an increased risk of rebleeding, it is not of sufficient risk itself to warrant operation. On the other hand, waiting until the patient rebleeds carries the risk of mortality from hypotension and impaired tissue perfusion. It is self-evident that early intervention is essential in those in whom a spurting vessel is seen at endoscopy and those with torrential haemorrhage.

Birmingham trial—timing of surgery

In a Birmingham trial designed to investigate the optimum timing of operative intervention for bleeding peptic ulcers (Morris et al, 1984), patients were stratified into groups older and younger than 60 years and randomized to receive either early or delayed operative intervention. The three most important criteria chosen to influence the timing of surgery were the age of the patient, the volume of blood or plasma expander required to restore haemodynamic stability and rebleeding in hospital. The transfusion index for emergency surgery is the volume required to restore haemodynamic stability and not to correct a low haemoglobin concentration. This distinction should be firmly maintained, although it is often blurred in individual patients.

In younger patients no advantage was found from early operation and an operation rate of 50% in this group was thought to be excessive. In the older group (60 years or more), mortality was significantly lower in patients receiving early surgery, being 4% compared with 15% ($p < 0.05$) in patients where surgery was delayed. In the presence of a bleeding gastric ulcer, the mortality of early surgery was zero compared with 24% ($p < 0.01$) for delayed surgery. Since 1984 we have no longer used endoscopic stigmata of recent haemorrhage (clot, oozing and visible vessel) as an indication for very early surgery (Table 3) because we thought that this was the principal reason for our high operation rate of 61% in patients over 60 years having early surgery. We have maintained a post-trial audit of our operation and mortality rate in the 5 years since the completion of the 'timing of surgery'. Exclusion of endoscopic criteria has not been associated with an increased mortality and there has been a significant reduction in operation rates to 26% (Table 4)

Using these criteria (Table 3), 76 patients had an operation over a 5-year period. The major indications (Table 5) were active bleeding on admission (13%), first rebleed (58%) and second rebleed (11%). Only 6 (8%) of the patients were operated upon for the volume replacement criteria.

TABLE 3

Current criteria for surgical intervention in bleeding peptic ulcer disease used at the General Hospital, Birmingham

Immediate surgery (all ages)
Exsanguinating haemorrhage: if the patient's condition cannot be stabilized during initial resuscitation because of continued blood loss
Spurting vessel at endoscopy

Patients older than 60 years
4 units of blood or plasma expander required on admission to secure haemodynamic stability
One recurrence of bleeding in hospital
Persistent bleeding requiring transfusion of 8 units/48 hours

Patients younger than 60 years
8 units of blood or plasma expander required on admission to ensure haemodynamic stability
Two recurrences of bleeding in hospital
Persistent bleeding requiring transfusion of 12 units/48 hours

TABLE 4

Outcome of patients admitted with bleeding peptic ulcer disease to the General Hospital, Birmingham, 1980–1988

(a) 1980–1983. Trial of surgery results (Morris et al, 1984)

Age group	Admissions	Total deaths	Operations	Operative mortality
Under 60	42	0	13 (31%)	0
Over 60	100	10 (10%)	44 (44%)	10 (22.7%)
Early surgery	47	2 (4.3%)	29 (61.7%)	2 (6.9%)
Late surgery	53	8 (15.1%)	15 (28.3%)	8 (53%)
All	142	10 (7%)	57 (40.1%)	10 (17.5%)

(b) 1984–1988

Age group	Admissions	Total deaths	Operations	Operative mortality
Under 60	132	1 (0.8%)	17 (12.9%)	1 (5.9%)
Over 60	228	14 (6.1%)	59 (25.9%)	2 (3.4%)
All	360	15 (4.2%)	76 (21.1%)	3 (3.9%)

Experience from other units on criteria for operation in peptic ulcer

Hunt (1984) uses a different selection pattern, advocating that all patients older than 50 years with concurrent disease or shock on admission should undergo surgery since these patients are particularly susceptible to organ failure. His

TABLE 5
Indications for surgery 1984–1988

Indication	Patients
Exsanguinating haemorrhage	5 (6.6%)
Spurting vessel	5 (6.6%)
First recurrence of bleeding	44 (58%)
Second recurrence of bleeding	8 (10.5%)
Continuous bleed	4 (5.3%)
Volume replacement	6 (7.9%)
Concomitant perforation	4 (5.3%)
Total	76

operation rate for peptic ulceration was 34% with an overall mortality of 5.8% and an operative mortality of 11.5%.

These indications are applicable to patients with well-defined chronic peptic ulceration. They do not apply to more diffuse processes, e.g. acute mucosal erosions, oesophagitis, cancer or bleeding varices. In patients with erosive or inflammatory mucosal disease, surgical control is poor and non-surgical therapy holds more prospect of controlling the bleeding process.

GENERAL PREOPERATIVE MEASUREMENTS

Intensive Therapy Unit care

Intensive therapy unit (ITU) care is often indicated in the perioperative phase in severely ill patients requiring substantial blood transfusion and those with portal hypertension or severe associated disease.

Prophylactic antibiotics

Gatehouse et al (1978) have shown that patients with an upper gastrointestinal bleed have abnormally high gastric bacterial counts and that there is a close correlation between counts of bacteria in gastric juice and the risk of postoperative sepsis. Therefore all patients having an operation for upper gastrointestinal bleeding should receive prophylactic antibiotics since the stomach or duodenum are invariably opened at operation with a risk of bacterial contamination.

Low dose heparin

In the series reported by Allan and Dykes (1976), an important potentially preventable cause of death was pulmonary embolism. It is possible that low dose heparin could be of value to decrease fatal postoperative thromboembolism (Kakkar et al, 1975). No such study has so far been done in upper gastrointestinal bleed patients. We have been using low dose heparin since 1979 with the marked absence of fatal pulmonary embolism and we have not recorded an increased incidence of postoperative bleeding complications. Contrary to common belief any bleeding episode is normally followed by a hypercoagulable state and not by a bleeding tendency (Blair et al, 1986); thus low dose heparin should not increase the postoperative rebleeding rate.

Endoscopy

Preoperative endoscopy helps to plan the operative approach and should always be done. Even in patients who have to be taken directly to theatre from casualty, on-table endoscopy is indicated to localize the bleeding and exclude bleeding varices.

TYPE OF SURGERY

Undiagnosed bleeding

Less than 5% of patients will present with a catastrophic persistent haemorrhage, so that they are too unstable to undergo preoperative endoscopy. These patients must be moved to the operating room without delay where after induction of anaesthesia, haemorrhage may decrease or cease altogether. With the airway protected, it is always advisable to perform on-table endoscopy and proceed with laparotomy only if a discrete lesion is located. If torrential haemorrhage persists after induction of anaesthesia, immediate laparotomy is required. Indeed in these circumstances there is usually so much clot in the stomach that endoscopy is often unrewarding.

Duodenal ulceration

Proximal gastric vagotomy

Over the last decade proximal gastric vagotomy (PGV) has become the preferred definitive surgical treatment of duodenal ulceration. Protagonists of PGV have also recommended its use for selected patients with bleeding duodenal ulceration, underrunning the ulcer via a duodenotomy. PGV was used in this way by Johnston et al (1973) in a series of 26 patients with no deaths. Despite these excellent results PGV is not widely accepted for this purpose as it is a more lengthy procedure and must only be done by an appropriately skilled surgeon; it is also associated with a high rate of ulcer recurrence.

Truncal vagotomy and pyloroplasty

For the majority of surgeons in the United Kingdom truncal vagotomy and pyloroplasty (TV&P) combined with underrunning of the bleeding vessel remains the operation of choice (Stringer and Cameron, 1988) and was the operation performed in more than half of our patients over the last 5 years (Table 6a). If the patient is not actively bleeding at the time of surgery it is advisable to start with the vagotomy, whereas in the presence of active bleeding, it is better to start by controlling blood loss by underrunning the ulcer. About 3 cm of each vagal trunk should be excised and the lower 5 cm of oesophagus carefully cleared of all vagal fibres. Care should be taken not to perforate the oesophagus. If a bleeding vessel is present, this should be separately tied off with figure of eight stitches proximal and distal to the bleeding point. Following this the mucosa could be approximated with a few deep stitches (Figure 2). Smaller ulcers without a vessel should be sutured with about three of these deep sutures. The common duct is usually safely away from these sutures, but great care should be taken to avoid its damage especially if there is gross duodenal deformity. The preferred suture material is any one of the synthetic absorbable materials. After underrunning the ulcer, the gastroduodenotomy is closed transversely as a Heinecke–Mickulicz pyloroplasty. With severe duodenal scarring due to anterior and posterior duodenal ulceration the pyloroduodenal incision may be closed as a Finney pyloroplasty to prevent gastric outlet obstruction.

TABLE 6
Type of surgery for bleeding ulcers and outcome at the General Hospital, Birmingham, 1984–1988

(a) Duodenal ulcers

Procedure	No.	Deaths	Rebleeds
Vagotomy, pyloroplasty and underrunning	22	0	1
Underrunning alone	5	1	0
PGV	1	0	1
Billroth II gastrectomy	5	0	0
Vagotomy and antrectomy	5	0	0
Total	38	1	2

(b) Gastric ulcers

Procedure	No.	Deaths	Rebleeds
Partial gastrectomy	15	0	0
Underrunning/excision with vagotomy	12	1	0
Underrunning/excision alone	11	1	1
Total	38	2	1

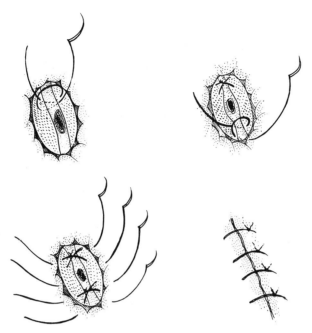

FIGURE 2 Technique of underrunning of a bleeding duodenal ulcer (Hunt, 1983, adapted by permission of the publishers, Butterworth & Co (Publishers) Ltd)

Truncal vagotomy and antrectomy

Herrington and Davidson (1987) advocate truncal vagotomy with antrectomy (TV&A) and Billroth I reconstruction, as well as underrunning of the bleeding ulcer for the good risk patient, provided the inflammatory process in the duodenum allows resection and a safe gastroduodenal anastomosis. They report an overall mortality for TV&A of 5.5% and an incidence of early rebleeding of less than 1% in a total of 250 emergency and semi-emergency operations. They advise TV&P for the high risk patient. Regrettably, there have been no controlled clinical trials to compare mortality, rebleeding rates and late morbidity of TV&P, TV&A and underrunning alone in patients with bleeding duodenal ulcers.

Billroth II gastrectomy

For a large duodenal ulcer a Billroth II gastrectomy may still be required to control bleeding especially after rebleeding following a more conservative operation. Suture line leakage and duodenal stump complications are major sources of morbidity and mortality, limiting the indications for this operation.

Mortality rates for all types of surgery vary widely in the literature. Venables (1981) reviewed several series of standard operative procedures and found an average mortality of 13% for gastric and 10% for duodenal ulceration. Mortality seemed independent of whether a gastric resection or a vagotomy had been performed. Many deaths are undoubtedly due to technical deficiencies (Hunt, 1984).

Underrunning alone

Already in 1976 Allan and Dykes suggested that the trend in surgery for upper gastrointestinal bleed patients should be towards more conservative operations since gastrectomy was associated with a high mortality, mainly due to anastomotic leaks. A recent development in the conservative surgical management for high risk patients is that of controlling bleeding by underrunning the bleeding vessel without performing any ulcer healing procedure. Ulcer healing is then achieved by long-term postoperative administration of H_2RAs. This approach is usually relatively simple and quick, thus limiting the duration of the operation as well as the length of the abdominal incision. The aim therefore is to minimize the early postoperative morbidity and mortality and to reduce the incidence of diarrhoea, dumping, bile vomiting and the long-term metabolic sequelae. The main disadvantages are the need for continued anti-ulcer therapy, possibly for life, and the risk of ulcer relapse. Underrunning of the vessel and postoperative medical ulcer therapy has previously been reserved for patients at an extremely high risk level for any surgery and has not been studied in fitter patients. A trial is in progress in the United Kingdom comparing this limited operation against standard procedures.

Where underrunning is performed without vagotomy, it can usually be done via a duodenotomy, leaving the pylorus intact (Figure 3). However, if exposure is poor, the pylorus must be transected. Reconstruction is done in the line of incision provided the duodenum is not grossly deformed, in which case there could be a hazard of postoperative gastric outlet obstruction (Johnston, 1977) (Figure 4). If there is a stricture limited to the duodenum, the duodenotomy should be closed as a duodenoplasty, avoiding pyloroplasty. The suture line should always be

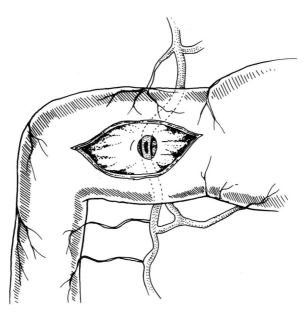

FIGURE 3 Duodenotomy for bleeding duodenal ulceration (Alexander-Williams, 1973, adapted by permission of the publishers, Butterworth & Co (Publishers) Ltd)

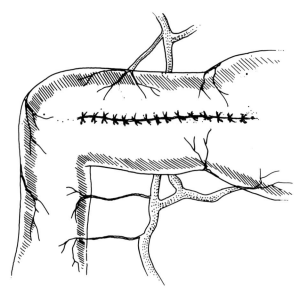

FIGURE 4 Longitudinal closure after control of bleeding (Alexander-Williams, 1973, adapted by permission of the publishers, Butterworth & Co (Publishers) Ltd)

tested with CO_2 for airtightness to prevent suture line leaks. Location of a duodenal ulcer may be difficult at surgery, in which case a Perspex proctoscope or vaginal speculum can be very useful.

Gastric ulceration

Conventional surgery

These patients form a particularly high risk group where surgical delay is particularly hazardous (Morris et al, 1984). The standard operation for a bleeding gastric ulcer has been gastrectomy, usually of the Billroth I type. This is associated with virtually no risk of rebleeding and low risk of ulcer recurrence (4%) but even in good hands has a relatively high mortality of 16% (Ovaska and Havia, 1988). It may have the advantage of adequately treating unsuspected early gastric carcinoma (Hunt et al, 1982). However, since many operations for bleeding gastric ulcers are performed on high risk elderly patients, gastrectomy can carry a mortality of well over 20% (Rogers et al, 1988). Furthermore, high gastric ulcers may present technical difficulties if treated by partial gastrectomy.

Largely for these reasons the practice of gastrectomy has been diminishing over recent years and truncal vagotomy with excision of the ulcer or underrunning of the vessel, biopsy and a pyloroplasty has become more widely used with a lower mortality (7%), higher rebleeding rate (7%) and recurrent ulceration in about 15% of patients (Herrington and Davidson, 1987).

PGV has little to offer in bleeding gastric ulceration and could be technically very difficult with high lesser curve ulcers.

Conservative surgery

Underrunning and biopsy or excision of the ulcer without any attempt at a curative procedure have in the past been reserved for the very high risk patient, but more recently some units have been advocating a more widespread use of this conservative approach. Early results from Rogers et al (1988) are impressive, with an operative mortality of 10% for underrunning alone, compared with 26% for partial gastrectomy and, remarkably, 45% for vagotomy and underrunning. Only one of the 20 patients treated by underrunning alone rebled but this study was not controlled and the patients were collected over 8 years. At the General Hospital in Birmingham our choice has been for a conservative surgical option in a third of the patients with bleeding gastric ulcer (Table 6b). Following non-resectional gastric surgery, all patients should be on a long-term follow-up programme. More conservative surgery for bleeding gastric ulcers should still be tested by a randomized clinical trial. A gastric ulcer should always be excised rather than biopsied to decrease the rebleeding rate and to prevent missing a cancer because of inadequate material for histological examination. Transgastric excision of a high gastric ulcer is the preferred procedure (Figure 5) as attempts to excise the ulcer by wedge excision from the lesser curvature endangers the nerves of Laterjet and may thus lead to antral stasis and recurrent ulceration (Johnston, 1985). The low Birmingham surgical mortality for gastric ulcers may be explained by well-timed surgery performed by senior registrars or consultants with the help of a senior anaesthetic team.

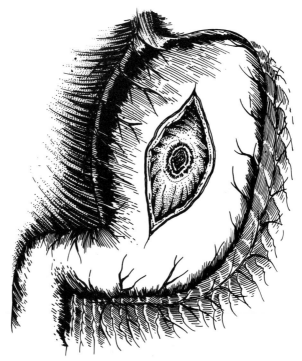

FIGURE 5 Transgastric ulcer excision of a posterior gastric ulcer (Johnston, 1983, adapted by permission of the publishers, Butterworth & Co (Publishers) Ltd)

Mallory–Weiss tears

Mallory–Weiss tears are diagnosed in about 5% of patients with upper gastrointestinal bleeding and are rarely associated with mortality. The diagnosis is suggested by a history of repeated retching followed by vomiting bright red blood: alcohol is a prominent precipitating factor. At endoscopy a linear mucosal tear is seen in the distal oesophagus, at the oesophagogastric junction or in the cardia; these are often associated with a hiatal hernia (Michel and Malt, 1986). Tears are multiple in 15% of patients and associated mucosal lesions are found in up to 80% of patients. These tears seldom endanger life and usually heal spontaneously, but vasopressin can be useful when bleeding is persistent. If an operation is required, exposure through a high longitudinal gastrotomy is satisfactory for oversewing the tear and a Perspex proctoscope may be very helpful to determine the extent of the lesions. One absolute indication for operation is in patients with a full thickness oesophageal tear with perforation into the mediastinum (Boerhave syndrome). These patients are gravely ill often presenting shocked with severe retrosternal and abdominal pain, surgical emphysema in the neck, radiological evidence of air in the mediastinum, neck and sometimes under the diaphragm. Treatment is directed to dealing with the perforation.

Stress bleeding

Due to the high standard of intensive care therapy, stress ulceration is becoming a rare condition. As the mortality of patients operated on for haemorrhage exceeds 30% (Cheung, 1981), attempts at decreasing the mortality are best directed at prevention. Antacid and H_2RA therapy has been shown to be beneficial for the prevention of these ulcers (Shuman et al, 1987) but their value in treatment is unclear (Cheung, 1981). Tranexamic acid has been proposed as effective treatment (Biggs et al, 1976). Increasing use of endoscopic injection with adrenaline and sclerosing agents for bleeding ulcers should be extended to this problem by those with the appropriate experience. If bleeding persists and operation is mandatory, the stomach should be opened and attempts made to underrun individual bleeding points, as deeper discrete lesions may be responsible for the haemorrhage. This should always be combined with vagotomy and pyloroplasty. For the patient with recurrent bleeding or multifocal bleeding, total gastrectomy may be indicated. In such situations the mortality may exceed 50% (Hubert et al, 1980).

Alcohol- and drug-induced gastritis

Conservative measures should normally suffice but if operation is required, vagotomy, pyloroplasty and underrunning of the bleeding points appears to be the most appropriate procedure.

Dieulafoy vascular malformations (exulceratio simplex)

This is a rare cause of upper gastrointestinal bleeding which can easily be overlooked at endoscopy and at operation as a cause of massive, often recurrent haematemesis. Bleeding is caused by an unusually large (1–3 mm) artery that runs in the submucosa in close contact with the mucous membrane. Massive bleeding can occur if the mucous membrane and arterial wall are eroded. The mucosal defect is usually only 2–5 mm and in more than 80% of patients the site of bleeding is found within 6 cm of the gastrooesophageal junction, usually along the lesser curve. It can occur at any age (mean age 52) and is twice as frequent in men as in women (Veldhuyzen van Zanten et al, 1986). A high mortality is associated with delayed diagnosis. The endoscopic appearances of the Dieulafoy lesion are variable. Sometimes no abnormality is seen and sometimes it is only after repeated endoscopies that active bleeding from a pinpoint mucosal lesion is seen. Sometimes there is a small erosive defect with a tiny visible vessel or adherent clot. If endoscopic treatment fails, wedge resection without vagotomy is recommended.

Cushing and Curling ulcers

Massive upper gastrointestinal bleeding from gastroduodenal ulceration may occur after head injury (Cushing ulcer) or following major burns (Curling ulcer). Management depends on the endoscopic findings. Discrete deep ulcers are likely to involve larger vessels and are usually treated in the same way as peptic ulcers. Diffuse shallow ulceration is best managed in a fashion similar to that outlined for stress ulceration.

Stomal and recurrent (postoperative) ulceration

Occasionally bleeding may occur from a stomal ulcer. This can usually be managed with H$_2$RAs as bleeding from stomal ulcers is rarely catastrophic. Indications for operation are more conservative than those outlined for peptic ulcers. As reoperation after previous gastrectomy may be technically extremely demanding especially under emergency conditions, only experienced surgeons should operate on these patients. The type of operation will depend upon the site of ulceration, the fitness of the patient and the nature of the original operation. Thus vagotomy or revagotomy, gastric resection or reresection or a combination of these with underrunning of the ulcer are each sometimes the most appropriate.

Tumours

Bleeding from a mesenchymal tumour, of which leiomyoma is the most common, is a relatively rare cause of massive upper gastrointestinal bleeding. It is usually a well-circumscribed submucosal tumour with ulceration of the overlying mucosa, causing the bleeding. The same criteria for surgical intervention are used as for peptic ulcers and local resection is sufficient. Tumours near the oesophagogastric junction can be treated by incising the overlying mucosa and enucleating the tumour.

Gastric lymphomas may present with bleeding and if possible should be managed by radical excision. Depending on the histologic type, adjuvant chemotherapy and radiotheraphy may be advisable.

The prognosis of patients with bleeding gastric adenocarcinoma is generally poor (Madden and Griffith, 1986). Most tumours are advanced and in only a few patients is radical excision justified. Bleeding duodenal or pancreatic cancers are almost never salvageable by surgery. It is important that ulcers with the appearance of cancer but negative histology and cytology be treated as a peptic ulcer. If it is clinically indicated surgery should not be witheld from these patients.

Aortoenteric haemorrhage

This serious cause of both minor and major upper gastrointestinal bleeding has an increasing incidence. The crucial issue for successful management is to suspect the diagnosis in any patient with a history of previous aortic surgery who presents with an upper gastrointestinal bleed. Ideally the patient should be endoscoped in the operating theatre possibly under general anaesthesia. If the diagnosis of aortoenteric fistula is confirmed or if in such a patient bleeding from another source in the oesophagus, stomach or duodenum is excluded, laparotomy should proceed immediately. If an aortoenteric fistula is found, the traditional approach is to oversew the aorta, remove the graft and perform an axillo-bifemoral bypass.

Haemobilia

Haemobilia is often overlooked and should be considered in all patients with right upper quadrant pain, jaundice, upper gastrointestinal bleeding and a history of recent trauma, liver instrumentation or liver tumour necrosis. Operation is best avoided and selective arterial catheterization with embolization is the treatment of choice.

Barrett ulcer

Though this is an uncommon finding, a peptic ulcer in the oesophagus is often complicated by massive haemorrhage. Conservative therapy is preferred as emergency surgery in these elderly patients is difficult with a high mortality.

RATIONAL MANAGEMENT OF PEPTIC ULCER BLEEDING

Over the last decade we have evolved a policy for the management of bleeding peptic ulcers, associated with acceptable rates for operative intervention (20%) and a low postoperative mortality (4%). This has produced an overall mortality for bleeding peptic ulceration at all ages of 4.2% and 6.1% for the over 60s. It is rare for well-managed patients less than 60 to die and the mortality rises progressively through each successive decade. The hypothesis that certain patients are too sick for operation is a fallacy; their already high level of risk is accentuated and not reduced by postponing surgical intervention.

No single factor is responsible for our good results which are due instead to the firm implementation of a composite policy by an efficient and coordinated team. Principles of management are simple and involve speedy resuscitation, the early use of diagnostic procedures, careful observation and monitoring, good communication between all staff and adherence to strict criteria for surgical intervention. We believe that adoption of these methods more widely could reduce by a half the number of patients dying from bleeding peptic ulcers, with little or no extra cost for equipment, nursing or medical care and little or no need for extra training.

(1) All patients should be admitted under the joint care of the receiving medical and surgical teams of the day.

(2) Prompt, effective resuscitation is essential. Crystalloids, plasma expanders and blood should be used to correct hypovolaemia. An initial volume requirement of 4 units of blood should be an indication for surgery, care being taken not to overtransfuse patients.

(3) All patients should be referred early to the endoscopist. Only endoscopists with specific training and experience in this area should be involved. Virtually all patients admitted with an upper gastrointestinal bleed should be endoscoped within 24 hours of admission. Less than 2% of our admissions proceed directly to operation because of bleeding too vigorous to allow time for endoscopy.

(4) All patients with other than trivial haemorrhage should be admitted to a designated gastrointestinal ward or the intensive care unit. An alternative to a designated gastrointestinal ward would be a high dependency ward near the intensive care unit. As the early diagnosis of rebleeding is very dependent on careful nursing observation of the patient, it is a great advantage to have nurses experienced in such monitoring and especially in the recognition of rebleeding.

(5) Strict criteria for timing of surgical intervention should be carefully adhered to. A real hazard appears to be unrecognized exsanguination and prolonged recurrent fluctuations in circulatory status. Careful selection of the small group who will inevitably require surgery with early intervention is the key to good results. Our own policy is to operate on all patients less than 60 years of age with an exanguinating haemorrhage, a spurting vessel at endoscopy, 8 units of blood or colloid needed in 24 hours to ensure cardiovascular stability or two rebleeds in hospital. Patients older than 60 years come to surgery if they have an exanguinating bleed, a spurting vessel at endoscopy, a single rebleed or if they need 4 units of blood in 24 hours to secure cardiovascular stability. If there is doubt, we tend to opt for surgical rather than conservative management. The choice of the actual type of operation is left to the surgeon, but there is a trend to avoid resection for gastric as well as duodenal ulcers. Non-curative surgery where the only goal is to control haemorrhage is currently under trial, backed by the use of H_2RAs.

(6)   All operations on bleeding ulcers should be performed by surgeons of senior registrar or consultant grade, with an anaesthetist of commensurate experience.

(7)   All patients undergoing operation for gastrointestinal haemorrhage should receive prophylactic subcutaneous heparin and an intravenous cephalosporin to reduce the incidence of postoperative pulmonary embolism and wound infections.

(8)   Combined medical and surgical care is important as many of the elderly have multiple underlying diseases.

(9)   All patients presenting with upper gastrointestinal haemorrhage should be presented each week to a combined medical/surgical gastroenterology meeting. Careful auditing of results is the key to early recognition of bad results and errors in management. Regular update of morbidity and mortality figures could then be provided to keep all involved personnel enthusiastic towards the management of these patients.

(10)   All patients admitted with a bleeding ulcer, whether treated medically or by conservative surgery, should be followed at an out-patient clinic to ensure ulcer healing.

(11)   Awareness and communication are the two attributes of our overall management policies hardest to quantify and to establish, but are the two factors most vital to good results. A large part of our success is due to the awareness of all doctors involved in the care of such patients regarding potential clinical and management problems and policies. Overall results are presented to all medical staff on an annual basis and all junior doctors are closely involved in the care of patients with upper gastrointestinal haemorrhage. Good communication between several doctors and nurses is a prerequisite of any successful management policy and can be the hardest objective to achieve and maintain.

CONCLUSIONS AND THE WAY FORWARD

Likely developments

The aim of further progress in this field must be to stop bleeding rapidly and to prevent it from recurring. In this way danger to the patient can be averted whilst powerful modern drugs heal the ulcer. There is no evidence that a pharmacological agent given orally or systematically can dramatically affect this problem. Evidence suggests that the H_2RAs and antiproteolytic agents such as tranexamic acid can make a marginal difference, but are unlikely to give the assurance necessary. The next few years should determine whether more powerful inhibition of acid secretion by omeprazole, or stronger antiproteolysis (e.g. aprotinin) will be more successful.

Currently the more promising approach that may avoid the need for surgery is endoscopic therapy directed to the bleeding point. Further trials of an increasing diversity of these techniques should determine whether the bleeding point can be rendered safe. If this can be established long enough it will allow us to take advantage of the powerful healing agents being produced by modern pharmacology.

Surgical technique has also improved substantially, but the major question now to be answered is whether emergency operation should be limited to stopping the bleeding, and as with endoscopic therapy leave healing to the physicians.

Mortality rates have dropped to a level where further significant improvement is difficult to show, but if the approaches outlined are successful, mortality rates of less than 5% might be achievable in the over 60 age groups.

Unanswered questions

(a) Is there a 'medical' way (drugs, endoscopic) to stop bleeding and/or prevent rebleeding?

(b) How can the patient who will inevitably require operation be identified accurately and early?

(c) What is the reason for the cardiovascular complications and thus how may they be prevented?

(d) Is minimal surgery an advantage?

REFERENCES

Alexander-Williams J (1973) Pyloroplasty. In Rob C & Smith R (eds) *Operative Surgery Abdomen*, 3rd edn, p 73. London: Butterworth.

Allan R & Dykes P (1976) A study of the factors influencing mortality rates from gastrointestinal haemorrhage. *Quarterly Journal of Medicine* **45**: 533–550.

Armstrong CP & Blower AL (1987) Non-steroidal anti-inflammatory drugs and life threatening complications of peptic ulceration. *Gut* **28**: 527–532.

Asby DW, Anderson J & Peaston JT (1963) Haemorrhage from peptic ulcer treated by continuous intragastric milk drip and early generous feeding. *Gut* **4**: 344–348.

Biggs JC, Hugh TB & Dodds AJ (1976) Tranexamic acid and upper gastrointestinal haemorrhage—a double blind trial. *Gut* **17**: 729–734.

Blair SD, Janvrin SB, McCollum CN & Greenhalgh RM (1986) Effect of early blood transfusion on gastrointestinal haemorrhage. *British Journal of Surgery* **73**: 783–785.

Bornman PC, Theodorou NA, Schuttleworth RD et al (1985) Importance of hypovolaemic shock and endoscopic signs in predicting recurrent haemorrhage from peptic ulceration: a prospective evaluation. *British Medical Journal* **291**: 245–247.

Brearley S, Morris DL, Hawker PC, Dykes PW & Keighley MRB (1985) Prediction of mortality at endoscopy in bleeding peptic ulcer disease. *Endoscopy* **17**: 173–174.

Brearley S, Hawker PC, Morris DL, Dykes PW & Keighley MRB (1987) Selection of patients for surgery following peptic ulcer haemorrhage. *British Journal of Surgery* **74**, 893–896.

Brook PM (1988) The side-effects of non-steroidal anti-inflammatory drugs. *Medical Journal of Australia* **148**: 248–251.

Callender ST (1981) Chronic blood loss. In Dykes PW & Keighley MRB (eds) *Gastrointestinal Haemorrhage*, pp 112–125. Bristol: Wright-PSG.

Cheung LY (1981) Treatment of established stress ulcer disease. *World Journal of Surgery* **5**: 235–240.

Clason AE, Macleod DA & Elton RA (1986) Clinical factors in the prediction of further haemorrhage or mortality in acute upper gastrointestinal haemorrhage. *British Journal of Surgery* **73**: 985–987.

Collins R & Langman M (1985) Treatment with histamine H₂ antagonists in acute upper gastrointestinal hemorrhage—implications of randomised trials. *New England Journal of Medicine* **313**: 660–666.

Cox HT, Poller L & Thomson JM (1967) Gastric fibrinolysis—a possible aetiological link with peptic ulcer. *Lancet* **i**: 1300–1302.

Dave P, Romeu J & Messer J (1983) Upper gastrointestinal bleeding in patients with portal hypertension: a reappraisal. *Journal of Clinical Gastroenterology* **5**: 113–116.

Devitt JE, Brown FN & Beattie WG (1966) Fatal bleeding ulcer. *Annals of Surgery* **164**: 840–844.

Duggan JM (1986) Ten year follow-up of gastrointestinal hemorrhage patients. *Australian and New Zealand Journal of Medicine* **16**: 33–38.

Engqvist A, Broström O, Feilitzen F et al (1979) Tranexamic acid in massive haemorrhage from the upper gastrointestinal tract: a double blind study. *Scandinavian Journal of Gastroenterology* **14**, 839–844.

Foster DN, Miloszewski KJA & Losowsky MS (1978) Stigmata of recent haemorrhage in diagnosis and prognosis of upper gastrointestinal bleeding. *British Medical Journal* **i**: 1173–1177.

Gatehouse D, Dimock F & Burdon DW et al (1978) Prediction of wound sepsis following gastric operations. *British Journal of Surgery* **65**: 551–554.

Helgstrand U (1983) Fibrinolysis and peptic ulcer. *Scandinavian Journal of Gastroenterology* (**supplement**): 39–41.

Henry DA & O'Connell DL (1989) Effects of fibrinolytic inhibitors on mortality from upper gastrointestinal haemorrhage. *British Medical Journal* **298**: 1142–1146.

Herrington JL & Davidson III JR (1987) Bleeding gastroduodenal ulcers: choice of operations. *World Journal of Surgery* **11**, 304–314.

Himal HS, Watson WW, Jones CW et al (1974) The management of upper gastrointestinal hemorrhage: A multiparametric computer analysis. *Annals of Surgery* **179**: 489–493.

Hubert JP, Kiernan PD, Welch JS, ReMine WH & Bears OH (1980) The surgical management of bleeding stress ulcers. *Annals of Surgery* **191**: 672–677.

Hunt PS (1983) Operative treatment for bleeding ulcer. In: Dudley H, Pories W & Carter D (eds) *Rob and Smith's Operative Surgery Alimentary Tract and Abdominal Wall: 1 Principles, Oesophagus, Stomach, Duodenum, Small Intestine, Abdominal Wall, Hernia* 4th edn, p 291. London: Butterworth.

Hunt PS (1984) The management of chronic peptic ulcer—a ten year prospective study. *Annals of Surgery* **199**: 44–50.

Hunt PS (1987) Bleeding gastroduodenal ulcers: Selection of patients for surgery. *World Journal of Surgery* **11**: 289–294.

Hunt PS, Hansky J & Korman MG (1979a) Mortality in patients with haematemesis and melaena: a prospective study. *British Medical Journal* **1**: 1238–1240.

Hunt PS, Korman MG, Hansky J et al (1979b) Bleeding duodenal ulcer: reduction in mortality with a planned approach. *British Journal of Surgery* **66**, 633–635.

Hunt PS, Hansky J & Korman MG (1982) Bleeding carcinomatous ulcer of the stomach (letter). *Medical Journal of Australia* **1**: 494.

Johnston D (1977) Division and repair of the sphincteric mechanism at the gastric outlet in emergency operations for bleeding peptic ulcer. *Annals of Surgery* **186**: 723–729.

Johnston D (1983) Highly selective vagotomy with excision of the ulcer for gastric ulceration. In Dudley H, Pories W & Carter D (eds) *Rob and Smith's Operative Surgery Alimentary Tract and Abdominal Wall: 1 Principles, Oesophagus, Stomach, Duodenum, Small Intestine, Abdominal Wall, Hernia*, 4th edn, pp. 226, 228. London: Butterworth.

Johnston D (1985) Duodenal and gastric ulcer. In Schwartz SI & Ellis H (eds) *Maingot's Abdominal Operations*, pp 767. Norwalk, CT Apple-Century-Crofts.

Johnston D, Lyndon PJ, Smith RB & Humphrey CS (1973) Highly selective vagotomy without a drainage procedure in the treatment of haemorrhage, perforation and pyloric stenosis due to peptic ulcer. *British Journal of Surgery* 60: 790–797.

Jones FA, (1956) Hematemesis and melena with special reference to causation and to the factors influencing the mortality from bleeding peptic ulcers. *Gastroenterology* 30: 166–190.

Kakkar VV, Corrigan TP, Fossad DP et al (1975) Prevention of fatal pulmonary embolism by low doses of heparin. An international multicentre trial. *Lancet* 2: 7924–7951

Langman MJS, Coggon D & Spieghalter D (1983) Analgesic intake and the risk of acute upper gastrointestinal bleeding. *American Journal of Medicine* 74(6A): 79–82.

Laurence BH & Cotton PB (1987) Bleeding gastroduodenal ulcers: Nonoperative treatment. *World Journal of Surgery* 11: 295–303.

Madden MV & Griffith GH (1986) Management of upper gastro-intestinal bleeding in a district general hospital. *Journal of the Royal College of Physicians of London* 20: 212–215.

Magnussen I, Ihre T, Johansson C et al (1985) Randomised double blind trial of somatostatin in the treatment of massive upper gastrointestinal haemorrhage. *Gut* 26: 221–226.

Michel L & Malt RA (1986) Mallory–Weiss syndrome. In Hunt PS (ed) *Clinical Surgery International. Volume 11—Gastrointestinal Haemorrhage.* Edinburgh: Churchill Livingstone.

Morris DL, Hawker PC, Brearley S, Simms M, Dykes PW & Keighley MRB (1984) Optimal timing of operation for bleeding peptic ulcer: a prospective randomised trial. *British Medical Journal* 288: 1277–1280.

Murray WR, Laferla G, Cooper G & Archibald M (1986) Doudenal ulcer healing after presentation with haemorrhage. *Gut* 27: 1387–1389.

Murrary WR, Cooper G, Laferia G et al (1988) Maintenance ranitidine treatment after haemorrhage from a duodenal ulcer. A 3-year study. *Scandinavian Journal of Gastroenterology* 23: 183–187.

Ovaska JT & Havia T (1988) Surgical treatment of high gastric ulcer. *Annales Chirurgiae et Gynaecologiae* 77: 6–8.

Rogers PN, Murray WR, Shaw R & Brar S (1988) Surgical management of bleeding gastric ulceration. *British Journal of Surgery* 75: 16–17.

Shuman RB, Schuster DP & Zuckerman GR (1987) Prophylactic therapy for stress ulcer bleeding: a reappraisal. *Annals of Internal Medicine* 106: 562–567.

Smart HL & Langman MJS (1986) Late outcome of bleeding gastric ulcers. *Gut* 27: 926–928.

Snook JA, Holdstock GE & Bamforth J (1986) Value of a simple biochemical ratio in distinguishing upper and lower sites of gastrointestinal haemorrhage. *Lancet* i: 1064–1065.

Snyman JH & Keighley MRB (1989) Acute non-variceal haemorrhage. *Current Practice in Surgery* 1: 2–9.

Söderlund C (1987) Vasopressin and glypressin in upper gastrointestinal bleeding. *Scandinavian Journal of Gastroenterology* 22 (supplement 137): 50–55.

Staël von Holstein CCS, Eriksson SBS & Källén R (1987) Tranexamic acid as an aid to reducing blood transfusion requirements in gastric and duodenal bleeding. *British Medical Journal* 294: 7–10.

Storey DW, Brown SG, Swain CP, Salmon PR, Kirkham, JS & Northfield TC (1981) Endoscopic prediction of recurrent bleeding in peptic ulcers. *New England Journal of Medicine* 305: 915–916.

Stringer MD & Cameron AEP (1988) Surgeons' attitudes to the operative management of duodenal ulcer perforation and haemorrhage. *Annals of the Royal College of Surgeons of England* 70: 220–223.

Taylor TV (1985) Deaths from peptic ulceration. *British Medical Journal* 291: 653–654.

Thon K, Stöltzing H, Ohmann C et al (1988) Decision-making and clinical problem solving in upper gastrointestinal bleeding. *Theoretical Surgery* **2**: 185–198.

Veldhuyzen van Zanten SJO, Bartelsman JFMW, Schipper MEI & Tytgat GNJ (1986) Recurrent massive haematemesis from Dieulafoy vascular malformations—a review of 101 cases. *Gut* **27**: 213–222.

Venables VW (1981) Gastroduodenal surgery. In Dykes P W & Keighley MRB (eds) *Gastrointestinal Haemorrhage*, pp 337–356. Bristol: Wright-PSG.

4

BLEEDING OESOPHAGEAL VARICES

R. Shields

Bleeding from oesophageal varices can present the clinician with one of the most challenging therapeutic problems. Bleeding may be rapid and exsanguinating, requiring urgent treatment for its control and resuscitation of the patient; the patient's general condition may be poor because of previous haemorrhage and impairment of renal and hepatic function. A first bleed carries a mortality of 40–60% and once bleeding is controlled, the patient stands a 60% chance of a second major haemorrhage within a year. Fortunately there are now available several methods of treatment, but it behoves the clinician to have a clear-cut management policy.

Conventionally, the management of oesophageal varices is divided into (a) the control of an acute bleeding episode and (b) the prevention of rebleeding in the future. It is with the first of these that this chapter will deal. However, the distinction between these two scenarios is blurred. Not all patients who are admitted as an emergency require immediate treatment to control the haemorrhage. In a comprehensive endoscopic study, Mitchell et al (1982) showed that, when endoscopic examination was carried out within 4 hours of an emergency admission, in only 25% of episodes was actual bleeding observed; in the remainder the bleeding had stopped spontaneously. Our own experience confirms this observation. Therefore the patient should be endoscoped on admission and, if bleeding has stopped, it is unnecessary and unwise to administer a vasoconstrictor or tamponade the oesophagus with a balloon, because both measures are associated with complications. However, of the patients who had stopped bleeding, about 60% had a further variceal haemorrhage during their stay in hospital, indicating that a definitive procedure should be planned and undertaken during the initial admission.

Most centres adopt a sequential management policy, employing the simplest, least invasive methods first. Unfortunately we do not have good indicators to predict the likelihood of continuing or recurrent bleeding, as, for example, the visible vessel in bleeding peptic ulcer. Increase in intravariceal pressure is the event most probably associated with variceal rupture, and therefore cherry red spots and haemocystic spots are possible endoscopic markers of impending variceal haemorrhage (Kleber et al, 1989). However, these signs are not sufficiently reliable to predict recurrent or persistent bleeding to allow us to pass over the simpler, but less effective measures, to more radical treatment, such as oesophageal transection.

RESUSCITATION

Resuscitation should be embarked upon immediately. The patient should be admitted to hospital. Blood, preferably fresh, should be transfused, but over-transfusion should be avoided by monitoring the central venous pressure. Fresh frozen plasma and platelets are often required to correct deficiencies in coagulation. Monitoring in a high dependency unit is usually necessary and occasionally a Swan Ganz catheter has to be passed if the patient has had an acute bleeding episode superimposed on chronic haemorrhage or cardiac disease.

ENDOSCOPY

Diagnostic endoscopy is essential to confirm that varices are present and are the source of bleeding. The varices are seen as bluish protrusions into the oesophageal lumen and are most clearly seen at, or just above, the gastro-oesophageal junction. Small varices may be confused with mucosal folds and gastric varices may be missed unless a flexible endoscope is carefully manipulated to view the fundus. It is important to ensure that there are no other causes of upper gastrointestinal haemorrhage, such as oesophagitis, duodenal ulcer and gastric erosions. Varices may be diagnosed as the certain source of bleeding if active bleeding is evident or fresh clot is adherent to the varices; in the absence of signs of recent bleeding, they are the likely source if no other pathology is seen in the upper gastrointestinal tract.

If varices are confirmed, the patient should be transferred to an appropriate centre once the bleeding has been controlled and resuscitation completed, because further measures are required to prevent its recurrence.

In some centres a vasoactive drug, e.g. vasopressin, is administered, with or without balloon tamponade, and endoscopy postponed until the following day. This is not our practice. Endoscopy on admission is mandatory and, if active bleeding is confirmed, treatment is begun immediately. Our own practice is to inject the oesophageal varices with sclerosant during the same endoscopic session. Endoscopic sclerotherapy is highly effective and immediate treatment avoids the use of vasoactive drugs, some of which have side effects, and balloon tamponade, which is frequently attended by complications. There is also evidence that immediate sclerotherapy is better than delayed treatment. However, vasoactive drugs and balloon tamponade will be considered first.

VASOACTIVE DRUGS

Vasopressin

Until recently, the most commonly used drug was vasopressin, a powerful systemic and splanchnic vasoconstrictor, which reduces portal pressure and flow. It is usually administered as a continuous intravenous infusion. The initial dose is 20 units in 100 ml 5% dextrose infused over 20 min, followed by continuous infusion of 0.2–0.4 units/min, up to 0.8 units/min if necessary. Unfortunately generalized vasoconstriction, which vasopressin produces, may cause undesirable side effects, such as coronary, cerebral and mesenteric vasoconstriction, predisposing to infarction of the related tissues and organs. Side effects may require that treatment is stopped in about 20% of cases. The treatment is not highly effective because bleeding is controlled in only 50–60% of episodes.

To reduce side effects and potentiate its haemodynamic effect on the portal circulation, vasopressin has been combined with nitroglycerin, administered intravenously, sublinguinally or transdermally. The usual recommendation is sublingual nitroglycerin, one tablet every half-hour for up to 6 h. The combination of the drugs may be more effective at reducing side effects than increasing efficacy.

An alternative agent is triglicyl vasopressin (glypressin), an analogue of vasopressin, which is given intravenously as a 2 mg bolus every 6 h. Again, the benefit may lie in reducing side effects rather than increasing effectiveness.

Somatostatin

The role of this 14 amino peptide in controlling acute variceal haemorrhage is currently under study. It seems to act by reducing the flow and pressure in the collateral circulation (e.g. oesophageal varices) rather than reducing portal pressure directly. Initial trials suggest that it is more effective than other drugs and placebos (Kravetz et al, 1984; Jenkins et al, 1985; Testoni et al, 1986) and may be equal to injection sclerotherapy.

The current high cost of the naturally occurring somatostatin may curtail its wider use. It is given by intravenous infusion 250 μg/h, with an initial bolus of 250 μg injected over 2 min, repeated daily to cover renewing the infusing syringe. The analogue octreotide (sandostatin, Sandoz) may be as effective and is much cheaper. In emergency circumstances it is given by intravenous infusion, 50 μg/h, with bolus supplements.

Other drugs

Other drugs have been used and are currently being evaluated, especially those which are said to produce their action by constricting the lower oesophageal sphincter, e.g. pentagastrin, metoclopramide and cisapride.

BALLOON TAMPONADE

Balloon tamponade can be an effective method in stopping bleeding in 70–80% of patients. It is, however, a stop-gap measure, allowing time for resuscitation and planning further management. Tamponade should be continued for 12–24 h only, to avoid necrosis of the oesophagus. After removal of the tube, there is a high rate of recurrence of bleeding. Continued haemorrhage during tamponade indicates bleeding from other sites, such as fundal varices, gastric ulcer, or perhaps problems associated with impaired coagulation. Serious complications are encountered in 10% of patients and include oesophageal necrosis and rupture, and aspiration pneumonia. So serious are these complications that balloon tamponade should not be used as an initial measure, but only in those who have failed vasoconstrictor therapy or injection sclerotherapy, or both.

Several different tubes are available but the most popular is the Minnesota modification of the Sengstaken–Blakemore tube. It has four channels: the longest one is used for aspirating the stomach, the second for inflating the gastric balloon, the third for inflating the sausage-shaped oesophageal balloon and the fourth channel for aspirating blood and swallowed saliva from the upper oesophagus.

Instructions for balloon tamponade

On each occasion a new tube should be used. Before use, each balloon is inflated to test for leaks. The balloons are then deflated and coated with a water-miscible lubricating jelly. The patient is placed on his left side with a head-down tilt to reduce the risk of aspiration. The tube should be passed by mouth, to prevent damage and obstruction to the nasal passages and to permit its rapid removal, if this is required. The passage of the tube is aided by careful folding of the oesophageal and gastric balloons around it. The tube should be passed until the 50 cm mark is reached. The position can be checked by X-ray or, alternatively, air can be insufflated down the gastric aspiration channel and the epigastrium auscultated. Suction is applied to the gastric and oesophageal aspiration channels to reduce the risk of regurgitation of gastric content, blood and saliva when the gastric balloon is inflated. The gastric balloon is inflated with air or saline solution containing a small quantity of radio-opaque contrast medium. After 250–350 ml have been instilled, the gastric balloon inlet is doubly clamped with rubber-shod clamps and firm traction is applied to the tube, until the resistance of the inflated gastric balloon can be felt firmly against the gastro-oesophageal junction. With minimal traction on the tube, its upper end is fixed to the side of the mouth. Alternatively a cord may be tied to the tube and led over pulleys to a 1–2 kg weight.

The stomach is then washed with isotonic saline solution until the aspirate is clear. If bleeding is not controlled, the oesophageal balloon should be inflated to a pressure of 35–40 mmHg, recorded on a blood pressure manometer attached to the oesophageal channel. The channel leading to the inflated oesophageal balloon is doubly clamped. The stomach should be aspirated at intervals to determine if bleeding is continuing. Continuous aspiration of the oesophagus above the oesophageal balloon is necessary to remove swallowed saliva.

The balloons should be kept inflated and on traction for no more than 24 h. After 12–18 h the oesophageal balloon is slowly deflated and, by aspiration through the oesophageal and gastric channels, checks are made for recurrence of the haemorrhage. If there is no bleeding, traction on the tube should be released and the gastric balloon deflated. If bleeding still remains stopped, the tube should be cautiously removed. If bleeding recurs during this sequence the balloons should be reinflated and traction applied for another 12 h. However, during this 12-h period, the risk of complications is greatly increased and preparation should be made for definitive treatment.

Nursing and medical staff looking after the patient should be completely familiar with the Sengstaken tube. Knowledge and scrupulous care in its use greatly reduce the incidence of complications. A pair of scissors should always be taped to the head of the patient's bed so that, if the oesophageal balloon migrates into the hypopharynx, or if respiratory distress develops, the attendants can remove the balloon as rapidly as possible. Traction on the tube and pressure in the oesophageal balloon should be checked every 4 h.

ENDOSCOPIC INJECTION SCLEROTHERAPY

Currently the most popular method of controlling acute variceal haemorrhage is the injection of sclerosant into, or alongside, the oesophageal varices. Between 80% and 90% of acute bleeds can be controlled by endoscopic sclerotherapy.

In some centres bleeding is controlled initially by vasoconstrictor drugs, with or without balloon tamponade, followed by injection sclerotherapy the following day. The advantage of this approach is that the endoscopist's field of vision is clear of blood. Alternatively, and this is our practice, immediate injection of the varix is undertaken at the initial endoscopy on the patient's admission. Considerable expertise in endoscopy is required because the varices may still be bleeding, but there is good evidence that such an approach is more successful (Westaby et al, 1986). Because of its high rate of success, sclerotherapy is preferable to balloon tamponade or vasopressin for the initial control of bleeding.

There are several variations in the technique of endoscopic sclerotherapy: intravariceal versus paravariceal injection; the type of sclerosant (alcohol, sodium morrhuate, ethanolamine oleate); volume of sclerosant; general anaesthesia or heavy sedation. The fact that there does not seem to be any great difference in outcome among these variants suggests that they are not important determinants of success. Our own practice is to use a flexible endoscope, passed into the oesophagus of the anaesthetized patient, so that the airway is under control and protected. We use an overtube, or sheath, so that the bleeding varices are allowed to protrude in turn into the lumen through a slot at its end. Using a flexible needle, we inject 3–5 ml ethanolamine oleate into each varix, just above the cardio-oesophageal junction. All visible varices are injected at this first session, and up to 20 ml sclerosant may be used. The results of several trials have recently been reviewed by Burroughs (1988a).

Complications, the rates of which vary from one reported series to another, are relatively uncommon. They include ulceration at the site of the injection (more common after paravariceal, rather than intravariceal, injection), oesophageal stricture (which is easily dilated) and, rarely, perforation of the oesophagus. A slight fever after the procedure is relatively common and the patient may complain of dull, retrosternal pain and discomfort for 24 h.

FURTHER MANAGEMENT

In about 10–15% of patients, bleeding may recur within hours or days of the initial treatment (either endoscopic sclerotherapy or somatostatin infusion), and may be significant, requiring blood transfusion. Further endoscopy should always be performed to determine the cause. There are at least four possible causes of recurrence of bleeding soon after apparently successful initial treatment: (a) recurrence of bleeding from oesophageal varices; (b) bleeding from gastric varices; (c) bleeding from oesophageal ulcer secondary to injection; (d) bleeding from oesophagitis, gastric erosion or portal hypertensive gastropathy.

Recurrent bleeding from oesophageal varices

If oesophageal varices which have previously been injected are the source of bleeding, somatostatin infusion should be set up; if, however, bleeding recurs from oesophageal varices after somatostatin treatment, endoscopic sclerotherapy should be undertaken. The success rate of those treated by a crossover to the alternative regimen is about 80–90%.

If bleeding is not controlled despite these attempts at sclerotherapy and infusion of somatostatin, definitive treatment is urgently required. There is little point in continuing with further attempts at sclerotherapy or infusion of a vasoconstrictor; further treatment should not be delayed by the use of balloon tamponade, except as a very brief stop-gap measure before surgical intervention. In this group of patients mortality is high and liver function is often severely impaired. If the patient's condition is good, with only mild to moderate impairment of liver function, operation should be undertaken expeditiously. The outlook will be poor if there is continuing delay and procrastination with repeated attempts at sclerotherapy, balloon tamponade or vasocontrictor treatment.

Bleeding from gastric varices

Bleeding from gastric varices can be temporarily controlled by balloon tamponade, provided the gastric balloon is well inflated with moderate traction, for gastric varices usually lie high in the fundus. Gastric varices can be injected with sclerosant, but there can be difficulties in positioning the endoscope. In many cases control of gastric varices will require operation (see later).

Bleeding from oesophageal ulcers

Bleeding may occur from oesophageal ulcers, usually secondary to necrosis of overlying mucosa after submucosal injection of the sclerosant. We have found that somatostatin infusion has been invariably successful in stopping a haemorrhage from this source.

Bleeding from portal hypertensive gastropathy

Recurrent bleeding may occur from erosions accompanying the congestive gastropathy of portal hypertension (McCormack et al, 1985). Usually these lesions are not the source of major haemorrhage and we have found that this bleeding can be controlled by somatostatin infusion. Bleeding can usually be prevented by propranolol, the non-selective beta-blocker.

EMERGENCY OPERATIONS

If bleeding from oesophageal varices recurs and is clearly not being controlled, the patient is a candidate for an emergency operation which should be undertaken sooner rather than later, before the risks of operation are increased by excess transfusions, fluid overload and the problems of aspiration of blood into the lung. A portasystemic shunt should be considered in the young non-alcoholic patient, because the results of such operations are good. The simplest and easiest procedures are either end-to-side portacaval shunt, or an H-graft portacaval shunt. Under other circumstances stapling oesophageal transection is preferred. A different approach is required for gastric varices.

The results of an emergency procedure in a jaundiced patient with hypo-albuminaemia, ascites and encephalopathy are poor. These patients, belonging to the Child C category of liver disease, will have an almost 100% mortality after any emergency operation.

Oesophageal transection

Stapling transection of the oesophagus is one of the simpler operations aimed at obliterating the gastro-oesophageal varices. Former operations, such as transthoracic oesophageal transection (Milnes–Walker operation), or high gastric transection (Tanner operation), in which the lower oesophagus or upper stomach was divided and reanastomosed to occlude the varices, were formidable procedures in an ill patient and were attended by a high rate of recurrent bleeding or leakage at the anastomosis. These complications were reflected in high morbidity and mortality.

The introduction of stapling instruments has enabled abdominal transection of the oesophagus to be performed with relative ease and safety (Spence and Johnston, 1985). The stapling instrument is inserted into the stomach through a small incision on its anterior wall. The head of the instrument is passed into the lower oesophagus. The vagal nerves are reflected out of the way and a linen thread is placed and tied around the shaft of the head of the instrument, which is then closed and fired. The oesophagus is simultaneously transected and reanastomosed and in this way, it is hoped, the varices are obliterated. Usually extrinsic devascularization is carried out at the same time, by ligating the left gastric vascular axis in continuity and by dividing and ligating prominent veins in the vicinity of the lower oesophagus and upper part of the stomach.

Varying results have been reported for this operation used in emergency circumstances. Mortality is high when oesophageal transection is delayed and undertaken late. Death in these circumstances is related to hepatic failure in patients with poor liver function, rather than recurrence of bleeding (Jenkins and Shields, 1989). On the other hand, three trials (Cell et al, 1982; Huizinga et al, 1985; Teves et al, 1987), have shown that oesophageal transection is as good as endoscopic sclerotherapy, in terms of short-term control of the bleeding and survival. Stapling transection also avoids the risk of encephalopathy which is associated with shunt operations. Most centres, it must be emphasized, continue to use sclerotherapy as the primary emergency treatment.

There are other operations in which a direct attack on the varices is the cardinal feature. The most extensive is the Sugiura procedure (Sugiura and Gutagawa, 1984), in which the spleen is removed, the oesophagus transected and there is extensive para-oesophageal devascularization up to the inferior pulmonary vein. The oesophagus and stomach are stripped of their venous collaterals. Although this operation has found favour in Japan, where the reported incidence of postoperative rebleeding is remarkably low, it has not become popular in Europe or the United States. The mortality rate in Western countries has been high (from 11% to 60%), with rebleeding in 20–50% of cases. The differences in results may be accounted for by variation in technique, but the main reason is probably the type of liver disease. In the Sugiura series, over 70% of patients had postnecrotic cirrhosis, whereas in the Western experience alcoholic cirrhosis predominates. Moreover, in the Japanese group, liver function was usually much better than that encountered in European or American patients.

The specific indication for devascularizing operations is continuing haemorrhage, despite lesser measures, in a patient with portal vein thrombosis, in whom portal systemic shunting is not possible. The surgeon should not too readily operate in a young patient because a child can tolerate frequent haemorrhage corrected by blood transfusion, on the basis that a collateral circulation may develop and the bleeding become less frequent.

Portasystemic shunt

An emergency portasystemic shunt is considered only if bleeding is not controlled by other measures and the patient's condition, especially liver function, is good. The aim of a shunt operation is to reduce portal pressure and so control the haemorrhage and prevent recurrent bleeding. The attainment of such an objective requires a major anastomosis between splanchnic and systemic veins. Lesser procedures to reduce portal flow, e.g. splenectomy (but see below), hepatic arterial ligation, or attempts to create diffuse shunts, e.g. omentopexy, are usually fruitless. While shunt operations are usually successful in stopping the haemorrhage and preventing its recurrence, the price to be paid is an increasing risk of hepatoportal encephalopathy and postoperative liver failure.

Portasystemic shunts are customarily divided into two types:

(a) *Total* portasystemic shunts, e.g. end-to-side portacaval shunt, H-graft portacaval shunt, mesocaval shunt and central splenorenal shunts. These shunts are so called because the entire splanchnic bed is decompressed. In end-to-side portacaval shunt (Figure 1) the liver is not decompressed because the portal vein cannot act as an outflow from the liver and so sinusoidal hypertension is maintained.

(b) *Selective* shunts in which the gastro-oesophageal varices are provided with a selective decompressive pathway, while portal hypertension is maintained in the rest of the splanchnic circulation. The theoretical advantage of these operations is that the venous blood flow to the liver is preserved and, because hepatic perfusion is unimpaired, liver function does not deteriorate after operation, at least not on account of the shunt. Examples of the selective shunts are distal spleno-renal shunt (Figure 2) and coronary-caval shunt.

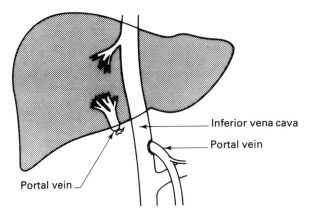

FIGURE 1   End-to-side portacaval shunt
(reproduced from Taylor et al, 1984, by kind permission of Heinemann Education Books Ltd).

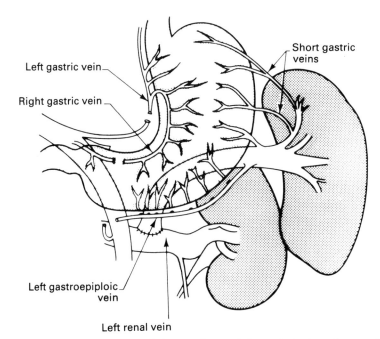

FIGURE 2   Distal spleno-renal shunt with partial devascularization of stomach
(reproduced from Taylor et al, 1984, by kind permission of Heinemann Educational Books Ltd).

If a portasystemic shunt is contemplated, the potency of the major veins must be confirmed. Angiography should include superior mesenteric and coeliac axis arteriography, with good venous phase studies, and inferior vena-cavography. There may not be an opportunity in the severely bleeding patient to perform these investigations, but ultrasound of the abdomen should be undertaken to confirm the patency of the portal vein.

The most commonly performed operation in emergency circumstances is the standard, end-to-side portacaval shunt (Figure 1). Bleeding will be controlled so long as the shunt remains patent; the chances are greater if the anastomosis is wide and synthetic graft is not used (for example, when dacron graft is interposed between the superior mesenteric vein and the inferior vena cava, there is a high incidence of graft thrombosis in the long term). Although bleeding is usually satisfactorily controlled, the incidence of encephalopathy is about 15%.

Controversy still exists about the role of portacaval shunt in the emergency control of bleeding. One extreme has been the performance of a shunt within 8 h of the diagnosis of variceal bleeding (Orloff and Bell, 1986). However, mortality is high, and it does seem unacceptable to subject all patients admitted to hospital with bleeding varices to a major operation, when simpler methods, e.g. endoscopic sclerotherapy, would bring the bleeding under control in the majority of occasions. The opposite view has been that portacaval shunt has little role in the emergency care of these patients. This is equally extreme. Results can be good in the younger, non-alcoholic patient with good liver function. Advice should be sought early in such patients, if bleeding is not controlled by two attempts at endoscopic sclerotherapy and somatostatin infusion.

The technique for end-to-side portacaval shunt will not be described and the interested reader should consult texts of operative surgery, or, preferably, observe the operation being undertaken by an experienced surgeon.

An alternative operation, marginally easier to perform, is the partial portacaval H-graft shunt, in which a synthetic graft, usually of polytetrafluoroethylene (PTFE), is inserted between the portal vein and inferior vena cava (Sarfeh, 1988). These grafts are of smaller diameter (8–10 mm) than those formerly used in the mesenteric caval shunt (18–20 mm) and are claimed to reduce portal pressure while preserving hepatic perfusion, so reducing the incidence of hepatoportal encephalopathy. These operations remain to be tested in long-term trials to determine if the grafts remain patent.

A central splenorenal shunt is now rarely employed, but can be undertaken in the treatment of gastric varices after the spleen has been removed. It is a technically demanding operation and there is a high risk of thrombosis, due to low flow through the narrow anastomosis.

The distal splenorenal shunt (Figure 2) has increased in popularity because it selectively decompresses the critical area at the cardio-oesophageal junction and maintains, at least in the short term, an adequate hepatic perfusion. The operation seems to be as successful as a total shunt in terms of the patient's survival and the control and prevention of recurrent bleeding. In some, but not all, reported trials the incidence of hepatoportal encephalopathy is reduced. An important component of the operation is preservation of the short gastric veins to the spleen and adequate gastric devascularization including coronary azygos disconnection.

Because the operation is technically more difficult than end-to-side portacaval shunt, and adequate preoperative investigations including angiography are necessary, it is more appropriately performed electively, when the venous anatomy and direction of venous flow can be defined. In emergency circumstances it should be performed only by those skilled in its use and certainly only in patients with good liver function (Child Groups A and B). The operation is contraindicated in the presence of ascites, portal vein occlusion and after splenectomy or left nephrectomy.

An advantage of distal splenorenal shunt is that it does not impede, to the same extent as other operations, liver transplantation whose indications in the management of these patients are increasing.

Without doubt recent reports have reawakened interest in emergency shunt operations (Warren et al, 1986; Shields, 1989). There is good evidence that portasystemic shunts may be more effective than sclerotherapy in preventing recurrence of bleeding with no difference in survival. Shunt operation should be considered much earlier in the management policy in those patients who do not respond to sclerotherapy.

Operations for gastric varices

Bleeding from gastric varices has been considered to be uncommon, but the conventional incidence of less than 10% is probably an underestimate. Bleeding gastric varices can be difficult to control and often operation is required (Greig et al, 1990). We try initially to control the gastric varices by injection sclerotherapy, but this can be difficult.

In our practice, two operations can be of help in different circumstances. The lesser operation (Ong, 1977) is carried out when the spleen is small. Through an abdominal incision, the anterior wall of the stomach is incised. Bleeding gastric varices can be seen in the posterior wall, radiating from the cardio-oesophageal junction. The varices are underrun with continuous, non-absorbed sutures. Extrinsic devascularization and stapling transection are undertaken at the same time. This procedure, however, is not successful—indeed may be hazardous—when the patient has a grossly enlarged spleen which embraces the greater curvature of the stomach, incorporating it into its hilum. These patients have large venous collaterals running between the splenic hilum and the stomach. Attempts to plicate gastric varices will lead to further haemorrhage. The operation of choice in these circumstances is a splenectomy—a difficult, often bloody, operation, which is, however, usually successful in stopping the bleeding.

Other procedures

Most other procedures such as percutaneous transhepatic obliteration of the varices have been abandoned and others have not yet been established as successful, e.g. laser coagulation, electrocautery, or endoscopic elastic banding of varices.

SUPPORTIVE TREATMENT

During the patient's stay in hospital, simultaneously with resuscitation and control of bleeding, measures should be undertaken to improve the patient's condition and prevent complications. More than lip service should be paid to these measures because their employment can considerably reduce morbidity and mortality.

(a) To minimize or prevent hepatoportal encephalopathy, lactulose and neomycin are given.

(b) Because of the high incidence of gastric erosions and peptic ulceration, especially in alcoholic cirrhotics, gastric acid production is reduced by giving H_2 blocking drugs, e.g. cimetidine or ranitidine.

(c) Prevention of renal failure is an important component of the patient's management. Previously normal kidneys can be rapidly and irreversibly damaged by severe and prolonged hypotension following an acute haemorrhage. Associated secretion of antidiuretic hormone can lead to intravascular retention of water. Resuscitation should be, therefore, with blood or salt-poor albumin, and plasma expanders such as haemocel should be avoided. Fluids should be restricted only when plasma concentration of sodium is less than 120 mmol/l. Diuretics should not be given in the presence of hypovolaemia or septic shock. Paracentesis of ascites is acceptable so long as there is simultaneous infusion of salt-poor albumin. To monitor the patient, an urethral catheter should be inserted for measurement of 24 h output of urine. Central venous pressure (CVP) should be maintained between +4 and +8 cm H_2O. A negative recording should be acted upon immediately by replacing with blood or salt-poor albumin.

(d) Coagulation defects should be identified and corrected by the administration of platelets and fresh frozen plasma.

(e) Infections should be meticulously searched for and treated, because unexpected deterioration in a patients' condition may be caused by infection in the urine, in the chest, in ascitic fluid or in intravenous lines.

CONCLUSIONS AND THE WAY AHEAD

It is strongly advocated that at the initial endoscopy, when the presence of bleeding varices is confirmed, emergency injection sclerotherapy or somatostatin infusion should be carried out. If bleeding recurs, endoscopy should be undertaken to confirm the source of the bleeding. If bleeding recurs from varices, further injection sclerotherapy or somatostatin infusion should be employed. If bleeding continues, oesophageal transection or portasystemic shunt should be performed. For bleeding from gastric varices, injection sclerotherapy should be tried, otherwise recourse should be taken to early operation. For bleeding from oesophageal ulceration, intravenous infusion with somatostatin is very effective. This treatment is also effective in dealing with bleeding from gastric or oesophageal erosions, associated with the portal hypertensive gastropathy. In our own practice, balloon tamponade is used much less frequently, because of the success of the above measures and because of the fear of complications. Vasoactive treatment, particularly somatostatin, is a valuable alternative to injection sclerotherapy where the patient is not fit, where injection sclerotherapy has been tried and has not been successful, or where the necessary expertise and equipment is not available.

With the rapid advances in the treatment of oesophageal varices, it is likely that, in the near future, new techniques will be successfully developed. There is a great need to improve the preoperative evaluation of patients and particularly to define markers which will predict those patients who will probably do well with the minimum of treatment, e.g. endoscopic sclerotherapy, and those in whom bleeding tends to recur despite seemingly adequate treatment. Early recourse to operation would be indicated in these patients. The majority of deaths occur usually in the first 5 days of admission to hospital and meticulous attention has to be paid to the treatment of the patient during this critical period.

Undoubtedly hepatic transplantation will become an increasingly important modality in the treatment of portal hypertension secondary to liver disease. Thus in patients with primary biliary cirrhosis hepatic transplantation should be a readily considered treatment option. However, the place of transplantation in the acute bleeding patient has yet to be resolved. Rather bleeding should be staunched by the means described in this chapter and recourse to transplantation taken to prevent recurrence and liver failure in the future. However, it is important that nothing is done during the acute stage which may frustrate the transplant surgeon in the future. For example, end-to-side portacaval shunt should be avoided and distal spleno-renal shunt is preferred.

It would, however, be preferable to prevent the development of varices and bleeding from them. The main way to prevent the former in western countries would be to ensure a marked reduction in alcohol intake. Prophylactic measures to prevent bleeding in the cirrhotic with varices which have not yet bled have been extensively investigated and it may very well be that the use of pharmacological agents, such as propranolol, will be of considerable benefit in the future (Burroughs, 1988b).

REFERENCES

Burroughs AK (1988a) The management of bleeding due to portal hypertension. Part 1. The management of acute bleeding episodes. *Quarterly Journal of Medicine* **67**: 447–458.

Burroughs AK (1988b) The management of bleeding due to portal hypertension. Part 2. Prevention of variceal bleeding and prevention of the first bleeding episode in patients with portal hypertension. *Quarterly Journal of Medicine* **68**: 507–516.

Cell J, Cras S & Trunkey D (1982) Endoscopic sclerotherapy versus transection in Childs class C patients with variceal hemorrhage. Comparison with results of portacaval shunt: preliminary report. *Surgery* **91**: 333–338.

Greig JD, Garden OJ, Anderson JR & Carter DC (1990) Management of gastric variceal haemorrhage. *British Journal of Surgery* **77**: 297–299.

Huizinga WKJ, Angorn PA & Baker WW (1985) Esophageal transection versus injection sclerotherapy in the management of bleeding esophageal varices in patients at high risk. *Surgery, Gynecology and Obstetrics* **160**: 539–546.

Jenkins SA & Shields R (1989) Variceal haemorrhage after failed injection sclerotherapy: the role of emergency oesophageal transection. *British Journal of Surgery* **76**: 49–51.

Jenkins SA, Baxter JN, Corbett W et al (1985) A prospective randomised controlled trial comparing somatostatin and vasopressin in controlling acute variceal haemorrhage. *British Medical Journal* **290**: 275–278.

Kleber G, Sauerbruch, T, Fischer G & Paumgartner G (1989) Pressure of intra-oesophageal varices assessed by fine-needle puncture: its relation to endoscopic signs and severity of liver disease in patients with cirrhosis. *Gut* **30**: 228–232.

Kravetz D, Bosch J, Teres J et al (1984) Comparison of intravenous somatostatin and vasopressin infusions in treatment of acute variceal hemorrhage. *Hepatology* **4**: 442–446.

McCormack TT, Sims J, Eyre-Brock I, Kennedy H, Goepel J, Johnson AG & Triger DR (1985) Gastric lesions in portal hypertension: inflammatory gastritis or congestive gastropathy. *Gut* **26**: 1226–1232.

Mitchell KJ, MacDougall BRD, Silk DBA & Williams R (1982) A prospective reappraisal of emergency endoscopy in patients with portal hypertension. *Scandinavian Journal of Gastroenterology* **17**: 965–968.

Ong GB (1977) Transgastric ligation of oesophageal varices. In: Dudley H, Rob C & Smith R (eds) *Operative Surgery. Abdomen.* London: Butterworths, 212–215.

Orloff MJ & Bell RH (1986) Long-term survival after emergency portacaval shunt for bleeding varices in alcoholic cirrhosis. *American Journal of Surgery* **151**: 176–180.

Sarfeh IJ (1988) Partial shunting for portal hypertension: surgical technique. *Contemporary Surgery* **32**: 11–16.

Shields R (1989) Variceal haemorrhage. *Current Practice in Surgery* **1**: 10–16.

Spence RAJ & Johnston GW (1985) Results in 100 consecutive patients with stapled esophageal transection for varices. *Surgery, Gynecology and Obstetrics* **160**: 323–329.

Sugiura M & Gutagawa S (1984) Esophageal transection with paresophagogastric devascularisation (The Sugiura Procedure) in the treatment of esophageal varices. *World Journal of Surgery* **8**: 673–682.

Taylor S, Chisholm GD, O'Higgins N & Shields R (eds) (1984) *Surgical Management.* Heinemann Educational Books.

Teres J, Baroni R, Bordas JM, Vias J, Pera C & Rodes J (1987) Randomized trial of portacaval shunt, stapling transection and endoscopic sclerotherapy in uncontrolled variceal bleeding. *Journal of Hepatology* **4**: 159–167.

Testoni PA, Masci E, Passaretti A et al (1986) Comparison of somatostatin and cimetidine in the treatment of acute bleeding oesophageal varices. *Current Therapeutic Research* **39**: 758–766.

Warren WD, Henderson JM, Millikan WJ et al (1986) Distal splenorenal shunt versus endoscopic sclerotherapy for long-term management of variceal bleeding. *Annals of Surgery* **203**: 454–462.

Westaby D, Hayes PC, Gimson AES, Polson R & Williams R (1986) Injection sclerotherapy for active variceal bleeding: a controlled trial. *Gut* **27**: A1246.

5

RECURRENT OBSCURE GASTROINTESTINAL HAEMORRHAGE

W. E. G. Thomas

INTRODUCTION

The term 'recurrent obscure gastrointestinal haemorrhage' applies to those patients who present with recurrent gastrointestinal bleeding for which no easily identifiable cause can be found after routine investigation. Such haemorrhage may be acute or chronic, and may present either as recurrent melaena, rectal bleeding or anaemia, and very occasionally as haematemesis. The underlying cause of gastrointestinal haemorrhage is identified in over 90% of patients using routine investigations such as endoscopy or barium studies, but in the remainder the diagnosis proves elusive. Fortunately such cases are uncommon but when they do occur, a disproportionate amount of time and resources is expended in attempting to achieve a diagnosis. Therefore a logical approach to investigation is required.

A majority of these causes have the origin of blood loss sited in the small bowel below the duodenal–jejunal flexure, or in the proximal colon, and diagnostic problems arise because the bleeding is often intermittent and the small bowel is relatively inaccessible and difficult to investigate. It is the most remote part of the bowel from both mouth and anus, and therefore endoscopy is technically complex and seldom possible except at laparotomy. Barium follow-through studies, although easy to perform, have a very low 'pick-up' rate and although enteroclysis (small bowel enema) has now superseded the standard follow-through study, it will fail to identify many cases of small bowel pathology. This difficulty in investigation, and the relative rarity of many of the conditions that may present as recurrent obscure bleeding, often results in a delay in diagnosis. Furthermore, laparotomy may not always provide an easy option for diagnosis, as many of the lesions that will be described are impalpable. It is therefore highly desirable that a preoperative diagnosis is achieved wherever possible. This should be arrived at by the judicious use of currently available investigative procedures and any attempt to employ the 'blunderbus' approach of throwing every available investigation at the suffering patient should be resisted.

The differential diagnosis of enteric haemorrhage is vast (Table 1) and includes any form of ulceration, tumour or vascular anomaly. The clinical picture therefore is variable, often with a fluctuating pattern of haemorrhage. Bleeding may be occult throughout, initially occult or intermittent and then subsequently overt or

TABLE I

Causes of gastrointestinal haemorrhage

Foregut	Small bowel	Large bowel
Oesophagitis/gastritis	Ulcers	Neoplasia
Peptic ulcer	Neoplasia	Inflammatory bowel disease
Neoplasia	Vascular anomalies	Diverticular disease
Vascular anomalies	Jejunal diverticula	Angiodysplasia
Haemobilia	Meckel's diverticulum	Suture lines
Telangiectasia	Crohn's disease	Ischaemia
Portal hypertension	Telangiectasia	Portal hypertension
Suture lines	Portal hypertension	Endometriosis
Chronic pancreatitis	Aorto-enteric fistula	Trauma
Trauma	Suture lines	Bleeding diathesis
Bleeding diathesis	Parasitic infestation	
	Endometriosis	
	Trauma	
	Bleeding diathesis	

sudden and dramatic. Severe bleeds may often precipitate urgent laparotomy, but it must be stressed once more that, even in this situation, every effort should be made to obtain a preoperative diagnosis. However investigative radiology should never take priority over resuscitation, and preferably they should proceed simultaneously.

The actual choice or sequence of investigations will depend on an accurate history and meticulous examination of the patient. These will often provide valuable clues as to the possible source or site of the bleeding, thus indicating how essential these established clinical principles are when chasing an obscure case of gastrointestinal haemorrhage.

CAUSES OF GASTROINTESTINAL HAEMORRHAGE (Table I)

Fortunately the majority are usually revealed by routine investigations, and only a minority are recurrent and obscure. The heterogeneous nature of the conditions that can present with bleeding means that the clinical picture is exceedingly variable. This may result in confusion in some cases, but in others a definite clinical picture may provide useful diagnostic clues.

Patients with clotting diatheses such as thrombocytopenic purpura, thrombocythaemia, Von Willebrand's disease, haemophilia or poorly controlled anticoagulation may present with gastrointestinal haemorrhage. However up to 25% of these patients also have a coexisting organic lesion of the gastrointestinal tract (Forbes et al, 1973). Other metabolic conditions such as uraemia may also result in occult bleeding.

Foregut

Most of the foregut causes of gastrointestinal bleeding will be apparent on oesophago-gastro-duodenoscopy. One trusts that conditions such as oesophageal varices, oesophagitis, gastritis, peptic ulceration and neoplasia would be identified at endoscopy, and therefore rarely are incriminated as being the cause of recurrent obscure gastrointestinal haemorrhage. However some vascular anomalies may not be recognized for what they are, such as telangiectasia or the Dieulafoy syndrome (Thomas, 1989), and therefore it may be worth repeating the endoscopy if the history suggests that the cause of the bleeding emanates from the foregut. The Dieulafoy lesion, a submucosal microaneurysm (Goldman, 1964), causes diagnostic problems as the lesion may be situated high on the greater curvature of the stomach and be covered by blood clot. The bleeding may be profuse, but is also intermittent, and when it is not actively bleeding the lesion is a small brown spot on the mucosa that may be indistinguishable from altered flecks of blood elsewhere in the stomach. Repeat endoscopy with mucosal washing may be productive as long as the possibility of such a lesion is borne in mind.

One further major pitfall in diagnosis is provided by haemobilia. This can so easily be overlooked and is often only diagnosed by angiography when lesions such as hepatic artery aneurysms are demonstrated (Thomas and May, 1981) (Figure 1). However in these cases valuable time can be saved by considering haemobilia within the differential diagnosis and, if the clinical picture indicates this as a possible cause for bleeding, one should proceed immediately to the appropriate investigation.

Chronic pancreatitis is a very rare cause of intestinal haemorrhage, but can present with obscure bleeding due to pseudoaneurysm formation (Hall et al,

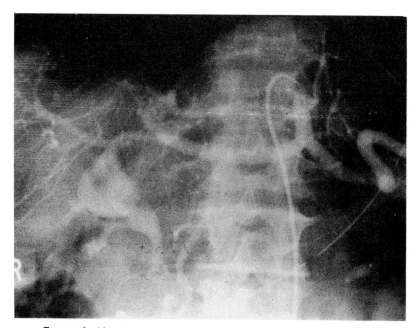

FIGURE I Hepatic artery aneurysm presenting with heavy haemobilia

1982). Other causes such as suture line haemorrhage, trauma and bleeding diatheses should be clinically apparent. Indeed in some cases it is the bleeding disorder that brings a gastrointestinal lesion to light.

Small bowel

By the very nature of the small bowel, this often harbours a considerable number of the conditions that present with recurrent obscure gastrointestinal haemorrhage (Table 2). This is because the small bowel is difficult to investigate and many of the lesions are uncommon and therefore not immediately considered.

Small bowel ulceration

Primary or idiopathic small bowel ulceration is uncommon (Guest, 1963; Thomas and Williamson, 1985). These lesions are sharp-bordered solitary ulcers with little or no surrounding inflammation (Figure 2). The aetiology of such ulcers remains obscure, although in the 1960s enteric coated potassium was implicated in certain cases (Morgenstern et al, 1965; Campbell and Knapp, 1966) and its administration to dogs produces comparable lesions (Boley et al, 1965). Non-steroidal anti-inflammatory agents may produce similar lesions (Lang et al, 1985) and in time other agents may be implicated although at present the majority of cases have no obvious precipitating cause. There appears to be a changing pattern to the clinical presentation of such ulcers in that early reports described a high incidence of perforation (Evert et al, 1948; Watson, 1963) but more recent studies document a higher incidence of haemorrhage (Thomas and Williamson, 1985) or obstruction (Boydstun et al, 1981). All reports tend to stress the delay in diagnosis usually resulting from a lack of awareness of the condition on the part of the clinician.

Secondary small bowel ulceration may be associated with a systemic disease such as systemic lupus erythematosis, rheumatoid arthritis, polyarteritis nodosa, Ehlers–Danlos syndrome, dermatomyositis, Henoch–Schönlein purpura and amyloidosis when it is usually the result of vasculitis. Some of these conditions may cause a non-specific anaemia which can further complicate the clinical picture. It is therefore important to confirm true gastrointestinal blood loss. It is also important to exclude other causes of ulceration such as Crohn's disease, ischaemia, trauma, nutritional problems and hormonal conditions such as the Zollinger–Ellison syndrome. When ulceration is associated with malabsorption, it is essential to exclude coeliac disease and intestinal lymphoma (Baer et al, 1980; Robertson et al, 1983). Geographical associations also need to be considered as typhoid and tuberculosis are common causes of enteric ulceration in tropical climates (Eggleston et al, 1979).

Neoplasia

Occult gastrointestinal bleeding may occasionally be the presenting symptom of a small bowel tumour. Such lesions include carcinoid tumour, adenocarcinoma, leiomyosarcoma, lymphoma and benign tumours such as leiomyoma and adenomatous polyps. Tumours rarely account for more than 2–3% of cases of

TABLE 2
Causes of small bowel ulceration and haemorrhage

Congenital	
Intestinal atresia	Vascular
Ectopic gastric mucosa	Embolic
Intestinal reduplication	Thrombotic
Meconium ileus	Intussusception
Meckel's diverticulum	Polyarteritis nodosa
Acquired	Thromboangiitis obliterans
Infected	Anomalies
Bacterial	Telangiectasia
Tuberculosis	A–V malformations
Typhoid	Angiodysplasia
Cholera	Phlebectasia
Shigella dysentery	Haemangioma
Syphilis	Aorto-enteric fistula
Viral	Inflammatory
Cytomegalovirus	Crohn's disease
Other enteropathic viruses	Endometriosis
Fungal	Coeliac disease
Histoplasmosis	Jejunal diverticulosis
Aspergillosis	Chronic pancreatitis
Protozoal	Postirradiation
Amoebiasis	Hormonal
Parasitic	Zollinger–Ellison syndrome
Ancylostomiasis	Phaeochromocytoma
Ascariasis	Neoplastic
Drug induced	Benign
Enteric coated potassium	Leiomyoma
Corticosteroids	Adenoma
Indomethacin	Malignant
Phenylbutazone	Adenocarcinoma
Immunosuppression	Lymphoma
Trauma	Carcinoid
External	Leiomyosarcoma
Bands	Malignant histiocytosis
Volvulus	Secondary tumour
Hernia	Metabolic
Luminal	Uraemia
Foreign bodies	Haematological
Bolus impaction	Thrombocytopaenic purpura
Gallstone ileus	Thrombocythaemia
Intubation	Haemophilia
	Von Willebrand's disease
	Poorly controlled anti-coagulation
	Idiopathic

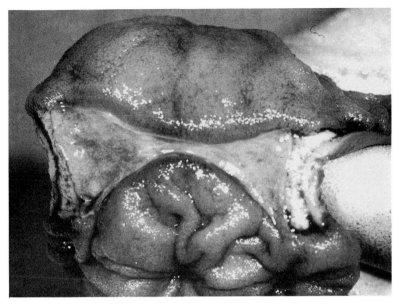

FIGURE 2 Idiopathic small bowel ulceration

gastrointestinal haemorrhage, but when it does occur the lesion is usually an adenocarcinoma (Schiller et al, 1970; Forrest and Finlayson, 1974). Carcinoid tumours and lymphomas are more common than adenocarcinomas but these are more likely to perforate or obstruct than to cause haemorrhage (Williamson et al, 1983). Benign lesions or polyps may ulcerate or initiate an intussusception which, if it becomes chronic or recurrent without causing overt obstruction, may result in enteric ulceration and occult bleeding. Such occult bleeding may also occur in Peutz–Jeghers syndrome (Figure 3) where the classical melanin pigmentation of the mucocutaneous junction provides a valuable clinical clue as to the diagnosis and cause of bleeding. Other polyposis conditions such as familial polyposis, Gardner's syndrome, juvenile polyps or benign lymphoid polyps may present in a similar manner.

Vascular anomalies

Small bowel vascular anomalies are particularly difficult to diagnose, but fortunately account for less than 1% of patients presenting with haematemesis and melaena (Forrest, 1982). The commonest vascular malformation causing gastrointestinal bleeding is undoubtedly colonic angiodysplasia, but small bowel arteriovenous malformations, phlebectasia and telangiectasia are becoming increasingly recognized. Telangiectasia may be found either as part of an hereditary condition such as the Osler–Weber–Rendu syndrome or more commonly as isolated flat intramucosal telangiectasia or true haemangiomas. These can be diffuse and occupy the whole thickness of the bowel wall, or cavernous and polypoid. Phlebectasia are small bluish submucosal lesions due to anomalies of the mesenteric veins. Angiomatosis is a diffuse vascular abnormality and can cause massive haemorrhage (Pierce and Davis, 1969).

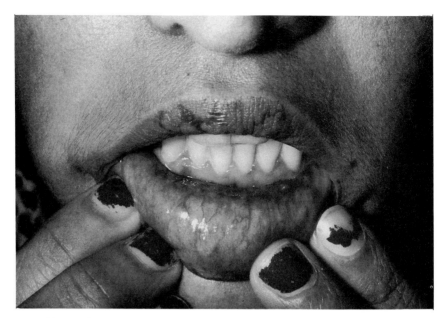

FIGURE 3   The muco-cutaneous pigmentation of Peutz–Jeghers syndrome

Diverticula

Meckel's diverticulum Up to 25% of patients with a Meckel's diverticulum present
with haemorrhage (Mackey and Dineen, 1983). This is the result of peptic
ulceration of the adjacent ileal mucosa due to acid secretion from ectopic gastric
mucosa. The pattern of bleeding ranges from occult loss (Williamson et al, 1984)
to the passage of large amounts of bright red blood per rectum (Mackey and
Dineen, 1983). In some cases the bleeding can be so profuse that the patient may
rapidly exsanguinate, and cases of intestinal obstruction secondary to intraluminal
thrombus have been reported (Neuss et al, 1986).

Jejuno-ileal diverticula Small bowel diverticulosis is an uncommon cause of intestinal
bleeding, but when it does occur the haemorrhage may be acute and severe
(Thomas et al, 1967) or chronic and occult (Geroulakis, 1987) as with a Meckel's
diverticulum. However most patients present with melaena which is uncommon
with Meckel's diverticulum. The haemorrhage results from ulceration at the
diverticular neck where the blood vessels penetrate the bowel wall and are
vulnerable due to the lack of the muscularis layer (Shackelford and Marcus, 1960).
Twenty-five per cent of patients who present with acute haemorrhage will have
had evidence of previous chronic blood loss (Taylor, 1969; Geroulakis, 1987), thus
presenting a similar pattern to that seen with colonic diverticulosis (Jones, 1974).

Miscellaneous small bowel conditions

Other disorders of the small bowel may cause obscure haemorrhage such as
endometriosis, postirradiation ileitis and aorto-enteric fistula. This latter condition
often gives cause for concern due to the delay in diagnosis that can range from 24
hours to 3 months (Thomas and Baird, 1986). It often presents with the

characteristic clinical picture of secondary haemorrhage with initial occult bleeding, eventually becoming overt and ending up with massive rapid exsanguination that can be fatal. The initial sentinel bleeds should be recognized for what they are, and any patient who has undergone previous aortic surgery and presents with any form of gastrointestinal haemorrhage should be assumed to have an aorto-enteric fistula until proved otherwise. These secondary fistulae tend to occur in about 1–2% of prosthetic graft reconstructions (Sheil et al, 1969), but can also occur after endarterectomy (Lamerton, 1984). The diagnosis is predominantly a clinical one, but other causes of haemorrhage such as peptic ulcers can coexist with vascular disease, and should be considered (Crowson et al, 1984). However even if another potential bleeding source is demonstrated, a fistula must be excluded or diagnosed early as it can carry a mortality of up to 45% (Reilly et al, 1984).

Large bowel

As with foregut conditions, most large bowel lesions presenting with gastrointestinal bleeding will be easily demonstrated on either colonoscopy or barium enema. Conditions such as neoplasia, inflammatory bowel disease, diverticular disease, ischaemia and suture line haemorrhage should be apparent and therefore rarely fall into the category of recurrent obscure intestinal bleeding. However there are other conditions that can still prove elusive. Right-sided colonic diverticula are much less common than sigmoid diverticular disease, and they may be single or multiple. They appear to have a predisposition to bleed, and at times angiography is required to demonstrate the actual bleeding site. In this situation extravasated contrast may often be seen within the diverticulum (Figure 4).

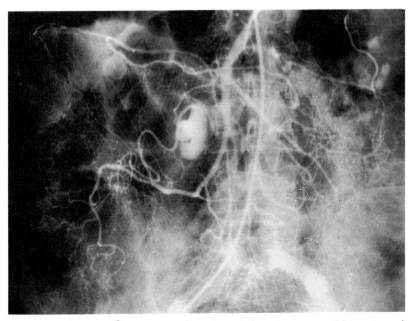

FIGURE 4 Extravasated blood in a colonic diverticulum demonstrated by angiography

Endometriosis may provide a further diagnostic problem in that when the lesion is not bleeding or in the right phase of the cycle, virtually no mucosal abnormality may be seen. The most frequently encountered colonic condition causing bleeding is angiodysplasia.

Angiodysplasia

Angiodysplasia is the commonest cause of recurrent obscure gastrointestinal haemorrhage in many series (Baum et al, 1977; Boley et al, 1977; Thompson et al, 1987) (Table 3). It can unfortunately be missed on colonoscopy, especially if the

TABLE 3
Diagnosis and investigation of 58 cases of recurrent obscure gastrointestinal haemorrhage

Diagnosis	Number	Endoscopy	Small bowel enema	Angiography	Isotope scan	Other	Laparotomy
Colonic angiodysplasia	17	7	–	9	–	–	1
Small bowel tumours	7	–	2	3	–	–	2
Small bowel ulcers	6	–	2	2	–	–	2
Small bowel vascular anomalies	4	–	–	2	–	–	2
Meckel's diverticulum	5	–	–	1	3	–	1
Jejunal diverticula	2	–	–	–	1	–	1
Osler's telangectasia	2	–	–	–	–	other lesions	–
Crohn's disease	2	–	1	–	–	–	1
Aorto-enteric fistula	2	–	–	1	–	–	1
Haemostatic disorders	2	–	–	–	–	clotting screen	–
Anti-coagulant abuse	1	–	–	–	–	clotting screen	–
Dieulafoy syndrome	1	–	–	–	–	–	1
Endometriosis	1	–	–	–	–	–	1
Chronic pancreatitis	1	–	–	–	–	ERCP	–
Haemobilia	1	–	–	1	–	–	–
Unexplained Intermittent	2	–	–	–	–	–	–
Occult	2	–	–	–	–	–	–
Total	58	7	5	19	4	4	13

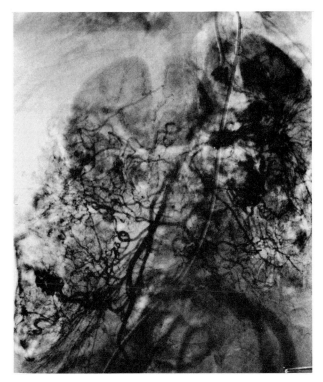

FIGURE 5 Angiodysplasia of the caecum
(by kind permission of Professor A P Hemingway)

bowel preparation is poor or the endoscopist does not get a good view of the caecum where this condition is most commonly found. Quite tiny areas of angiodysplasia, about 2 mm in size, are capable of producing severe haemorrhage and so meticulous bowel cleansing is essential. If oral total gut irrigation is used for this purpose an added benefit may be experienced. The brisk antegrade flow of bowel contents provides little opportunity for blood to reflux retrogradely, and so in patients who have been bleeding recently, the point where the lumen becomes blood free at colonoscopy gives a good indication of the proximal limit of the bleeding lesion. Colonoscopy thus remains the investigation of choice for demonstrating angiodysplasia, as not only is it diagnostic but it also may provide access for therapeutic manoeuvres such as diathermy coagulation. When colonoscopy fails to exclude angiodysplasia, and yet it is high on the list of differential diagnoses, angiography is required.

The incidence of angiodysplasia and other vascular anomalies increases with age (Boley et al, 1977) and in one series, 80% of patients over 60 years presenting with obscure intestinal bleeding had colonic angiodysplasia (Thompson et al, 1987). Angiography is therefore recommended for older patients in whom angiodysplasia is suspected and yet colonoscopy has been unproductive for whatever reason. The angiographic appearances include an early filling feeding artery, vascular lakes, prominent intramural veins and an early filling but late emptying draining vein (Figure 5). However having found an area of angiodysplasia, it is important not to overlook a second lesion, and up to 10% of

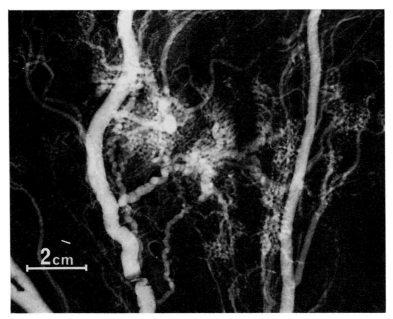

FIGURE 6 Microradiograph of angiodysplasia
(by kind permission of Professor A P Hemingway)

patients may have two or more potential or actual causes of haemorrhage. Accurate localization of any area or areas of angiodysplasia is essential as they are totally impalpable to the operating surgeon, and even after resection, the specimen looks most unimpressive to the pathologist. Injection techniques of the specimen, possibly accompanied by microradiographs, are the only reliable way of demonstrating the resected abnormality (Figure 6).

Finally there remain cases in which patients suffer from iron deficiency anaemia with positive occult blood for which no identifiable cause can be found. A similar pattern has been described in marathon runners who may develop iron deficiency anaemia with occult gastrointestinal bleeding but with no delineated cause being demonstrable for this phenomenon (Stewart et al, 1984).

DIAGNOSIS

Symptoms

A full and detailed history is essential, and although it may not provide a definite diagnosis in most cases, it often presents some valuable information and may indicate which is likely to be the most productive investigation. The age of the patient is important. For example, a Meckel's diverticulum is more likely to present in children or young adults, while angiodysplasia is more common in the elderly (Mackey and Dineen, 1983; Thompson et al, 1987). Pain may be an accompanying feature, and its site and nature are important in that colicky abdominal pain may indicate an element of intestinal obstruction caused by a stricture, tumour, or intussusception, etc. Postcibal pain and weight loss may indicate mesenteric ischaemia, while cyclical pain in a woman with positive faecal occult blood may suggest a diagnosis of endometriosis. Other symptoms such as nausea, vomiting, dysphagia, altered bowel habit or weight loss may provide further clues as to the level or nature of the lesion.

The pattern of bleeding should be noted as to whether it is occult, intermittently overt, or rapid and massive from the outset (Thomas, 1989). In some cases, as has already been described for an aorto-enteric fistula, the bleeding may initially be occult, eventually become overt and end up as massive rapid haemorrhage that can be fatal (Reilly et al, 1984). In spite of the well-recognized clinical picture, a worrying feature in nearly all published series of aorto-enteric fistulae is the delay in diagnosis, with a median of 2 weeks in our own series (Thomas and Baird, 1986). This is because many clinicians are not as aware of this condition as are those surgeons who are routinely involved with vascular reconstructions. It is well recognized that other potential causes of bleeding may coexist such as peptic ulceration (Crowson et al, 1984), but the discerning clinician will always be wary of accepting such a diagnosis as the cause of bleeding, if there is the scar of previous vascular surgery.

Other factors in the past medical history should be studied carefully, with particular reference to any previous trauma, gastrointestinal disease or surgery. A history of travel abroad may indicate a parasitic infestation which is a common cause of chronic intestinal blood loss world-wide. A drug history should be taken in order to exclude the effect of non-steroidal anti-inflammatory agents, steroids, anticoagulants, immunosuppressive agents, and enteric coated potassium preparations. A history of alcohol abuse should be sought that may have resulted in cirrhosis, portal hypertension or chronic pancreatitis. Family history may bring to light the possibility of a bleeding diathesis or Osler–Weber–Rendu hereditary telangiectasia.

Signs

All too often examination of the patient may be unproductive. Nevertheless, a meticulous examination of the patient may reveal valuable subtle physical signs such as clinical evidence of anaemia, telangiectasia, stigmata of Peutz–Jeghers syndrome (Figure 3), scars of previous surgery, and abdominal tenderness or masses. It will also demonstrate any clinical evidence of acute blood loss. Rectal examination may confirm the presence or absence of melaena and sigmoidoscopy and proctoscopy may exclude any lower rectal lesion. It must be pointed out that although melaena usually indicates upper gastrointestinal haemorrhage, red rectal bleeding may also originate high in the bowel if the rate of bleeding is rapid enough, although in this case the indices of acute blood loss, such as tachycardia and hypotension, should be obvious. Having taken an accurate history and performed a thorough examination, a decision has to be taken as to which investigation is likely to be most productive. Figure 7 indicates a possible course of action dependent on the clinical picture and the strengths and limitations of the following investigations.

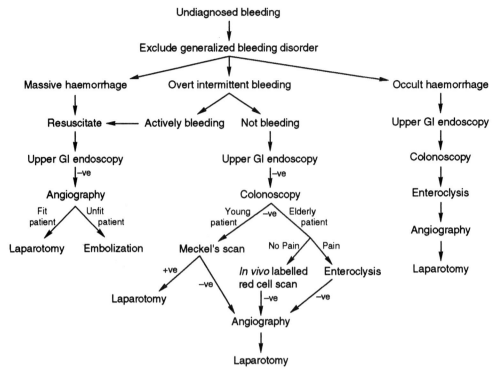

FIGURE 7 Suggested course of action for investigating obscure gastrointestinal haemorrhage

METHODS OF INVESTIGATION

Occult blood tests

The first essential investigations, especially in those cases in which the patient presents with iron-deficiency anaemia, are aimed at confirming gastrointestinal bleeding. Faecal occult blood tests were initially designed for screening purposes looking for colorectal neoplasia (Gnauck, 1980), but they now have a wider application in identifying blood loss throughout the gastrointestinal tract. It has been calculated that normal subjects may have a blood loss of up to 2 mg haemoglobin/g stool which is equivalent to 2 ml/day for a stool weight of 150 g (Macrae and St John, 1982). Early tests had a poor reputation for a high incidence of false positive results (Irons and Kirsner, 1965; Ostrow et al, 1973) but modification of these tests using Haemoccult, which is less sensitive than the standard guaiac tests, produces a positive result with a haemoglobin content of over 10 mg haemoglobin/g stool (Ostrow et al, 1973). This can tend to produce more false negative results (Vellacott et al, 1981) which can be as high as 30% (Doran and Hardcastle, 1982; Macrae and St John, 1982). Rehydration may reduce this false negative rate to 9% but this is not officially advised as it also increases the false positive rate. In order to try and overcome these problems, immunofluorescent techniques have been devised (Vellacott et al, 1981). These use fluorescein-labelled rabbit anti-human haemoglobin serum, which undoubtedly increases the specificity of the test. These techniques also have the advantages of not cross reacting with animal haemoglobin, minimize observer error and permit the adjustment of sensitivity.

Endoscopy

Oesophago-gastro-duodenoscopy

The value of endoscopy in investigating gastrointestinal haemorrhage is well established. Indeed oesophago-gastro-duodenoscopy will demonstrate the cause of bleeding in the vast majority of cases of upper gastrointestinal haemorrhage. When the initial endoscopy is negative, a repeat may be indicated, but is seldom productive. This fact is confirmed in our own series of cases of recurrent obscure haemorrhage (Table 3) in that upper gastrointestinal endoscopy was not effective in achieving a diagnosis in a single case, and even a gastric vascular anomaly (Dieulafoy syndrome) in the fundus of the stomach was not recognized for what it was, in spite of repeated endoscopies by different endoscopists. It is important therefore to be aware that such anomalies do occur, and to be vigilant for other uncommon conditions such as telangiectasia or haemobilia, although the latter is difficult to diagnose unless the patient is actually bleeding at the time of endoscopy. In patients with rapid overt bleeding in whom time does not allow a formal preoperative endoscopy, this procedure may be performed in the operating theatre immediately before laparotomy. Pre-endoscopy gastric lavage has been used to remove gastric blood clot, but it is often unproductive. These patients seldom prove such a diagnostic problem as the bleeding site is usually apparent. However it is essential to exclude oesophageal variceal bleeding.

Endoscopic-retrograde-cholangio-pancreatography

ERCP may be of limited value in such cases, but will diagnose cases of chronic pancreatitis, which can occasionally present with bleeding due to pseudoaneurysm formation (Hall et al, 1982). Haemobilia is easier to see when using a side-viewing duodenoscope at ERCP.

Colonoscopy

Colonoscopy is of proven value in the diagnosis of colonic angiodysplasia, which is one of the most common causes of recurrent obscure haemorrhage from the bowel (Thompson et al, 1987; Thomas, 1989) (Table 3) but it is well recognized that cases of angiodysplasia can very easily be missed at endoscopy (Thompson et al, 1987). Colonoscopy is also useful in providing access for therapeutic manoeuvres, such as polypectomy or laser and heater probes for angiodysplasia and other vascular malformations (Rogers and Adler, 1976).

Small bowel endoscopy

In cases where upper and lower gastrointestinal endoscopy are negative, one is left with bleeding from the small bowel that is relatively inaccessible to the endoscope, and yet can harbour bleeding ulcerated lesions representing a wide variety of clinical conditions (Table 2). In ideal circumstances the gastroscope may be advanced into the proximal jejunum and the colonoscope passed into the distal 50 cm of the terminal ileum (Shinya and McSherry, 1982), but this still leaves the vast majority of the small bowel unexamined.

Recently three types of small bowel endoscopes have been described in an attempt to traverse the whole length of the small intestine with the aim of examining the lumen during withdrawal of the endoscope (Shinya and McSherry, 1982; Tada and Kawai, 1984). The 'push type' is simply an extremely long duodenoscope which is advanced as far as possible but in reality rarely proceeds further than 90 cm into the jejunum. The 'rope-way type' depends on a previously passed transintestinal string which is retrieved per anum and this then pulls the endoscope through the bowel. This technique requires a general anaesthetic as it is most uncomfortable for the patient and there is a danger of damaging the bowel by a 'cheese-wire' form of injury. The 'sonde type' endoscope works on the same principle as the Miller–Abbott or Cantor tube. The endoscope has a distal balloon cuff which is inflated once the endoscope has been swallowed and has reached the distal duodenum. The endoscope is then allowed to migrate through the small bowel, but this takes time and is not always successful. In all three techniques, the examination of the lumen is undertaken on withdrawal, but these methods are unreliable, time consuming, and not routinely available.

Intra-operative enteroscopy

Intra-operative gastrointestinal endoscopy has been widely practised (Lau et al, 1986; Apelgren et al, 1988), and has proved particularly useful in identifying vascular anomalies within the small bowel. It has the advantage of being able to detect occult lesions not found on gross examination fo the bowel and can also confirm that any lesion found is actually the source of bleeding. In the case of multiple lesions it can identify which lesion or lesions are actually the source of bleeding and it also indicates the required extent of enteric resection. In order to optimize the results of operative enteroscopy, certain practical considerations need to be considered.

Adequate bowel preparation is essential and in those cases in which there is any question of the adequacy of bowel clearance, then total gut irrigation is recommended. In the emergency situation where enteroscopy is required during surgery and there has not been adequate time for preoperative preparation, it is possible to carry out total gut irrigation intra-operatively, but this is not recommended unless absolutely necessary as it leaves the bowel very moist, and is messy and time consuming.

The patient is operated on in the lithotomy position and a thorough laparotomy performed. Once enteroscopy has been considered necessary, a colonoscope is introduced via the mouth and passed into the small bowel. The operating surgeon needs to help the endoscopist pass the instrument through the small bowel to its full length, feeding the bowel over the endoscope in a concertina manner. Great care should be taken not to allow a large loop of the endoscope to form along the greater curvature of the stomach as this can create great tension and result in tearing of the short gastric vessels. Having reached the furthest limitation of the endoscope, a marker suture is inserted in the bowel wall and the lumen of the intestine examined during withdrawal and any abnormality again marked by a stay suture. The remainder of the intestine can then be examined by introducing the colonoscope into the lumen of the small bowel via an enterotomy, but this technique is 'messy', and thus most prefer to introduce it per anum and manipulate it proximally with the help of the operating surgeon until the entire small bowel has been adequately examined.

During examination it is advisable to turn all the operating lights off. This is an advantage to the endoscopist, but also allows the operating surgeon to obtain an excellent view of the transilluminated bowel wall. This is particularly useful for identifying small vascular anomalies (Thomas, 1989). At the end of the procedure it is advisable to decompress the bowel during withdrawal, otherwise the distension may make it difficult to close the abdomen.

Intra-operative endoscopy is thus a most valuable addition to the diagnostic options available to the clinician engaged in chasing obscure gastrointestinal haemorrhage. However it requires both an experienced surgeon and an experienced endoscopist. It is impossible in patients with marked adhesions from previous surgery and in those with extraluminal tumour deposits or other pathology that limits the passage of the endoscope.

Barium studies

Before the advent of routine endoscopy, barium contrast studies were the mainstay of gastrointestinal imaging. However endoscopy has now taken over as the primary investigation for gastrointestinal haemorrhage and if adequate upper and lower intestinal endoscopy fails to reveal the source of bleeding, then it is unlikely that a standard barium meal or enema will be of any added value, and therefore they are not recommended.

Barium studies of the small bowel have tended in the past to depend on the follow-through technique (Nolan, 1981), but this has now been found to be inadequate in most cases, especially for delineating cases of small bowel ulceration. Maglinte and Antley (1984) suggested that it is only the infrequency of small bowel lesions that has disguised the inadequacies of the barium follow-through for so long. Barium enemas are also inadequate for examination of the terminal ileum, since reflux through the ileocaecal valve only occurs in about 25% of patients (Gurian et al, 1982).

Enteroclysis (small bowel enema) is now the technique of choice for radiological examination of the small bowel and has significantly improved the diagnostic yield of small bowel abnormalities (Sellink, 1974). It involves the passage of a 12Fr tube to the duodeno-jejunal flexure and then barium is infused under pressure to distend all segments of the bowel (Maglinte et al, 1984). Intermittent compression fluororadiography is then undertaken looking at each segment of jejunum and ileum in turn. The diagnostic rate can be further improved by the simultaneous infusion of methylcellulose, water or air down the tube. It can be a time-consuming investigation, and may be uncomfortable for the patient (Reddie et al, 1982), although those workers involved in performing a considerable number of small bowel enemas stress that it is easy to perform, safe and quick (Maglinte et al, 1984). In certain series enteroclysis produced over 90% positive diagnoses (Keddie et al, 1982) and it is frequently successful in situations in which a follow-through study has failed to demonstrate any abnormality (Maglinte et al, 1984). A barium follow-through should now be reserved for patients in whom duodenal intubation cannot be achieved.

In recurrent obscure gastrointestinal bleeding a small bowel study may be instrumental in identifying such causes as small bowel tumours, ulcers, strictures (Figure 8) or jejunal diverticula (Figure 9), but it is unreliable for demonstrating vascular anomalies or Meckel's diverticulum. It is therefore an investigation which is worth considering if upper and lower gastrointestinal endoscopy are negative and the patient presents with any symptoms referrable to the small bowel, such as central abdominal colicky pain. In our series it was instrumental in diagnosing only 10% of cases, so its role in recurrent obscure gastrointestinal bleeding is a limited one. Furthermore it is important to avoid barium studies if angiography or CT scanning is being considered as residual barium within the intestine obscures angiographic detail or produces distortion on scanning, and may remain in the bowel for several days.

Angiography

In certain centres angiography is rapidly becoming the most effective investigation for identifying the cause of recurrent obscure gastrointestinal haemorrhage (Thompson et al, 1987). All patients presenting for angiography should have had upper and lower gastrointestinal endoscopy, but it must be stressed again that lesions such as colonic angiodysplasia, especially in the caecum, can be missed on colonoscopy. The role of angiography depends on the nature of the bleeding. In acute rapid blood loss, angiography seeks to demonstrate the actual site of haemorrhage by the confirmation of intraluminal extravasation of contrast medium, while in chronic haemorrhage, any abnormal vascular patterns are sought that may represent tumours or vascular anomalies.

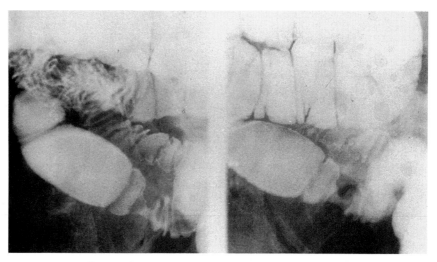

FIGURE 8   A small bowel stricture seen by enteroclysis
(by kind permission of *World J. Surgery*)

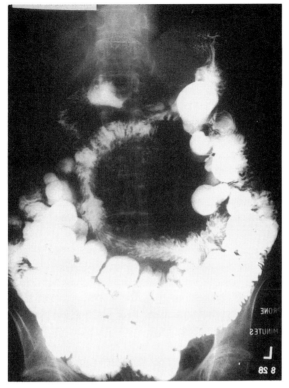

FIGURE 9 Multiple jejunal diverticula

Acute haemorrhage

Selective visceral angiography is preferred, and in acute haemorrhage, the vessel thought most likely to be the source on clinical grounds is catheterized first followed by the others if the initial study proves negative. Unfortunately all too often the bleeding has stopped by the time the patient undergoes angiography, but if the bleeding is active at the time of the investigation, then the actual bleeding site can be delineated. Intraluminal extravasation can be demonstrated from a wide variety of sources, for example arteriovenous malformations, ulcers, tumours, suture lines or diverticula. Occasionally contrast can be seen pooling in an adjacent diverticulum that was the underlying cause of the haemorrhage (Figure 4).

Having identified a site of bleeding it is important to attempt to localize the site of the lesion in the bowel. With care and patience a side winder catheter can be manipulated into most of the distal arteries of the mesentery, and this not only improves the localization of any lesion, but also improves the success rate for identifying intraluminal extravasation. For an aortic injection a lesion needs to be bleeding at a rate of 5–6 ml/min to be identified (Jaffe et al, 1965), but for selective visceral catheterization the rate required is only 0.5–2 ml/min (Balint and Sarfeh, 1977). In cases of massive haemorrhage the success rate is therefore high, but this pick-up rate falls off as the bleeding rate diminishes or becomes intermittent in nature. In one series only 7% of patients were actively bleeding at the time of angiography (Thompson et al, 1987).

In certain cases of active bleeding, angiographic techniques may also be of therapeutic value. Local infusions of vasopressin directly into the feeding artery may result in cessation of bleeding, while in carefully selected cases embolization has also been used. Embolization is not recommended for the large bowel as the collateral circulation is poor, but in the small bowel adequate collaterals usually prevent infarction. In a review of reported cases, four out of 18 patients embolized developed some degree of ischaemic damage (Palmaz et al, 1984), but many still prefer this technique to vasopressin infusions (Chalmers et al, 1986). Embolization is also of value in treating certain non-enteric cases of gastrointestinal haemorrhage arising from the coeliac or hepatic artery such as intrahepatic or pancreatic bleeding. These cases may present a daunting surgical prospect and embolization may have a role in controlling such haemorrhage.

Chronic haemorrhage

In intermittent or chronic blood loss, it is recommended that the inferior mesenteric artery is catheterized first to allow good views of the sigmoid colon and rectum, before the urinary bladder becomes filled with contrast, thus obscuring

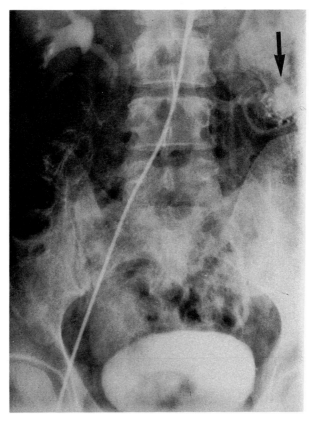

FIGURE 10   A tumour blush seen on angiography (arrowed)

the view of this area. This is then followed by the superior mesenteric artery and coeliac axis studies, the latter being particularly important for demonstrating sources of haemobilia such as hepatic artery aneurysms (Thomas and May, 1981) (Figure 1) or intrahepatic vascular malformations. Some vascular anomalies, namely venous abnormalities (phlebectasia), may not be picked up by angiography and often are only diagnosed by intra-operative enteroscopy.

In cases of chronic haemorrhage, attempts are made to identify a tumour blush (Figure 10) or vascular malformation. Angiographic features of angiodysplasia, the commonest cause of recurrent obscure gastrointestinal haemorrhage, include an early filling artery, vascular lakes and prominent intramural veins with delayed emptying (Figure 5), usually being seen in the caecum or ascending colon.

Having identified a bleeding source or vascular anomaly, efforts should again be made to localize the lesion as accurately as possible. Even when the exact arterial branch has been identified angiographically, it is sometimes still difficult for the surgeon at laparotomy to locate the lesion if it is not visible or palpable. In situations like this intraoperative angiography with marker clips on the bowel wall or supraselective arterial injections of methylene blue may facilitate identification of the lesion.

Radionuclide scanning

Radionuclide techniques for demonstrating the source of recurrent gastro-intestinal bleeding have recently gained in popularity as they appear to have no morbidity and are becoming increasingly reliable. Such techniques have the advantage over angiography in that images can be taken over several hours, thus increasing the likelihood of detecting the bleeding point.

Quantifying blood loss

In order to attempt to quantify the degree of blood loss, autologous red blood cells may be labelled with 1 MBq of ^{51}Cr and then reinjected intravenously. Stool samples are then collected for several days and a blood sample taken 10 min after reinjection and at the end of the examination. The half-life of ^{51}Cr is 28 days, so the degree of blood loss over a period of 5 days can be calculated by comparing the radioactivity of the stool samples with those of the two blood samples. A normal subject will lose up to 3 ml of blood a day into the bowel, although the actual figure for most people will be considerably less.

Localizing blood loss

There are two radionuclide techniques available for demonstrating blood loss from sites within the gastrointestinal tract. Any radioactivity present in the circulation at the time of bleeding will appear within the lumen of the bowel. Therefore any colloid suitable for reticuloendothelial scintigraphy may be effective. ^{99m}Tc-sulphur colloid was the first to be used in this context (Alavi et al, 1977), and as almost all administered colloid is cleared by the reticuloendothelial system within 10–15 min, any remaining blush of activity in the mid- or lower abdomen outside the liver, spleen and marrow would represent a site of haemorrhage. It has been estimated that bleeding rates below 1 ml/min may be detected by this method (Alavi, 1962) and rates as low as 0.1 ml/min have been reported (Merrick, 1988). However this technique is again limited by the intermittent nature of the blood loss, and bleeding sites in the upper abdomen are concealed by the liver and spleen.

The circulating level of radioactivity may be prolonged by labelling red blood cells *in vivo* with either ^{51}Cr as sodium chromate, ^{99m}Tc-methylene diphosphonate, ^{99m}Tc-pertechnetate stannous chloride or ^{111}indium. These methods allow extended studies for up to 24 h and using this technique, some workers claim up to 100% success rates for identifying bleeding sites (Winzelberg et al, 1982), compared with 65% with conventional angiography.

Meckel's diverticulum

Meckel's diverticulum is an important cause of intestinal bleeding, both acute (Mackey and Dineen, 1983) and chronic (Williamson et al, 1984), and yet is rarely demonstrated on barium studies. The incidence in the general population is up to 2% but only a minority are symptomatic. In children and adolescents it is a not uncommon source of intestinal bleeding and radionuclide scanning is now the investigation of choice for identifying haemorrhage from such a diverticulum. Scintigraphic studies do not depend upon demonstrating active bleeding but upon the trapping of ^{99m}Tc-pertechnetate by the ectopic gastric (oxyntic) mucosa found in a Meckel's diverticulum. It is the acid produced from such mucosa that causes ulceration of the adjacent small intestinal mucosa resulting in haemorrhage.

Pertechnetate imaging gives a reported sensitivity of 75% (Berquist et al, 1976), and the ease of visualization can be further improved by number of drugs or agents (Anderson et al, 1980). Pentagastrin may increase the uptake of pertechnetate, but also accelerates gastric emptying which decreases the probability of diagnosing a Meckel's diverticulum by increasing the amount of activity in the small bowel. Glucagon will reduce gastric motility, so when both agents are given together, the accuracy of the technique is improved (Yeker and Buyukunal, 1984). However H_2 blocking agents reduce acid secretion and intraluminal release of pertechnetate without impairing its uptake, and so have become the agents of choice (Baum, 1981). Using such techniques, the accuracy of Meckel's diverticulum imaging in children may be as high as 90% (Sfakianakis et al, 1981).

The patient is starved for 12 h to reduce gastric acid secretion and then 100–200 MBq of sodium pertechnetate is injected intravenously. Gamma camera images are recorded sequentially for 1 h. After injection of pertechnetate, activity is usually visible in the stomach within 2 min, and within 15–30 min activity is seen in the small bowel, which may be enough to obscure a Meckel's diverticulum. However if such a diverticulum is present it is usually represented by an area of activity below and to the right of the midline that appears within 5 min (Figure 11). The rate of development of activity can be compared with that of the stomach (Figure 12), as ectopic gastric mucosa has a similar rate of uptake as normal stomach, and this will distinguish it from most other structures or areas of activity such as the renal areas, ureters or bladder. False positives include ectopic gastric mucosa or uptake in tissues other than a Meckel's diverticulum such as reduplications, intussusception and infarction, but as these conditions also

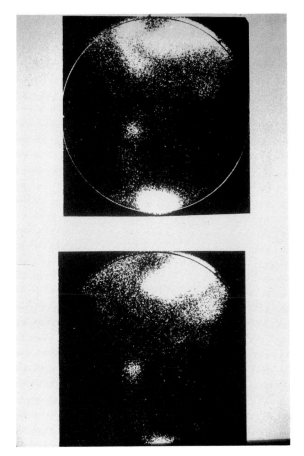

FIGURE 11 Technetium scan with activity in the right lower abdomen consistent with a Meckel's
diverticulum (by kind permission of *Hospital Update*)

MECKEL'S STUDY

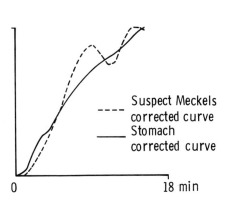

Suspect Meckels
corrected curve
Stomach
corrected curve

0   18 min

FIGURE 12 Graph of isotope activity in a suspected Meckel's diverticulum compared with activity in
the gastric parietal cells (by kind permission of *Current Practice in Surgery*)

require laparotomy such problems are rarely clinically significant. Further false positive results are seen occasionally representing activity in the ureter or the uterus during certain phases of the cycle in young women. However meticulous technique, lateral views and uptake studies should exclude these possibilities. In spite of these limitations this investigation is a valuable diagnostic tool as it is non-invasive, cheap, simple to perform and administers a much smaller dose of irradiation than enteroclysis or angiography.

Miscellaneous diagnostic techniques

In every case of recurrent obscure gastrointestinal haemorrhage, it is important to exclude any bleeding diathesis or drug-induced bleeding tendency, and therefore a haematological screen is essential. Such cases are usually obvious, but most series, including our own, tend to include one or two cases of unsuspected bleeding tendencies.

Staining techniques have also been employed in the past. A string test has occasionally been reported to be of value (Haynes et al, 1960). In this test a weighted string is passed by mouth and screened until it reaches the distal small bowel. An intravenous injection of fluoroscein is then given and the string subsequently retrieved and the level of fluoroscein staining identified. The distance from the mouth will give a very approximate level of any bleeding lesion, but this technique has largely been superseded by accurate angiography and scintigraphy techniques.

Intra-operative staining with methylene blue or indigo carmine (Crawford et al, 1980) has been used to provide segmental staining. However this depends upon superselective angiographic catheterization preoperatively. Once a lesion has been identified at angiography, the catheter is manipulated as distally as possible and left *in situ*. At the time of laparotomy, if the lesion is impalpable, the dye is injected down the catheter and will thus stain the affected segment and allow easy recognition. However care must be taken to observe the area at the time of injection as there is a tendency for the whole bowel to become stained as time passes.

Other forms of imaging have a limited role in investigating obscure haemorrhage. The applications of ultrasound scanning are growing all the time, but at present it remains somewhat unreliable for the small bowel due to its gas content. CT scanning may help identify a lesion in the liver or pancreas and its main role is in excluding an extra-enteric cause of bleeding.

MANAGEMENT (Figure 7)

When a specific bleeding source has been demonstrated preoperatively such as a vascular anomaly, tumour, stricture, ulcer or diverticulum, the management of the patient becomes straightforward in most cases. Surgical excision of the lesion is usually curative, unless the condition by its very nature recurs, or as in the case of tumours, has disseminated. For multiple lesions such as jejunal diverticula when all the lesions cannot be excised, it is essential that the lesion actually responsible for the haemorrhage is removed. This may well require intra-operative enteroscopy.

The main challenge in these difficult cases is when no preoperative diagnosis has been achieved, and when laparotomy reveals no obvious pathology. A thorough laparotomy by an experienced surgeon is necessary, not only examining the serosal appearance of the bowel but also feeling the texture of the bowel wall, which may reveal small ulcers or polyps. Mobilization of the duodenum and duodenojejunal flexure is also required. When the diagnosis is still in doubt, then one should proceed to intra-operative enteroscopy, with both an experienced surgeon and endoscopist present. Unless both are available, such difficult cases should not be embarked upon. In those few occasions when technical considerations exclude this course of action, such as marked adhesions, intra-operative angiography may be needed, but this requirement must be anticipated by the surgeon and an angiographic catheter inserted pre-operatively and the patient placed on a correct table..

Rapid and massive haemorrhage

In cases of rapid and massive haemorrhage, resuscitation and investigation should proceed simultaneously. Investigation should never take priority over resuscitation. A wide bore intravenous cannula should be inserted, and it is advantageous to have a central venous line for monitoring central venous pressure. Adequate transfusion and resuscitation should be undertaken before the patient is allowed to undergo any form of specialized investigation away from the ward.

The majority of causes will be demonstrated by urgent upper gastrointestinal endoscopy, but occasionally a stomach full of blood clot may obscure the bleeding site. This in itself is strong evidence of a gastric source, especially if the oesophagus and duodenum are normal, and although gastric washouts are of limited value, a repeat endoscopy, possibly even in the operating theatre prior to surgery, may eventually reveal the source.

In cases of massive bleeding in which upper gastrointestinal endoscopy is negative, the value of emergency colonoscopy is limited by the difficulty of achieving adequate bowel preparation and so urgent angiography is recommended. The yield from this investigation in these circumstances is high and may also allow therapeutic options such as embolization or vasoconstrictor infusions to be utilized. If this facility is not immediately available, an isotope colloid scan may be useful, although this may not be freely available out of hours. In our own series, angiography failed in two cases of massive haemorrhage, one being an aorto-enteric fistula and the other the case of a gastric vascular anomaly (Dieulafoy syndrome). The reason for failure was that although the bleeding was rapid and profuse in both cases, it was also intermittent and no actual angiographic abnormality was seen. Indeed a strong argument can be made for not performing an arteriogram in patients in whom an aorto-enteric fistula is suspected. Upper gastrointestinal endoscopy is mandatory in these cases to exclude or confirm a second bleeding lesion, but one may proceed straight to surgery as very often no angiographic abnormality is seen, although in a few cases a false aneurysm may be demonstrated at the anastomosis. In other cases in which no cause is found on angiography and yet the bleeding continues, laparotomy with on table intra-operative enteroscopy is the next step.

In a few unfortunate cases when intra-operative enteroscopy has been unsatisfactory or is not possible, the source of bleeding may still prove elusive. In this situation some surgeons have utilized temporary stomas in an attempt to isolate the affected segment of bowel (Eaton, 1981). This is unsatisfactory and excessively aggressive, and if the patient is indeed bleeding at such a marked rate, dividing the bowel into segments with soft non-crushing clamps may achieve the same result. Others have advocated a 'blind' right hemicolectomy as often an undetected bleeding source may lurk in the caecum, such as a bleeding diverticulum or angiodysplasia (Boley et al, 1977). However histological examination is often unable to confirm the presence of any vascular anomaly without formal arterial injection and microradiographic studies of the fresh specimen, but in many anecdotal cases the bleeding ceases. Fortunately, with the improved angiographic and endoscopic techniques, the need for such surgical options rarely arises, and such practices should not be necessary or encouraged.

In those cases in which laparotomy should be avoided if possible, then any rapid exsanguinating haemorrhage identified at angiography should be treated by super-selective intra-arterial vasopressin infusion or embolization (Balint and Sarfeh, 1977; Palmaz et al, 1984) using such material as sterile absorbable gelatin sponge (Gelfoam) or human dura mater (Lyodura) (Allison et al, 1982). In cases of life-threatening haemorrhage a form of glue, isobutyl-2-cyanoacrylate, has been used.

Overt intermittent haemorrhage

Cases of intermittent bleeding should be managed as for rapid massive bleeding, if they can be investigated during an active or overt phase. However in practice this is all too often difficult to organize in spite of the best of intentions. Once again upper gastrointestinal endoscopy is the first investigation of choice but if it is negative the patient's age should be taken into consideration. When the patient is young a Meckel's isotope scan may prove positive, but if the patient is elderly colonoscopy is indicated looking for lesions such as angiodysplasia, carcinoma or diverticular disease. If these investigations fail to achieve a diagnosis, angiography should be the next investigation, unless there are definite small bowel symptoms, in which case enteroclysis may pick up small bowel tumours, strictures, lymphomas, Crohn's disease or diverticula. However before ordering enteroclysis, it should be realized that once this has been performed, if negative, it will delay angiography because of residual barium in the bowel. Angiography will detect a lesion in about 50% of cases (Thompson et al, 1987) and remains the only way of making a preoperative diagnosis in cases of small bowel vascular anomalies and hepatic or splenic artery aneurysms. If this and a labelled red cell scan still prove inconclusive, then laparotomy, possibly with intra-operative enteroscopy, remains the only option. Lesions can then be seen both intraluminally and transmurally, identified, marked and excised. In a few cases of intermittent bleeding no actual cause is found in spite of extensive investigation. If the bleeding does not recur, then these cases may remain a mystery and there were two such cases in our series. However if bleeding should recur then complete reinvestigation from first principles is required.

Occult haemorrhage

Such patients present with iron-deficiency anaemia and positive faecal occult blood for which there is no apparent cause. It is important to exclude systemic conditions, infective conditions and all causes of small bowel ulceration as listed in Table 2. In certain parts of the world, parasitic infestation is a common cause of chronic gastrointestinal blood loss and stool samples should be examined for ova and cysts. Foreign bodies and trauma should also be excluded.

Upper gastrointestinal endoscopy is again the first investigation of choice to exclude peptic ulceration, haemorrhagic gastritis, oesophagitis, varices or neoplasia. If this investigation is negative, the next step is either a double contrast barium enema or colonoscopy. Our own preference is to go straight to colonoscopy, as it is mandatory anyway if a barium enema is negative. It also has the added advantage of allowing biopsies to be taken of any lesions encountered, and it will demonstrate any mucosal vascular anomaly such as angiodysplasia which would not be seen on a barium enema study.

If both upper and lower gastrointestinal endoscopy are negative, small bowel enteroclysis is advised to look for small bowel tumours, diverticula, strictures, ulceration or Crohn's desease, but it will rarely demonstrate a Meckel's diverticulum. As this lesion can be the cause of occult bleeding (Williamson et al, 1984), in younger patients a technetium scan should be performed. Angiography may demonstrate a tumour blush, but the yield is otherwise low, as the rate of blood loss is so slow that only significant vascular abnormalities will be detected.

Certain small lesions that are within range of the endoscope and are multiple, such as telangiectasia, may be amenable to endoscopic treatment. Application of laser or heater probes may be valuable in treating such lesions especially in the stomach or duodenum.

When all investigations are negative, then laparotomy with intra-operative enteroscopy is required in order to exclude small bowel vascular anomalies. However it is important to correct an iron-deficiency anaemia before operation. In spite of great care and diligence in investigation, there remains a very small number of patients in whom no causes for slow occult bleeding is found even after careful angiography and laparotomy. These patients should be treated with iron therapy. In the two cases in our series, no cause has yet come to light, and at a follow-up of 2 and 6 years, both remain in apparent good health.

CONCLUSIONS AND THE WAY FORWARD

Recurrent obscure intestinal haemorrhage is fortunately uncommon, because these patients do present diagnostic problems. Unless a careful clinical and logical approach is adopted, these patients may undergo multiple unnecessary and unproductive investigations and still remain a diagnostic mystery. It has been suggested that early careful laparotomy should be considered in young people and that angiography be reserved for older patients (Thompson et al, 1987). If expert angiography is not freely available, this policy would seem justified. However it is recommended that for the few very difficult cases, referral should be considered to a centre where high quality angiography is available as well as a surgeon experienced at dealing with these difficult diagnostic conundrums. There still remain pitfalls that can trap the unwary, such as multiple different potential bleeding sources, or inadequate investigations that are labelled as being negative, and these can easily influence the clinician resulting in erroneous conclusions and an inadequate line of management which all serve to compound the problem to the detriment of the patient. Regrettably, even after the application of extensive and meticulous investigations, about 5% of cases will remain undiagnosed.

The overall prognosis for these patients depends on the underlying cause. In the majority of cases, surgical resection of the causative pathology is curative, but the price paid by both patient and hospital resources may be high.

With regard to future developments in management of these difficult cases, our aims and endeavours should be focused on providing an earlier and more accurate diagnosis. In order for expertise to develop, such patients should be treated in centres where there is a high degree of expertise especially on the radiographic side. Arteriography has become exceedingly sophisticated, but more highly selective catheterization with magnification and microradiographs demonstrating finer detail may provide more accurate information in the future. However such a development would require some form of localization as it would be impossible to catheterize all distal branches of the three main arterial systems of the gastrointestinal tract. Greater definition on radionuclide scanning may provide this information especially if the patient is bleeding at the time. This raises an important logistical aspect of management. A major step forward in the management of these patients would be for there to be an out-of-hours emergency service both for radionuclide scanning and arteriography. If these services were to be available, as soon as any patient shows signs or symptoms of bleeding an immediate scan may give some indication of the approximate location of the blood loss and an arteriogram with selective cannulation and microradiographs may be able to identify very small lesions. Small bowel endoscopy must also be an area in which developments are overdue. It is not easy to see how advances are going to materialize in this technique other than gaining in experience with one of the methods described in the endoscopy section of this chapter. These techniques are not in wide use and are not very satisfactory and therefore new concepts would be welcome. Intra-operative endoscopy is here to stay, but the actual practical technique is being refined all the time as experience is being acquired. The future must rest with better diagnostic accuracy so that the surgeon may be able to operate on these patients knowing what is he going to find and what resection is going to be required. Hopefully the negative laparotomy for bleeding will soon become a procedure of the past.

REFERENCES

Alavi A (1982) Detection of gastrointestinal bleeding with Tc99m sulphur colloid. *Seminars in Nuclear Medicine* **12**: 126.

Alavi A, Dann RW, Baum S & Biery DN (1977) Scintigraphic detection of acute gastrointestinal bleeding, *Radiology* **124**: 753.

Alison DJ, Hemingway AP & Cunningham DA (1982) Angiography in gastrointestinal bleeding. *Lancet* **ii**: 30.

Anderson GF, Sfakianakis G, King DR et al (1980) Hormonal enhancement of technetium-99m pertechnetate uptake in experimental Meckel's diverticulum. *Journal of Pediatric Surgery* **15**: 900.

Apelgren MM, Vargish T & Al-Kawas F (1988) Principles for use of intra-operative enteroscopy for hemorrhage from the small bowel. *American Surgeon* **54**: 85.

Baer AM, Bayless TM & Yardley JH (1980) Intestinal ulceration and malabsorption syndromes. *Gastroenterology* **79**: 754.

Balint JA & Sarfeh IJ (1977) *Gastrointestinal Bleeding. Diagnosis and Management*, pp 31–41. New York: Wiley.

Baum S (1981) Pertechnitate imaging following cimetidine administration in Meckel's diverticulum of the ileum. *American Journal of Gastroenterology* **76**: 464.

Baum S, Athanasoulis CA, Waltman AC et al (1977) Angiodysplasia of the right colon: a cause of gastrointestinal bleeding. *A.J.R.* **129**: 789.

Berquist TH, Nolan NG, Stephens DH et al (1976) Specificity of 99mTc-pertechnitate in scintigraphy diagnosis of Meckel's diverticulum. Review of 100 cases. *Journal of Nuclear Medicine* **17**: 465.

Boley SJ, Schultz L, Krieger H, Schwartz S, Elguezabal A & Allen AC (1965) Experimental evaluation of thiazides and potassium as a cause of small bowel ulcer. *Journal of the American Medical Association* **192**: 763.

Boley SJ, Sammartano R, Adams A et al (1977) On the nature and etiology of vascular ectasias of the colon (degenerative lesions of ageing). *Gastroenterology* **72**: 650.

Boydstun JS, Gaffey TA & Bartholomew LG (1981) Clinicopathologic study of non-specific ulcers of the small intestine. *Digestive Disease Science* **26**: 911.

Cambell JR & Knapp RW (1966) Small bowel ulceration associated with thiazide and potassium therapy: review of 13 cases. *Annals of Surgery* **163**: 291.

Chalmers AG, Robinson PJ & Chapman AH (1986) Embolisation in small bowel haemorrhage. *Clinical Radiology* **37**: 379.

Crawford ES, Roehm JOF & McGavran MH (1980) Jejuno-ileal arteriovenous malformation. Localisation for resection by segmental bowel staining techniques. *Annals of Surgery* **191**: 404.

Crowson M, Fielding JWL, Black J et al (1984) Acute gastrointestinal complications of infrarenal aortic aneurysm repair. *British Journal of Surgery* **71**: 825.

Doran J & Hardcastle JD (1982) Bleeding patterns in colorectal cancer: the effect of aspirin and the implications for faecal occult blood testing. *British Journal of Surgery* **69**: 711.

Eaton AC (1981) Emergency surgery for acute colonic haemorrhage—a retrospective study. *British Journal of Surgery* **68**: 109.

Eggleston FC, Santoshi B & Singh CM (1979) Typhoid perforation of the bowel. *Annals of Surgery* **190**: 31.

Evert JA, Black BM & Dockerty MB (1948) Primary non-specific ulcers of the small intestine. *Surgery* **23**: 185.

Forbes CD, Barr RD, Prentice CRM & Douglas A (1973) Gastrointestinal bleeding in haemophilia. *Quarterly Journal of Medicine* **42**: 503.

Forrest JAH (1982) Gastrointestinal bleeding. In Shearman DJC & Finlayson NDC (eds) *Diseases of the Gastrointestinal Tract and Liver*, p 204. Edinburgh: Churchill Livingstone.

Forrest JAH & Finlayson NDC (1974) The investigation of acute upper gastrointestinal haemorrhage. *British Journal of Hospital Medicine* **12**: 160.

Geroulakis G (1987) Surgical problems of jejunal diverticulosis. *Annals of the Royal College of Surgeons of England* **69**: 266.

Gnauck R (1980) Occult blood tests. *Lancet* **1**: 822.

Goldman RL (1964) Submucosal arterial malformation (aneurysm) of the stomach with fatal hemorrhage. *Gastroenterology* **46**: 589.

Guest JL Jr (1963) Non-specific ulceration of the intestine. *International Abstracts of Surgery* **117**: 409.

Gurian L, Jendrzejewski J, Katon R, Bilbao M, Cope R & Melnyk C (1982) Small bowel enema. An underutilised method of small bowel examination. *Digestive Disease Science* **27**: 1101.

Hall RI, Lavelle MI & Venables CW (1982) Chronic pancreatitis as a cause of gastrointestinal bleeding. *Gut* **23**: 250.

Haynes WF, Pittmann FE & Christakis G (1960) Localisation of site of upper gastrointestinal tract hemorrhage by the fluorescein string test. *Surgery* **48**: 421.

Irons GV & Kirsner JB (1965) Routine chemical tests of the stool for occult blood: an evaluation. *American Journal of Medical Science* **249**: 247.

Jaffe BF, Youker JE & Margoulis AR (1965) Artographic localisation of controlled gastrointestinal hemorrhage in dogs. *Surgery* **58**: 984.

Jones PF (1974) Jejunal and ileal diverticula. In: *Emergency Abdominal Surgery*, p 550. Oxford: Blackwell.

Keddie N, Watson-Baker R & Saran M (1982) The value of the small bowel enema to the general surgeon. *British Journal of Surgery* **69**: 611.

Lamerton AJ (1984) Iliaco-appendiceal fistula complicating endarterectomy alone. *British Journal of Surgery* **71**: 501.

Lang J, Bjarnason I, Levi AJ & Price AB (1985) Pathology of iatrogenic ileal strictures caused by non-steroidal anti-inflammatory drugs. *Gut* **26**: A542.

Lau WY, Fan ST, Chu KW et al (1986) Intra-operative fibre optic enteroscopy for bleeding lesions in the small intestine. *British Journal of Surgery* **73**: 217.

Mackey WC & Dineen P (1983) A fifty year experience with Meckel's diverticulum. *Surgery Gynecology and Obstetrics* **156**: 56.

Macrae FA & St John DJB (1982) Relationship between patterns of bleeding and hemoccult sensitivity in patients with colorectal cancer or adenoma. *Gastroenterology* **82**: 891.

Maglinte DD & Antley RM (1984) Radiology of the small bowel: enteroclysis and the conventional follow-through. *Gastroenterology* **86**: 383.

Maglinte DDT, Hall R, Miller RE et al (1984) Detection of surgical lesions of the small bowel by enteroclysis. *American Journal of Surgery* **147**: 225.

Merrick MV (1988) The small intestine. In Rhys Davies E & Thomas WEG (eds) *Nuclear Medicine: Applications to Surgery*, p 69. Tunbridge Wells: Castle House.

Morgenstern L, Freilich M & Parish JF (1965) The circumferential small-bowel ulcer: Clinical aspects in 17 patients. *Journal of the American Medical Association* **191**: 637.

Neuss MN, Garbutt JT, Leight GS et al (1986) Intraluminal thrombus and bowel obstruction in acute leukemia due to bleeding Meckel's diverticulum. *American Journal of Medicine* **80**: 1194.

Nolan DJ (1981) Barium examination of the small intestine. *Gut* **22**: 682.

Ostrow JD, Mulvaney CA, Hansell UR & Rhodes RS (1973) Sensitivity and reproducibility of chemical tests for fecal occult blood with an emphasis on false positive reactions. *American Journal of Digestive Diseases* **18**: 930.

Palmaz JC, Walter JF & Cho KJ (1984) Therapeutic embolisation of the small bowel arteries. *Radiology* **152**: 377.

Pierce WS & Davis AV (1969) Massive bleeding from a diffuse vascular malformation of the small intestine. *Archives of Surgery* **98**: 336.

Reilly LM, Altman H, Lusby RJ et al (1984) Late results following surgical management of vascular graft infection. *Journal of Vascular Surgery* **1**: 36.

Robertson DAF, Dixon MF, Scott BB, Simpson FG & Losowsky MS (1983) Small intestinal ulceration: diagnostic difficulties in relation to coeliac disease. *Gut* **24**: 565.

Rogers BHG & Adler F (1976) Hemangiomas of the cecum. *Gastroenterology* **71**: 1079.

Schiller KFR, Truelove, SC & Williams DG (1970) Haematemesis and melaena with special reference to factors influencing the outcome. *British Medical Journal* **2**: 7.

Sellink JL (1974) Radiologic examination of the small intestine by duodenal intubation. *Acta Radiologica, Diagnosis* **15**: 318.

Sfakianakis GN, Anderson GF & King DR (1981) The effect of intestinal hormones on the Tc99m pertechnetate imaging of ectopic gastric mucosa in experimental Meckel's diverticulum. *Journal of Nuclear Medicine* 22: 678.

Shackelford RT & Marcus WY (1960) Jejunal diverticula—a cause of gastrointestinal hemorrhage. A report of three cases and review of the literature. *Annals of Surgery* 151: 930.

Sheil AGR, Reeve TS, Little JM et al (1969) Aorto-intestinal fistulas following operations on the abdominal aorta and iliac artery. *British Journal of Surgery* 56: 840.

Shinya H & McSherry C (1982) Endoscopy of the small bowel. *Surgical Clinics of North America* 62: 821.

Stewart JG, Ahlquist DA, McGill DB et al (1984) Gastrointestinal blood loss and anemia in runners. *Annals of Internal Medicine* 100: 843.

Tada M & Kawai K (1984) Small bowel endoscopy. *Scandinavian Journal of Gastroenterology* **19 (Supplement 102)**: 39.

Taylor MT (1969) Massive hemorrhage from jejunal diverticulosis. *American Journal of Surgery* 118: 117.

Thomas CS, Tinsley EA & Brockman SK (1967) Jejunal diverticula as a source of massive upper gastrointestinal bleeding. *Archives of Surgery* 95: 89.

Thomas WEG (1989) Recurrent obscure gastrointestinal haemorrhage. *Current Practice in Surgery* 1: 17.

Thomas WEG & Baird RN (1986) Secondary aorto-enteric fistulae: towards a more conservative approach. *British Journal of Surgery* 73: 875.

Thomas WEG & May RE (1981) Hepatic artery aneurysm following cholecystectomy. *Postgraduate Medical Journal* 57: 393.

Thomas WEG & Williamson RCN (1985) Non-specific small bowel ulceration. *Postgraduate Medical Journal* 61: 587.

Thompson JN, Salem RR, Hemingway AP et al (1987) Specialist investigations of obscure gastrointestinal bleeding. *Gut* 28: 47.

Vellacott KD, Baldwin RW & Hardcastle JD (1981) An immunofluorescent test for faecal occult blood. *Lancet* 1: 18.

Watson MR (1963) Primary non-specific ulceration of the small intestine. *Archives of Surgery* 87: 600.

Williamson RCN, Welch CE & Malt RA (1983) Adenocarcinoma and lymphoma of the small intestine. *Annals of Surgery* 197: 172.

Williamson RCN, Cooper MJ & Thomas WEG (1984) Intussusception of invaginated Meckel's diverticulum. *Journal of the Royal Society of Medicine* 77: 652.

Winzelberg GG, McKusick KA, Froelich JW et al, (1982) Detection of gastrointestinal bleeding with Tc99m-labelled red blood cells. *Seminars in Nuclear Medicine* 12: 139.

Yeker D & Buyukunal C (1984) Radionuclide imaging of Meckel's diverticulum: cimetidine versus pentagastrin plus glucagen. *European Journal of Nuclear Medicine* 9: 316.

6

ACUTE LIVER FAILURE

John G. O'Grady and Roger Williams

INTRODUCTION AND DEFINITIONS

A broad definition of acute liver failure (ALF) is severe hepatic dysfunction which is manifest by either encephalopathy or a coagulopathy and develops within 6 months of the onset of symptoms related to liver disease. There are a number of temporally based systems which subdivide ALF to reflect variations in the natural history, prognosis and clinical features. Fulminant hepatic failure (FHF) describes the subgroup with the most rapid progression and it is variously defined as the onset of encephalopathy within 4 weeks (Mathieson et al, 1980), 6 weeks (EASL, 1979) and 8 weeks (Trey and Davidson, 1970) of the onset of symptoms, or alternatively within 2 weeks of the onset of jaundice (Bernuau et al, 1986a). The patients with a more protracted clinical course are designated by the terms subacute or late-onset hepatic failure (LOHF) (Gimson et al, 1986) or subfulminant hepatic failure (Bernuau et al, 1986a). All of the above definitions require the presence of encephalopathy, although it has been argued that a coagulopathy is adequate evidence of severe hepatic dysfunction. Consequently, the term severe acute liver failure was proposed to describe the latter patients with a coagulopathy before the onset of encephalopathy, but unfortunately no discriminatory tests or values were included (Bernuau et al, 1986a).

A further problem with the clinical definitions is the classification of patients who present with the clinical features of ALF but have occult chronic liver disease. An example of this is the acute or fulminant presentation of Wilson's disease when cirrhosis is established at the time of diagnosis. Similarly, chronic hepatitis B surface antigen (HBsAg) carriers may develop ALF as a consequence of superinfection with delta or non-A, non-B (NANB) viruses. The clinical behaviour of these patients resembles that of other causes of ALF, rather than episodes of acute decompensation occurring in patients with chronic liver disease (often precipitated by some complication, e.g. gastrointestinal bleeding, sepsis or electrolyte abnormalities), which is best referred to as acute-on-chronic liver failure. For the purposes of this review three terms will be used—ALF covering all variants including the acute presentation of Wilson's disease, etc., FHF (as per Trey and Davidson, 1970) and LOHF using the interval between the onset of symptoms and encephalopathy as the distinguishing parameter.

AETIOLOGY AND DIAGNOSIS

The main causes of ALF vary geographically and the UK is almost unique in having paracetamol as the commonest aetiology (Figure 1). On a world-wide basis, viral hepatitis heads the list but the proportion of cases due to the different viruses also shows geographical variation (Table 1).

Viral hepatitis

ALF due to viral hepatitis A (HAV) is relatively uncommon, occurring in 0.14–0.35% of hospitalized cases. In the UK, the proportion of cases of ALF due to HAV is relatively high. This appears to be due to exposure to the virus in later life when the risks are increased, and 71% of 138 recorded deaths from hepatitis A in England and Wales between 1979 and 1985 were aged over 50 years (Forbes and Williams, 1988). While it was previously assumed that HAV was a directly

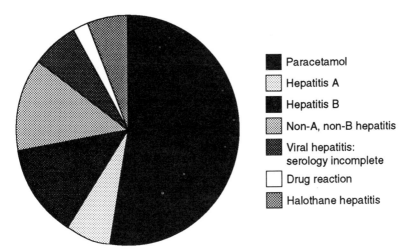

■ Paracetamol
▨ Hepatitis A
■ Hepatitis B
▨ Non-A, non-B hepatitis
▨ Viral hepatitis:
  serology incomplete
□ Drug reaction
▨ Halothane hepatitis

FIGURE I Relative incidence of causes of acute liver failure in 620 patients admitted to King's College Hospital 1973–1985

TABLE I
Relative frequencies of viral aetiologies in series of patients with fulminant hepatic failure

	HAV	HBV	NANB
United Kingdom	20%	44%	36%
France	6%	60%	34%
Denmark	20%	32%	48%
Greece	2%	74%	24%
United States	2%	60%	38%
Japan	2%	74%	24%

cytopathic virus, there is now evidence emerging that it is an immunopathologic process, possibly involving cytolytic T cells (Lemon, 1985; Vallbracht et al, 1986). The diagnosis of HAV ALF is based on detection of the IgM antibody in serum, which appears soon after infection and can persist for up to 200 days.

The risk of developing ALF is higher with hepatitis B (HBV), occurring in 1–4% of hospitalized patients, and appears to be increased when there is coinfection with the hepatitis D or delta virus (HDV). Evidence of HDV infection was found in 34–43% of patients with HBV FHF (58–79% due to superinfection in chronic HBV carriers and the remainder as a consequence of acute coinfection) as compared to 4–19% of less severe cases (Smedile et al, 1982; Govindarajan et al, 1984). HBV is not a directly cytopathic virus and the pathogenesis of liver damage appears to involve immunological mechanisms associated with accelerated clearance of the HBV (Trepo et al, 1976; Woolf et al, 1976). The demonstration of the IgM antibody to HBV core antigen in serum is the basis for establishing the diagnosis of HBV ALF. HBsAg is cleared rapidly from serum in these patients and was undetectable in 12–55% of cases at the time of presentation (Gimson et al, 1983; Brechot et al, 1984; Papaevangelou et al, 1984). Viral replication has usually ceased by the time of presentation; HBeAg was found in 12% and 37% of patients in two series, and in the latter HBV DNA was present in only 9% (Gimson et al, 1983; Brechot et al, 1984). Coinfection or superinfection with delta virus is diagnosed by the demonstration of delta antigen or IgM antibody to delta in serum. Females are at increased risk of developing HBV FHF and there is some evidence that homosexuals have a decreased risk (Bernuau et al, 1986a, b).

The presence of HBsAg in serum does not necessarily implicate HBV in the pathogenesis of the ALF. In one series, 15% of HBsAg-positive cases were attributed to NANB hepatitis on the basis of the absence of IgM antibodies to HAV, core antigen and delta (Papaevangelou et al, 1984). However, a recent Taiwanese study of 76 similar cases developing acute hepatitis (but not ALF) superimposed upon previously unrecognized asymptomatic HBsAg carriers suggested that most cases occurring in HBeAg-positive patients (88%) represented immune clearance of HBeAg in the natural course of chronic HBV infection (Chu et al, 1989). Whether this mechanism can cause ALF remains to be established.

The diagnosis of presumed NANB viral hepatitis is currently made when there is no serological evidence of other viral infections or history of exposure to hepatotoxic drugs or chemicals. However, a new assay for circulating antibodies to what is now called hepatitis C virus (HCV) has been described (Kuo et al, 1989), and it is becoming commercially available (Ortho Diagnostics). The initial report suggests this test is positive in 80–90% of chronic post-transfusion NANB hepatitis patients and in 58% of sporadic cases. However, its diagnostic value in ALF patients is uncertain as only 15% of acute post-transfusion patients were positive. The extent to which HCV accounts for patients currently designated as NANB ALF remains to be seen.

The risk of developing NANB FHF is 2.3–4.7% of hospitalized cases. NANB hepatitis is the predominant cause of LOHF, accounting for over 90% of cases in one series (Gimson et al, 1986). Almost all cases of NANB ALF are sporadic, and in one series of 515 cases of transfusion-related NANB hepatitis none developed ALF (Dienstag, 1983). In the Indian subcontinent, a water-borne variety of NANB viral hepatitis is recognized which causes FHF in up to 10% of cases and is especially virulent in advanced pregnancy (Khuroo, 1980; Wong et al, 1980). A virus particle of approximately 27 nm diameter has recently been identified in faeces from a patient with this variety of NANB hepatitis (Arankalle et al, 1988).

Unusual causes of viral ALF include herpes simplex 1 and 2, varicella zoster, Epstein–Barr virus and cytomegalovirus. An important differential diagnosis in Epstein–Barr virus infections is the virus-associated hemophagocytic syndrome, pathognomonic features of which may be demonstrable on examination of the bone marrow, including benign lymphohistiocytic proliferation and hemophagocytosis (Risdall et al, 1979). Disseminated intravascular coagulation is a prominent feature and treatment with interferon may be effective.

Paracetamol (Acetaminophen)

Paracetamol overdose is usually taken with suicidal or parasuicidal intent, but instances of ALF secondary to appropriate therapeutic usage have been reported in chronic alcohol consumers and patients concomitantly taking enzyme-inducing drugs, particularly antiepileptic therapy. Metabolism of paracetamol by the cytochrome P_{450} system results in the formation of a toxic, unstable metabolite (N-acetyl-p-benzoquinone imine) which is normally rapidly inactivated by conjugation with glutathione. Saturation of the detoxifying system is thought to result in the accumulation of this metabolite leading to lipid peroxidation and consequently hepatocyte injury (Davis, 1986).

Drug reactions

Halothane hepatitis is one of the more frequently occurring idiosyncratic drug reactions, and it accounted for 5% of the overall number of cases of FHF in our series between 1973 and 1985. Typically, FHF develops within 5–15 days after the second or subsequent exposure to halothane, and usually effects obese, atopic, middle-aged females. While the diagnosis was previously made on clinical criteria, a specific halothane antibody test has been described (Neuberger et al, 1983) and it may prove to be a sensitive discriminator of halothane hepatitis from other causes of ALF after anaesthesia. The drugs that most frequently cause ALF idiosyncratically include isoniazid, monoamine oxidase inhibitors, non-steroidal anti-inflammatory drugs, gold, sodium valproate, disulphiram, cotrimoxazole, sulphonamides and ketoconazole.

Miscellaneous causes

Poisoning with *Amanita phalloides* occurs particularly on continental Europe between September and November. Carbon tetrachloride has been implicated in some cases of ALF, and can independently cause renal failure. Acute fatty liver of pregnancy develops in the latter stages of pregnancy, usually with a male fetus, and is characterized by severe microvesicular steatosis which is often detectable on radiologic scanning. ALF in pregnancy may also result from pre-eclampsia, septicemia or viral hepatitis.

The acute or fulminant presentation of Wilson's disease is characterized by the coexistence of a Coomb's negative haemolytic anaemia, and Kayser–Fleischer rings may be present. The serum caeruloplasmin level is low and urinary copper excretion is greatly increased. ALF is an unusual presentation of the Budd–Chiari syndrome and malignancy (especially myeloproliferative disorders).

CLINICAL FEATURES AND MANAGEMENT

Encephalopathy

The severity of encephalopathy is graded clinically on a scale of 0–IV (Table 2). The grade of encephalopathy may fluctuate in the early phases, especially in LOHF. Many cases do not progress beyond grades I–II and in these patients the prognosis is excellent. Once grade III–IV encephalopathy develops, the patient is at particular risk of developing other complications and the outcome is much less certain. In paracetamol patients encephalopathy develops 3–4 days after drug ingestion and progresses through the different stages over periods as short as 24–48 hours. In viral hepatitis, the onset of encephalopathy is more variable and may even on occasions precede the onset of jaundice.

The mechanisms underlying the encephalopathy are as yet unsolved and may be multifactorial. Ammonia, phenols, fatty acids, middle molecular weight substances and mercaptans have all been proposed as possible causative agents, and although none provides a totally independent explanation they may act synergistically or contribute to the overall process. Such toxins interfere with neuronal energy metabolism, and may also contribute to alterations in blood–brain barrier (BBB) permeability by direct toxicity and inhibition of Na^+, K^+-ATPase activity. Considerable recent interest has been focused on the inhibitory neurotransmitter γ-amino-butyric acid (GABA). This is synthesized by gut flora and increased circulating levels have been documented in ALF, some of which could permeate across a damaged BBB. However, cerebral or cerebrospinal fluid GABA levels have not been found to be elevated in patients with encephalopathy. Attention has switched to possible mechanisms upregulating the GABA receptor, and one such mechanism could involve the benzodiazepine receptor, which forms a supramolecular complex with the GABA receptor on neuronal plasma membranes. The most recent evidence suggests that

TABLE 2

Clinical features of grade of encephalopathy

Grade	
I	Mild or episodic drowsiness, impaired intellect, concentration and psychomotor function, but rousable and coherent
II	Increased drowsiness with confusion and disorientation. Rousable and conversant
III	Very drowsy, disorientated, responds to simple verbal commands, often agitated and aggressive
IV	Responds to painful stimuli at best, but may be unresponsive. May be complicated by evidence of cerebral oedema

an endogenous benzodiazepine ligand, with a molecular weight of less than 10 000 daltons, is present in the cerebrospinal fluid of patients with hepatic encephalopathy (Mullen et al, 1988). This has potential therapeutic implications because of the development of benzodiazepine antagonists like flumazenil which might reverse or ameliorate the encephalopathy. A beneficial role for such drugs has not yet been established, but it would appear that they should not be administered to patients with grade IV encephalopathy as their use may aggravate coexisting cerebral oedema. Other suggested mechanisms for the encephalopathy for which data have at times been reported, but whose importance in the overall process have not been established, include the development of false neuro-transmitters in serum and brain, e.g. octopamine, and imbalances in the ratios of plasma and intracerebral amino acids.

Whatever the mechanisms of the encephalopathy, it is aggravated by the absorption of nitrogenous substances from the gut, and in early encephalopathy the withdrawal of dietary protein and the administration of lactulose may be beneficial. In more advanced stages however, there is little evidence to suggest that these measures are advantageous. A number of haemoperfusion systems have been used to reduce the load of circulating toxins, and these are discussed later.

Cerebral oedema

This develops in 75–80% of patients with FHF in grade IV encephalopathy, irrespective of aetiology, and is one of the major causes of death (O'Grady et al, 1988a). In contrast, only four (9%) of 47 patients with LOHF developed cerebral oedema (Gimson et al, 1986). The pathogenesis of the cerebral oedema appears to be a combination of both vasogenic (extravasation of protein and extracellular oedema in the presence of a damaged BBB) and cytotoxic (intracellular edema) mechanisms, together with a two- to threefold increase in cerebral blood flow as a consequence of vasodilatation (Ede and Williams, 1986). The clinical features of increased intracranial pressure include systemic hypertension, 'decerebrate' posturing, hyperventilation, abnormal pupillary reflexes and ultimately impairment of brain stem reflexes and functions (papilloedema however is rarely seen). In the initial stages the signs of cerebral oedema are usually paroxysmal and are often precipitated by tactile stimuli or manoeuvres that cause haemodynamic instability. Later, the episodes of cerebral oedema become more frequent and spontaneous and finally the signs become more sustained. Cerebral oedema usually persists for no more than 4 days, even if grade IV encephalopathy persists.

The management of cerebral oedema is in part expectant and susceptible patients should be nursed in a quiet environment with the trunk at a 45° angle and subjected to the minimum of tactile stimulation. The cerebral perfusion pressure (mean arterial pressure – intracranial pressure) should be maintained above 50 mmHg where possible, and potent aggravating factors like hypotension, hypoxia and hypercapnia should be avoided. The optimal management of cerebral oedema requires the insertion of a subdural transducer once grade IV encephalopathy develops. This gives direct measurements of intracranial pressure, thus allowing for earlier and more accurate detection of cerebral oedema, especially in the ventilated patient in whom most of the clinical signs (except systemic hypertension and pupillary reflexes) are masked. Experience with intracranial pressure monitoring in our unit suggests it is safe despite the presence of a coagulopathy. In the absence of direct intracranial pressure monitoring, continuous measurement of systemic blood pressure is the most reliable method of detecting paroxysms of cerebral oedema, and systolic pressures in excess of 150 mmHg ought to be interpreted and treated accordingly. The main differential diagnosis for systemic hypertension in this setting is a lighter grade of encephalopathy than anticipated in a paralysed patient, and it indicates the need for sedation if continued mechanical ventilation is needed.

In order to obtain the best possible control of cerebral oedema with the use of available therapies, it has been suggested that a low threshold for instituting treatment should be employed (Ede and Williams, 1986), and a level of 20–25 mmHg intracranial pressure is proposed (normal < 12 mmHg). Mannitol (0.3–0.4 mg/kg) by rapid bolus infusion is the first line treatment for raised intracranial pressure and can be repeated hourly if necessary. If the administration of mannitol does not induce a diuresis in patients with normal renal function, the plasma osmolarity should be measured and the mannitol dose repeated only if the osmolarity is less than 320 mOsm. In patients with coexisting oliguric renal failure, the administration of mannitol needs to be coupled with the removal of about three times the given volume by ultrafiltration 15–30 min later. Some recent evidence from our unit suggests that cerebral oedema which is resistant to mannitol and other measures may respond to sodium thiopentone, using initial bolus doses of 185–500 mg (median 250 mg) over 15 min followed by infusions of 50–250 mg/h for up to 4 h (Forbes et al, 1989). Side effects with this regimen were few, mainly hypotension reversible by dose reduction, but it should be used with care to minimize haemodynamic disturbances and possible impairment of white cell function. Hyperventilation as a therapeutic manoeuvre is beneficial in reducing intracranial pressure in acute events, but in a controlled trial involving 55 patients, sustained hyperventilation did not reduce the incidence or severity of the cerebral oedema (Ede and Williams, 1986). Furthermore, the prophylactic use of dexamethasone was not found to be effective in reducing cerebral oedema (Canalese et al, 1982).

Although the majority of patients who survive cerebral oedema revert to normal neurologic function, two cases with a residual deficit (one involving the brain stem, the other the cerebral cortex) have been reported (O'Brien et al, 1987). This is presumably a reflection of the severity and extent of the cerebral damage in patients who now survive with intensive therapy, but who previously would have succumbed to this complication.

Renal failure

Oliguric renal failure, as defined by a urine output < 300 ml/24 h and serum creatinine > 300 μmol/l in the presence of adequate intravascular pressures, develops in about 75% of patients with grade IV encephalopathy following a paracetamol overdose and 30% of other cases (O'Grady et al, 1988a). Renal failure after paracetamol overdose appears to be in part a consequence of direct renal toxicity, as it is usually established before the development of advanced encephalopathy and, even though a 'functional' phase (urinary sodium < 10 mmol/l, urine/plasma (U/P) osmolarity ratio > 1.1) may be seen, the urinary characteristics are normally those of tubular damage (urinary sodium > 10 mmol/l, U/P osmolarity ratio < 1.1). In addition, cases of isolated renal failure and minimal evidence of liver damage after paracetamol ingestion are well documented. In contrast, patients with other causes of ALF develop impairment of renal function when liver failure is more advanced, and it is usual to progress through a stage of 'functional' renal failure before finally demonstrating the characteristics of tubular damage. The pathogenesis of the renal impairment has not yet been elucidated, but may involve abnormalities in eicosanoid metabolism and/or activation of the sympathoadrenal/renin angiotensin system. The serum creatinine level should be used to monitor renal function in patients with ALF as impaired urea synthesis results in a considerable disparity between serum urea and creatinine levels.

Hypovolaemia and reduced intravascular filling pressures secondary to vasodilatation are common in ALF and may be contributing factors to deteriorating renal function. An accurate assessment of haemodynamics, coupled with appropriate treatments as discussed below, is therefore of great importance. The continuous infusion of dopamine (2–4 μg/kg/h) may reverse or slow down the deterioration in renal function by increasing renal blood flow, but this is unlikely to be effective in paracetamol patients with anuria. The use of high dose frusemide is not advised, and considerable care is indicated when using other potentially nephrotoxic drugs, including mannitol in high doses and aminoglycosides. The contention that ALF complicated by renal failure is associated with a particularly poor prognosis (Wilkinson et al, 1977; Ring-Larsen and Palazzo, 1981) is no longer valid as recent survival figures for such patients treated in our unit show survival rates of 50% in paracetamol patients and 30% in viral hepatitis A and B (O'Grady et al, 1988a). Further analysis indicated that much of the impact of renal failure was to reduce the efficacy of mannitol in the treatment of cerebral oedema, rather than the consequences of renal failure *per se*. This improvement occurred during a period when a policy of early and aggressive haemodialysis was in operation and when, in addition to the conventional indications, e.g. hyperkalaemia, acidosis and fluid overload, dialysis was performed daily if the serum creatinine exceeded 400 μmol/l.

Haemodialysis is reasonably well tolerated unless the patient is haemodynamically unstable. Despite the coexisting coagulopathy, heparin is necessary to protect the remaining coagulation factors and requirements are usually higher than in uncomplicated renal failure. Prostacyclin and regional citration are alternatives to heparin in patients with a significant clinical coagulopathy. It has been suggested that the rapid removal of urea and other solutes during haemodialysis may precipitate hypo-osmolar cerebral oedema, and in unstable patients the fall in systemic blood pressure often observed early during dialysis may also aggravate cerebral oedema. In such patients, the newly developed technique of continuous arteriovenous haemodiafiltration (CAV HD) has theoretic advantages and these are currently being evaluated. Peritoneal dialysis does not appear to be an effective alternative to other forms of dialysis. Renal failure may persist for up to 6 weeks after reversal of the hepatic encephalopathy, and during this period the risk of bacterial and fungal sepsis is considerably increased.

Metabolic disorders

Hypoglycaemia is a consequence of increased circulating insulin levels, impaired gluconeogenesis and inability to mobilize glycogen stores. It occurs in most cases and may precede the onset of grade III encephalopathy, and thus hypoglycaemia should be considered during any precipitous deterioration in mental state. In established encephalopathy the clinical signs and symptoms of hypoglycaemia are masked and the blood glucose levels should be monitored hourly and 50 ml of 50% glucose administered intravenously when the level falls below 3.5 mmol/l (63 mg%).

Metabolic acidosis is present in about 30% of patients developing ALF after a paracetamol overdose and is associated with a particularly high mortality—greater than 90% if the pH of arterial is less than 7.30. This acidosis is characteristically found 24–72 h after the drug overdose, and thus precedes the encephalopathy and is independent of renal function. In contrast, a metabolic acidosis is found in less than 10% of patients with other causes of ALF, where an alkalosis is the usual acid–base abnormality. Increased serum lactate levels have been documented in patients with a metabolic acidosis, but this is not necessarily the principal causative factor (Bihari et al, 1986). The increased serum lactate levels were interpreted as indicators of tissue hypoxia resulting from impaired oxygen extraction caused by microvascular shunting of blood away from actively respiring tissues. The latter may be due to changes in microvascular tone, increased capillary permeability or fibrin and cellular aggregate microemboli (Wendon et al, 1989). Impaired tissue oxygen extraction is associated with a poor prognosis. Treatment is directed at maintaining a cardiac index of $4.5 \, l/min/m^2$, oxygen delivery $> 600 \, ml/min/m^2$ and oxygen uptake $> 170 \, ml/min/m^2$. Prostacyclin has been shown to increase oxygen extraction in ALF (Bihari et al, 1986) but an improvement in survival associated with its use has yet to be established. However, treatment modalities directed at the manifestations of tissue hypoxia in blood, e.g. sodium bicarbonate and haemodialysis, are clearly ineffective.

The alkalosis is probably a combination of respiratory and metabolic abnormalities, and it is often associated with hypokalaemia. Hyponatraemia is also commonly encountered in ALF and appears to be mainly dilutional in origin. Hypophosphataemia occurs (Dawson et al, 1987), especially in patients with normal renal function, and while replacements may be indicated to improve diaphragmatic contractility, it should be remembered that levels will rise rapidly if renal impairment develops.

Cardiovascular system and haemodynamics

The haemodynamic abnormalities seen in ALF are similar to those observed in septic shock and are typified by a high cardiac output in association with low peripheral vascular resistance. The systolic systemic blood pressure may be increased in association with paroxysms of increased intracranial pressure, normal or low, but the diastolic blood pressure is almost invariably decreased. Relative hypovolaemia as a consequence of vasodilation results in decreased central venous, pulmonary artery and left atrial end-disatolic pressures. Volume replacement in such cases should be with blood if the haemoglobin is reduced, and otherwise with a combination of colloid (plasma or human albumin solutions) and crystalline (5–10% dextrose solutions). Persistent hypotension in patients with adequate intravascular volumes, and the consequent need to use inotropes, is associated with a very poor prognosis. However inotropes are useful to facilitate a therapeutic procedure, e.g. orthotopic liver transplantation or haemodialysis, which may alter the course of the disease. Dopamine and dobutamine are relatively ineffective, but transient increases in systemic blood pressure can be achieved with infusions of noradrenalin, adrenalin or vasopressin.

Cardiac arrythmias are said to be common in ALF, but in our experience they are usually due to a definable precipitating event, e.g. hypo- or hyperkalaemia, acidosis, hypoxia, or cardiac irritation by a catheter, especially Swan–Ganz catheters. Thus primary treatment should be directed at correction of any underlying cause before anti-arrythmic drugs are administered. Progressive bradycardia over a period of some hours is a common terminal event, with the pulse rate falling in steady increments until asystole supervenes.

Respiratory complications

These may be either neurogenic or pulmonary in origin. Hyperventilation is commonly observed in association with other signs of cerebral oedema, causing hypocapnea and contributing to the alkalosis described above. Advanced cerebral oedema which is unresponsive to treatment results in respiratory depression and finally apnoea. Assisted mechanical ventilation may be indicated either for fatigue complicating hyperventilation or respiratory depression.

Arterial hypoxaemia is often multifactorial in aetiology. The risk of aspiration of gastric contents is not inconsiderable in patients with grade II–III encephalopathy who frequently vomit, and airway protection with an endotracheal tube combined with gastric drainage is advised, particularly before transporting such patients. Radiologically evident bacterial infection was diagnosed in 20% of one series of patients from this unit, while pathogens were cultured from sputum in 46–50% of patients. Pulmonary oedema was diagnosed in 32% of patients and was largely non-cardiogenic in origin (pulmonary capillary wedge pressure < 18 mmHg), and was especially frequent in patients following a paracetamol overdose who had a coexisting metabolic acidosis. Intrapulmonary haemorrhage and atelectasis are other factors which may contribute to the arterial hypoxaemia. In some patients, the hypoxaemia occurs in association with a normal chest radiograph and is attributed to a ventilation/perfusion mismatch consequent on intrapulmonary vascular shunting.

The hypoxaemia is managed with assisted mechanical ventilation using adjuvant positive end-expiratory pressures, unless this accentuates haemodynamic instability. Bronchoscopy and lavage may be beneficial in selected cases to establish the cause of infection and aid in the selection of appropriate antibiotics. The role of physiotherapy in managing these patients may be curtailed by coexisting cerebral oedema, unless guided by direct monitoring of intracranial pressures during therapy.

Coagulopathy

The liver plays a central role in haemostasis and ALF results in a very complex coagulopathy. The liver synthesizes most of the coagulation factors with the exception of Factor VIII, and in ALF circulating levels of fibrinogen, prothrombin and Factors V, VII, IX and X are reduced. The prothrombin time is a very widely used indicator of the severity of liver damage, although Factor V has the shortest half-life and is theoretically a more sensitive yardstick for assessing synthesis of coagulation factors, and is favoured by some groups. Circulating levels of antithrombin III (AT III), an inhibitor of coagulation, are also reduced in ALF, and this has the clinical effect of shortening the half-life of heparin. In addition to decreased synthesis of these factors by the liver, there appears to be increased peripheral consumption. While overt disseminated intravascular coagulation (DIC) is unusual, sensitive techniques point to the presence of a low-grade process in most patients (O'Grady et al, 1986). Both quantitative and qualitative defects in platelet function are well described in ALF. In one study, platelet counts of less than $100 \times 10^9/l$ were documented in 69% of patients. Platelet aggregation is impaired, but there is an increase in platelet adhesiveness, a pattern that may be due to increased levels of circulating von Willebrand factor in ALF.

In an early study, haemorrhage was documented in 73% of 132 patients with FHF and was described as severe in 30% (O'Grady et al, 1986). However, the clinical impact of the coagulopathy has been reduced by the use of fresh frozen plasma and platelet concentrates. The deficiency of coagulation factors alone does not correlate with the risk of bleeding, and haemorrhage is most likely when there is an associated thrombocytopenia, and especially in the minority with a frank DIC syndrome. Gastrointestinal haemorrhage is especially common and is related to the development of gastric erosions, although the incidence and severity has been decreased by the prophylactic use of H_2 antagonists (Macdougall and Williams, 1978). More recently, the use of H_2 antagonists has been linked with an increased incidence of nosocomial respiratory infections and advantages have been suggested for using cytoprotective agents which do not inhibit gastric acid secretion. The other main sites include nasopharynx, lungs, kidneys, retroperitoneum and skin puncture sites. Ideally blood losses should be replaced with fresh blood, but if stored blood is used fresh frozen plasma is needed to replace coagulation factors. The prophylactic administration of fresh frozen plasma in the absence of bleeding was not associated with a reduction in either morbidity or mortality in one study (Gazzard et al, 1975). Because of the combined quantitative and qualitative defects in platelet function, platelet transfusions are indicated in patients with severe haemorrhage, and to maintain levels above $50 \times 10^9/l$ before invasive procedures are performed.

Sepsis

Patients with ALF are at increased risk of infections because of broadly compromised immune function, including impaired neutrophil and Kupffer cell function, and deficiency of opsonins, e.g. complement components and fibronectin. One early study in FHF demonstrated a bacteraemia rate of 22%, which was calculated as twice the expected rate for similarly ill patients without liver disease. However, covert infection may be difficult to detect and a high index of suspicion for sepsis is necessary. In a recent prospective study of infections in 50 patients with ALF and at least grade II encephalopathy, bacterial infection was diagnosed in 40 patients (80%) on the basis of positive cultures (Rolando et al, 1990). In a further five patients, bacterial infection was suspected. The source of positive culture was blood in 14 (isolated bacteraemia in six), urine in 12, sputum in 25 and indwelling cannulae in two patients. The predominant isolated organisms were *Staphylococcus aureus*, streptococci and coliform bacteria. In the same series, fungi were cultured from 16 (32%) patients, the majority being *Candida* species, usually later in the hospital course. These infections were particularly difficult to diagnose and were detected ante-mortem in only 50% of cases. The coexistence of renal failure results in an increased risk of developing both bacterial and fungal sepsis.

Daily cultures of all available specimens is indicated to maintain tight surveillance for emerging infection. Positive cultures should be treated with appropriate antibiotics, but the question of prophylactic administration of broad spectrum antibiotics has not yet been resolved. Studies are also in progress to assess the value of selective small bowel decontamination in reducing the incidence of infections. However, antibiotics and possibly antifungal agents should be commenced in patients who appear to be recovering from ALF but in whom a downward trend in prothrombin time is arrested before normal values are attained. This pattern in our experience is almost invariably associated with underlying sepsis.

SPECIFIC ASPECTS OF MANAGEMENT

While liver-orientated intensive care is the mainstay of the management of ALF, other therapies directed at reducing the toxin load or promoting hepatocyte regeneration need consideration. There is no role for corticosteroid therapy in FHF, and indeed data available from controlled studies suggest this treatment is contraindicated. Some patients with LOHF are steroid responsive, but these are not readily identifiable (by the presence or absence of autoantibodies), and the use of corticosteroids, as in FHF, increases the risk of sepsis. Continuous infusions of insulin and glucagon have been used to promote hepatic regeneration, and in one uncontrolled series an increase in survival from 14.4% to 22.6% was noted in a subgroup of patients whose encephalopathy developed between 11 and 30 days of the onset of symptoms (Takahashi, 1983). Circulating interferon levels were found to be markedly reduced in one study of 15 patients with viral FHF, and seven of nine patients treated with interferon for 3 or more days survived (Levin and Hahn, 1985). However in another series, only two of 12 patients treated with α_{2c} interferon survived (Sanchez-Tapias et al, 1987), and no controlled studies have been reported to date.

Charcoal haemoperfusion is the most extensively assessed of the proposed methods to reduce the load of circulating toxins in ALF. Charcoal is an effective absorbent of a wide range of water-soluble molecules including mercaptans,

GABA, middle molecules, aromatic amino acids and inhibitors of Na^+, K^+-ATPase. Significant reductions in the circulating levels of these latter substances have been demonstrated in patients with FHF receiving charcoal haemoperfusion, and both studies in animal models of hepatic failure and the initial results in humans suggested improved survival with this treatment. A biocompatible system for charcoal haemoperfusion was perfected using prostacyclin (Gimson et al, 1980), and a subsequent study in 76 patients suggested a significant increase in survival with haemoperfusion if it was commenced when the patient was in grade III rather than grade IV encephalopathy (Gimson et al, 1982). Subsequently, controlled trials to assess the efficacy and optimal duration of haemoperfusion were carried out in 137 patients. Seventy-five patients with grade III encephalopathy were randomized to receive 5 or 10 h of haemoperfusion daily, and there was no difference in survival between the two groups with respective survival rates of 51.3% and 50.0%. Sixty-two patients with grade IV encephalopathy were randomized to receive either no haemoperfusion or 10 h of haemoperfusion daily, and survival rates were similar in the two groups at 39.3% and 34.5%, respectively (O'Grady et al, 1988a). Although the study design was limited by the lack of a no-haemoperfusion control in patients with grade III encephalopathy (considered unethical on the basis of earlier results), these studies suggest that in our current practice charcoal haemoperfusion does not improve survival rates over those achieved with liver-orientated intensive care. However, it must be emphasized that the survival rates obtained in these studies exceed not only those reported in all other series but also those achieved at earlier times in our unit. This improvement in survival with time has been attributed to advances in liver-orientated intensive care (in particular the aggressive treatment of cerebral oedema), coupled with the expertise derived from treating relatively large numbers of such patients.

Preliminary studies with an albumin-coated resin column (Amberlite XAD-7) designed to remove protein toxins have established its biocompatibility in serial perfusions, and further evaluation is awaited (Hughes and Williams, 1986). Plasmapheresis and exchange transfusions have also been used. A temporary improvement in encephalopathy may be observed and some authors have been convinced of the benefits.

Early management of paracetamol overdose

The most important aspect of early management is to determine the time of overdose as accurately as possible, and administer the 'antidote' to appropriate cases. The current recommendation is to give n-acetylcysteine intravenously to patients with paracetamol blood levels above the 'treatment line' at 4–16 h after drug ingestion. n-Acetylcysteine should be commenced immediately in cases of doubt and later discontinued if the levels suggest there is little risk of developing liver damage, as there is little evidence it is toxic when administered in the recommended dose. It is possible that n-acetylcysteine may be useful if given later than 16 h, and trials are currently in progress to clarify this issue. Oral methionine is an alternative to n-acetylcysteine, but its bioavailability is less certain as it may be vomited.

Cases presenting more than 24 h after drug ingestion need early assessment of acid–base balance, renal and liver function. An arterial pH less than 7.30 is associated with a very poor prognosis, and is the earliest indication of the need for urgent liver transplantation. Serum creatinine and urine output should be measured to assess renal function. The prothrombin time is the best indicator of the degree of liver damage, and levels in excess of 40 s at 48 h or 50 s at 72 h indicate the need for referral to a specialized liver unit. Serum transaminases are of no value in determining outcome, even if they are increased in multiples of thousands. During this early period of observation, intravenous fluid replacement should be with 5% dextrose. Hypoglycaemia may cause a precipitous deterioration in mental state (before the onset of encephalopathy), and is treated with a bolus of 50 ml of 50% dextrose. Dietary protein withdrawal, H_2 antagonists and lactulose are usually given during this period. The development of encephalopathy should also precipitate referral to appropriate specialized units.

ASSESSMENT OF PROGNOSIS

The availability of orthotopic liver transplantation as a management option in ALF has increased the need for methods of accurately assessing prognosis as early as possible in the clinical course. The underlying aetiology has a major influence on outcome, and patients subdivide into two subgroups on this basis. The first comprises those with paracetamol-induced ALF and viral hepatitis A and B, where the insult to hepatocytes is of relatively short duration, recovery is possible and the eventual outcome is influenced by the pattern of complications that develop. In these patients survival rates of 39–67% are achieved with liver-orientated intensive care (O'Grady et al, 1988a). The second group consists of NANB hepatitis, idiosyncratic drug reactions, halothane hepatitis and the acute presentation of Wilson's disease, where the mortality exceeds 80% and has not been greatly improved by developments in the medical management of the resulting complications. In these patients there is a failure of net hepatic regeneration, either as a consequence of continued hepatocyte damage or inhibition of regeneration.

However, aetiology alone is insufficiently discriminatory and other early indicators of prognosis are needed. In non-paracetamol cases, the duration between the onset of jaundice and the development of encephalopathy is an important prognostic indicator. Analysis of factors affecting survival in patients with FHF treated in our unit showed that the best survival figures were attained in patients where this interval is 7 days or less (O'Grady et al, 1989). Age is also important and the highest mortality occurs in patients under 10 and over 40 years. Of the commonly used laboratory parameters, serum bilirubin and prothrombin time correlated best with outcome, and respective levels above 300 μmol/l (17.6 mg%) and 50 s (control 15 s) were associated with a particularly poor prognosis. In paracetamol cases, the pH of arterial blood was the strongest predictor of outcome (pH < 7.30 associated with 85% mortality), followed by the prothrombin time (O'Grady et al, 1989). Separate studies have found the absence of HBsAg in serum and elevated alpha-fetoprotein to be indicators of good prognosis in HBV FHF (Bernuau et al, 1986b). Other more specialized tests which are thought to have prognostic import include galactose and antipyrine clearance studies, bile acid conjugation and estimations of hepatocyte volume (Tygstrup and Ranek, 1986).

LIVER TRANSPLANTATION

Orthotopic liver transplantation is now well established as a therapeutic option in all variants of ALF, and survival rates of 54–74% were reported in early series (Bismuth et al, 1987; Peleman et al, 1987; O'Grady et al, 1988b; Vickers et al, 1988). The aetiologies particularly associated with a poor prognosis account for the majority of patients transplanted in our programme, but some patients with hepatitis A and paracetamol overdose have been so treated (Figure 2). The optimal selection process should identify suitable candidates as soon as possible in the disease process, thereby increasing the period of time available to find a donor organ. On the basis of the prognostic factors described above, we developed a model for selecting patients for transplantation using three static (aetiology, age and duration of jaundice before the onset of encephalopathy) and two dynamic (prothrombin time and serum bilirubin) variables in non-paracetamol patients (Table 3). The equivalent medical indications for transplantation after a paracetamol overdose involve the arterial pH, prothrombin time, serum creatinine and in some instances the grade of encephalopathy (Table 3).

Technically, the transplant operation is considerably 'easier' than anticipated, probably because of the lack of collateral circulations as a consequence of long-standing portal hypertension. Repletion with coagulation factors, and platelets where necessary, prior to surgery adequately reverses the clinical coaguolopathy in most cases and excessive haemorrhage is not frequently encountered. The presence of cerebral oedema is not a contraindication to transplantation, but it persists both during and up to 12 h after a successful transplant, so that continuous monitoring of intracerebral pressure during this period in susceptible

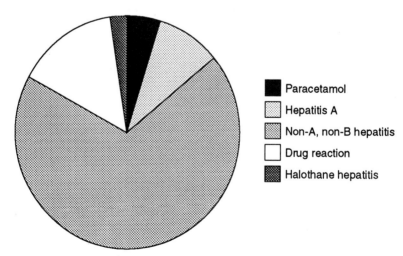

FIGURE 2 The causes of acute liver failure in patients transplanted in the Cambridge/King's College Hospital programme

TABLE 3

Criteria used at King's College Hospital for selection of patients with fulminant hepatic failure for liver transplantation

Paracetamol induced
1. pH < 7.30 (irrespective of grade of encephalopathy)

   or

2. Prothrombin time > 100 s and serum creatinine > 300 μmol/l in patients with grade III or IV encephalopathy

Patients other than paracetamol induced
1. Prothrombin time > 100 s (irrespective of grade of encephalopathy)

   or

2. Any three of following variables (irrespective of grade of encephalopathy):

   a. Age < 10 or > 40 years
   b. Aetiology—NANB hepatitis, halothane hepatitis, idiosyncratic drug reactions
   c. Duration of jaundice before onset of encephalopathy > 7 days
   d. Prothrombin time > 50 s
   e. Serum bilirubin > 300 μmol/l

patients is strongly advised. The risk of sepsis, including fungal infection, also persists post-transplantation and the management policy described above should be extended into this period.

CONCLUSIONS AND THE WAY FORWARD

Acute liver failure, once considered a rare and almost invariably fatal condition, is now a challenge which should result in 60–70% survival rates for all patients if optimally managed. The key to a successful approach is a clear treatment plan for each patient from the time of initial presentation, so that the recent advances in medical management and liver transplantation can be appropriately applied. This is facilitated by the development of early and simple prognostic indicators which identify most patients in need of urgent liver transplantation. Medical management and liver transplantation are however complementary disciplines as many patients require considerable periods of intensive medical care while awaiting the availability of a donor liver. Continued research and development are still required in both areas to push the currently attainable survival rate ever closer to 100%, and at the present rate of progress it would be disappointing if survival rates in specialized centres did not exceed 90% by the end of this century.

The clinical complications that require greatest attention in terms of continued research are cerebral oedema, haemodynamic instability and susceptibility to infection. Another area of investigation likely to contribute to improved results is factors influencing hepatocyte regeneration. The complexity of the functions of the liver renders attempts at the development of liver support systems very difficult but computerized systems to monitor and modulate the amino acid and soluble contents of plasma are not beyond the bounds of imagination. Greater progress may be achieved however in the development of support systems using matrices of human hepatocytes as the functioning unit. In the interim, further attention should be given to the use of auxiliary liver transplantation as a means of providing effective hepatocyte function over a limited period of time.

REFERENCES

Arankalle VA, Ticehurst J, Sceenivasan MA et al (1988) Aetiological association of a virus-like particle with enterically transmitted non-A, non-B hepatitis. *Lancet* **i**: 550–554.

Bernuau J, Rueff B & Benhamou J-P (1986a) Fulminant and subfulminant liver failure: definitions and causes. *Seminars in Liver Disease* **6**: 97–106.

Bernuau J, Goudeau A, Poynard T et al (1986b) Multivariate analysis of prognostic factors in fulminant hepatitis B. *Hepatology* **6**: 648–651.

Bihari DJ, Gimson AES & Williams R (1986) Cardiovascular, pulmonary and renal complications of fulminant hepatic failure. *Seminars in Liver Disease* **6**: 119–128.

Bismuth H, Samuel D, Gugenheim R et al (1987) Emergency liver transplantation for fulminant hepatitis. *Annals of Internal Medicine* **107**: 337–341.

Brechot C, Bernuau J, Thiers V et al (1984) Multiplication of hepatitis B virus in fulminant hepatitis B. *British Medical Journal* **288**: 270–271.

Canalese J, Gimson AES, Davis C, Mellon PJ, Davis M & Williams R (1982) Controlled trial of dexamethasone and mannitol for the cerebral oedema of fulminant hepatic failure. *Gut* **23**: 625–629.

Chu C-M, Liaw Y-F, Pao C-C & Huang M-J (1989) The etiology of acute hepatitis superimposed upon previously unrecognised asymptomatic HBsAg carriers. *Hepatology* **9**: 452–456.

Davis M (1986) Protective agents for acetaminophen overdose. *Seminars in Liver Disease* **6**: 138–147.

Dawson DJ, Babbs C, Warnes TW & Neary RH (1987) Hypophosphatemia in acute liver failure. *British Medical Journal* **295**: 1312–1313.

Dienstag JL (1983) Non-A, non-B hepatitis. I. Recognition, epidemiology and clinical features. *Gastroenterology* **85**: 439–462.

Ede RJ & Williams R (1986) Hepatic encephalopathy and cerebral edema. *Seminars in Liver Disease* **6**: 107–118.

European Association for the Study of the Liver (1979) Randomised trial of steroid therapy in acute liver failure. *Gut* **20**: 620–623.

Forbes A & Williams R (1988) Increasing age—an important adverse prognostic factor in hepatitis A virus infection. *Journal of the Royal College of Physicians of London* **22**: 237–239.

Forbes A, Alexander GJM, O'Grady JG et al (1989) Thiopental infusion in the treatment of intracranial hypertension complicating fulminant hepatic failure. *Hepatology* **10**: 306–310.

Gazzard BG, Henderson JM & Williams R (1975) Early changes following a paracetamol overdose and a controlled trial of fresh frozen plasma therapy. *Gut* **16**: 617–620.

Gimson AES, Langley PG, Hughes RD et al (1980) Prostacyclin to prevent platelet activation during charcoal haemoperfusion in fulminant hepatic failure. *Lancet* **i**: 173–175.

Gimson AES, Braude S, Mellon PJ et al (1982) Earlier charcoal haemoperfusion in fulminant hepatic failure. *Lancet* **ii**: 681–683.

Gimson AES, Tedder RS, White YS, Eddleston ALWF & Williams R (1983) Serological markers in fulminant hepatitis B. *Gut* **24**: 615–617.

Gimson AES, O'Grady J, Ede RJ et al (1986) Late-onset hepatic failure: clinical, serological and histological features. *Hepatology* **6**: 288–294.

Govindarajan S, Chin KP, Redeker AG & Peters RL (1984) Fulminant B viral hepatitis: role of delta agent. *Gastroenterology* **86**: 1417–1420.

Hughes R & Williams R (1986) Clinical experience with charcoal and resin hemoperfusion. *Seminars in Liver Disease* **6**: 164–173.

Khuroo MS (1980) Study of an epidemic of non-A, non-B hepatitis; possibility of another human hepatitis virus distinct from post-transfusion non-A, non-B type. *American Journal of Medicine* **68**: 818–824.

Kuo G, Choo Q-L, Alter HJ et al (1989) An assay for circulating antibodies to a major etiologic virus of human non-A, non-B hepatitis. *Science* **244**: 362–364.

Lemon SM (1985) Type A viral hepatitis: new developments in an old disease. *New England Journal of Medicine* **313**: 1059–1067.

Levin S & Hahn T (1985) Interferon deficiency syndrome. *Clinical and Experimental Immunology* **60**: 267–273.

Macdougall BRD & Williams R (1978) H$_2$-receptor antagonist in the prevention of acute upper gastrointestinal hemorrhage in fulminant hepatic failure. *Gastroenterology* **74**: 164–165.

Mathieson LR, Shivoj P, Nielsen JP, Purcell RH, Wong D & Ranek L (1980) Hepatitis type A, B and non-A, non-B in fulminant hepatitis. *Gut* **21**: 72–77.

Mullen KD, Martin JV, Mendelson WB et al (1988) Could an endogenous benzodiazepine ligand contribute to hepatic encephalopathy. *Lancet* **i**: 457–459.

Neuberger J, Gimson A, Davis M & Williams R (1983) Specific serological markers in the diagnosis of fulminant hepatic failure following halothane anaesthesia. *British Journal of Anaesthesia* **55**: 15–19.

O'Brien CJ, Wise RJS, O'Grady JG & Williams R (1987) Neurological sequelae in patients recovered from fulminant hepatic failure. *Gut* **28**: 93–95.

O'Grady JG, Langley PG, Isola LM et al (1986) Coagulopathy of fulminant hepatic failure. *Seminars in Liver Disease* **6**: 159–163.

O'Grady JG, Gimson AES, O'Brien CJ et al (1988a) Controlled trials of charcoal hemoperfusion and prognostic factors in fulminant hepatic failure. *Gastroenterology* **94**: 1186–1192.

O'Grady JG, Alexander GJM, Thick M, Potter D, Calne RY & Williams R (1988b) Outcome of orthotopic liver transplantation in the aetiological and clinical variants of acute liver failure. *Quarterly Journal of Medicine* **69**: 817–824.

O'Grady JG, Alexander GJM, Hallyar KM & Williams R (1989) Early indicators of prognosis in fulminant hepatic failure. *Gastroenterology* **97**: 439–445.

Papaevangelou G, Tassopoulos N, Roumeliotou-Karayannis A & Richardson C (1984) Etiology of fulminant viral hepatitis in Greece. *Hepatology* **4**: 369–372.

Peleman RR, Gavaler JS, Van Thiel D et al (1987) Orthotopic liver transplantation for acute and subacute hepatic failure in adults. *Hepatology* **7**: 484–489.

Ring-Larsen H & Palazzo U (1981) Renal failure in fulminant hepatic failure and terminal cirrhosis: a comparison between incidence, types, and prognosis. *Gut* **22**: 585–591.

Risdall RJ, McKenna RW, Nesbit ME et al (1979) Virus-associated hemophagocytic syndrome: a benign histiocyte proliferation distinct from malignant histiocytosis. *Cancer* **44**: 993–1002.

Rolando N, Harvey FAH, Brahm J et al (1989) Prospective study of bacterial infection in acute liver failure: an analysis of 50 patients. *Hepatology* **11**: 49–53.

Sanchez-Tapias JM, Mas A, Costa J et al (1987) Recombinant α$_{2c}$-interferon therapy in fulminant viral hepatitis. *Journal of Hepatology* **5**: 205–210.

Smedile A, Farci P, Verme G et al (1982) Influence of delta infection on severity of hepatitis B. *Lancet* **ii**: 945–947.

Takahashi Y (1983) Acute hepatic failure—in special relation to treatment. *Japanese Journal of Medicine* **22**: 140–145.

Trepo CG, Robert D, Motin J, Trepo D, Sepetjian M & Prince AM (1976) Hepatitis B antigen (BHsAg) and/or antibodies (anti-HBs and anti-HBc) in fulminant hepatitis: pathogenic and prognostic significance. *Gut* **17**: 10–13.

Trey C & Davidson LS (1970) The management of fulminant hepatic failure. In Popper H & Schaffner F (eds) *Progress in Liver Disease*, pp. 282–298. New York: Grune and Stratton.

Tygstrup N & Ranek L (1986) Assessment of prognosis in fulminant hepatic failure. *Seminars in Liver Disease* 6: 129–137.

Vallbracht A, Gabriel P, Maier K et al (1986) Cell-mediated cytotoxicity in hepatitis A virus infection. *Hepatology* 6: 1308–1314.

Vickers C, Neuberger J, Buckels J, McMaster P & Elias E (1988) Transplantation of the liver in adults and children with fulminant hepatic failure. *Journal of Hepatology* 7: 143–150.

Wendon J, Gimson AE & Potter D (1989) Oxygen uptake and delivery in fulminant hepatic failure. *Care of the Critically Ill* 5: 55–59.

Wilkinson SP, Weston MJ, Parsons V & Williams R (1977) Dialysis in the treatment of renal failure in patients with liver disease. *Clinical Nephrology* 8: 287–292.

Wong DC, Purcell RH, Sreenivasan MA et al (1980) Epidemic and endemic hepatitis in India: evidence for a non-A, non-B virus aetiology. *Lancet* ii: 876–879.

Woolf I, Sheikh N, Cullens H et al (1976) Enhanced HBsAb production in pathogenesis of fulminant viral hepatitis type B. *British Medical Journal* 2: 669–671.

7

ACUTE PANCREATITIS

David C. Carter

Acute pancreatitis remains a common, unpredictable and potentially dangerous condition. The disease has a broad spectrum of severity; at one end of the spectrum is the patient with mild disease in whom there is little systemic upset and rapid resolution of pain while at the other is the patient with fulminant disease and rapid progression to multiple organ failure and local complications with all their attendant threat to life. The danger of acute pancreatitis is attested by its continued high mortality rate. In the decade to 1979 the mortality rate in Bristol was 19.6% (Corfield et al, 1985a), a figure little different to that of the previous two decades. In Glasgow Royal Infirmary the overall mortality rate in the decade prior to 1970 was 21.4% although with developing interest in the condition and prospective study by general surgeons, the mortality rate appeared to have fallen to 9% in the period 1974–1984. However, this figure is misleading in that a more comprehensive review of the hospital uncovered additional cases of acute pancreatitis, many dealt with by units other than general surgical units and some diagnosed for the first time at autopsy. In addition to 73 deaths in patients diagnosed as having acute pancreatitis in general surgical units, another 53 deaths were discovered in which acute pancreatitis had not been diagnosed in life (Wilson et al, 1988a). These additional deaths raised the overall mortality rate from 9% to 12.9% and it seems likely that even this figure may be an underestimate, given the relatively low modern autopsy rate. It is clear that there is no room for complacency regarding our ability to diagnose and deal with acute pancreatitis.

DIAGNOSIS OF ACUTE PANCREATITIS

Determination of serum amylase concentrations remains the mainstay as far as confirmation of the clinical diagnosis of acute pancreatitis is concerned. However, the majority of patients in whom the diagnosis is suspected do not come to operation or autopsy, and until the relatively recent availability of alternative means of diagnosis such as high resolution CT scanning, it has been extremely difficult to determine the true diagnostic accuracy of serum amylase measurement. Limitations of serum amylase as a marker of acute pancreatitis include the following.

(1) Limited sensitivity: the sensitivity of serum amylase measurement in the

diagnosis of acute pancreatitis is currently estimated to be only about 80% (Clavien et al, 1989). It is now generally accepted that venous, lymphatic and transperitoneal absorption of enzyme released from the inflamed gland raises plasma amylase levels within 24 h of onset of inflammation. However, levels frequently return to normal within 5 days and may fall particularly quickly in patients with mild disease. Patients with severe pancreatitis and extensive destruction of the gland may have only modest hyperamylasaemia as the capacity for amylase production ceases. In general, patients with alcohol-associated acute pancreatitis produce lower levels of hyperamylasaemia than those with gallstone-associated disease, probably because of the reduced secretory capacity of the gland. In the past it was estimated that some 5% of cases of acute pancreatitis were associated with normal serum amylase levels, but recent CT scanning studies suggest that the true figure for normoamylasaemic pancreatitis may be close to 20% (Clavien et al, 1989).

(2) Limited specificity: a large number of conditions other than acute pancreatitis may increase the total serum amylase concentration (Table 1). Although electrophoretic techniques allow separation of pancreatic isoamylase from amylase produced from other sources (and indeed can

TABLE 1
Causes of hyperamylasaemia other than acute pancreatitis

Abdominal causes
Biliary tract disease
Perforated peptic ulcer
Acute perforated appendicitis
Peritonitis
Intestinal obstruction
Afferent loop syndrome
Mesenteric infarction
Pancreatic cancer
Dissecting aortic aneurysm
Pregnancy
Ruptured ectopic pregnancy
Prostatic disease
Pancreatic cancer
Non-abdominal causes
Myocardial infarction
Pulmonary embolism
Pneumonia
Metastatic carcinoma of the lung
Breast cancer
Postoperative causes
Abdominal operations
Cardiac by-pass procedures
Miscellaneous causes
Burns
Diabetic ketoacidosis
Drugs, e.g. opiates, azathioprine, phenylbutazone

separate three different subspecies of pancreatic isoamylase), the approach is impractical for routine diagnostic purposes. However, the method has allowed examination of the specificity of conventional serum amylase measurement and it appears that as many as one-third of patients with hyperamylasaemia and abdominal pain do not have high circulating levels of pancreatic amylase and are not suffering from acute pancreatitis (Weaver et al, 1982; Moossa, 1984).

(3) Problems associated with hyperlipidaemia: the relationship between hyperlipidaemia and acute pancreatitis is well recognized in that between 10% and 38% of patients with acute pancreatitis are reported as having high serum lipid concentrations (Garden et al, 1985). Such hyper-lipidaemia can interfere with the reliability of colorimetric amylase assays by causing marked turbidity. The problem is complicated further by the fact that alcohol, a major cause of acute pancreatitis, can cause hypertriglyceridaemia without producing pancreatic inflammation. Estimation of urinary amylase may help to determine whether acute pancreatitis is indeed present but marked hyperlipidaemia in a patient with severe abdominal pain should be taken as strongly suggestive of acute pancreatitis whether or not hyperamylasaemia is detected.

(4) Macroamylasaemia: this may affect 1–2% of the normal population and denotes the presence of amylase bound to an abnormal protein to form a molecule too large to be excreted by the kidney. Its significance is unknown and its importance lies in the fact that serum amylase levels are raised in the absence of urinary amylase excretion. It is therefore a potential cause of confusion in that hyperamylasaemia may be present in patients who do not have acute pancreatitis. Macroamylasaemia can be confirmed by specific assay and other markers of pancreatitis, such as serum lipase levels, are usually normal.

Given the limitations of serum amylase determination, other methods of diagnosing pancreatitis deserve consideration. Urinary amylase measurement has received impetus by the development of a rapid colorimetric test, the Rapignostic test, which is thought by some to be a valuable screening method (Thompson et al, 1987). However other workers report that the test is not specific and consider that its sensitivity may also be less than 70% (Burkitt, 1987). In theory, measurement of the amylase:creatinine clearance ratio offers advantages in diagnosis. Sadly, its early promise appears to have been short lived. It has not found application in routine clinical practice although it may occasionally be useful in evaluating patients with hyperlipidaemia, macroamylasaemia or renal failure.

Serum lipase values also rise in acute pancreatitis but the diagnostic values of this test has been restricted by the technical difficulties of the assay. However, rapid methods are now available and in one recent report, only six false positive elevations and no false negative results were found in 417 patients with acute abdominal pain (Moller-Petersen et al, 1986). Serum lipase is currently regarded as complementary to serum amylase estimations in the diagnosis of acute pancreatitis but may yet come to be seen as the screening investigation of choice. It is certainly one of the most specific tests (with a specificity of about 90%); furthermore, its levels rise more than those of amylase in alcoholic as opposed to biliary pancreatitis and remain elevated for longer.

For the moment, serum amylase seems likely to retain primacy in diagnosis in most centres but its limitations must be borne clearly in mind.

ASSESSMENT OF SEVERITY OF ACUTE PANCREATITIS

Severe acute pancreatitis may be defined as an attack in which there is a fatal outcome, or the development of major complications such as pseudocyst, pancreatic abscess or haemorrhage. Beger (1989) has provided a clinically useful stratification of acute pancreatitis into four clinically and morphologically distinct varieties (Table 2). Acute oedematous pancreatitis accounts for approximately three-quarters of the cases in the Ulm experience and is usually a mild self-limiting condition which seldom requires urgent surgical intervention. Necrotizing pancreatitis is a more severe disease which can progress rapidly to a fatal outcome, particularly if necrosis is extensive and the necrotic tissue becomes infected. Pancreatic abscess is relatively uncommon and is defined by Beger (1989) as a collection of pus surrounded by an inflammatory wall generated by the tissue harbouring the bacteria; by the time it becomes manifest the patient frequently has no morphological, clinical or laboratory signs of continuing acute pancreatitis. Pancreatic pseudocyst is approximately twice as common as abscess and consists of a fluid collection which may be sterile or infected and which is contained in a fibrous pseudocapsule. In practice, the key to effective early management depends on the prompt separation of patients into those with mild (oedematous) pancreatitis and those with severe (necrotizing) disease.

The large body of literature dealing with the early assessment of severity testifies to the difficulty of the problem, and as McMahon et al (1980) have pointed out, only one in every three cases of severe pancreatitis is recognized as such at the time of admission. In some patients the severity of the attack is obvious from the circulatory collapse, respiratory failure, abdominal distension and body wall ecchymosis. The presence of body wall discoloration in the flanks (Grey–Turner's sign) or umbilicus (Cullen's sign) is still regarded as having ominous prognostic significance. However, Dickson and Imrie (1984) report that 63% of a series of 23

TABLE 2
Types of acute pancreatitis treated in University Hospital, Ulm
(May 1982 to June 1987; from Beger, 1989)

Type of pancreatitis	No. of patients	% frequency
Oedematous/intestitial pancreatitis	567	76.2
Acute necrotizing pancreatitis	130	17.5
Conservative management	20	
Operative management	110	
Pancreatic abscess	14	1.9
Pancreatic pseudocyst	33	4.4

patients with such staining survived, although admittedly many of the survivors did develop complications such as pseudocysts.

Unfortunately, the serum amylase levels on admission are not a good index of severity although failure of levels to return to normal within 5–10 days should certainly alert the clinician to the likelihood that complications are developing. Attempts to use other single clinical or biochemical parameters as an index of severity have proved unsuccessful but there is current interest in the potential link between severity and the generation of trypsinogen activation peptides (Gudgeon et al, 1990). Such peptides are normally produced when trypsinogen is activated by enterokinase in the small intestine; in severe acute pancreatitis it has been suggested that they may be liberated within the pancreas and become detectable by radioimmunoassay following their absorption into the blood stream.

Clinical and biochemical scoring systems

In the absence of a single reliable indicator of severity, a number of multiple factor scoring systems have been devised. Such systems have three aims. Firstly, the clinician is alerted to the presence of severe disease and the likelihood of complications; to put this in perspective the mortality rate of attacks judged to be severe is 25–30% whereas that of mild disease is between zero and 3% (Mayer et al, 1985). Secondly, scoring systems allow comparison between different patient populations. Thirdly, the systems may aid in the selection of patients for more aggressive management and as a basis for defining entry of patients to trial of new forms of treatment.

After statistical analysis of 43 parameters, Ranson and his colleagues in New York developed an 11-factor scoring system (Table 3; Ranson et al, 1974). In a subsequent prospective study, severity was predicted correctly in 93% of 200 patients (Ranson and Pasternack, 1977); only one of the 162 patients thought to have mild disease turned out to have a severe attack, as opposed to 24 of the 38 patients graded as having severe illness on admission. Ranson's original scoring system was developed in a patient population in which males and alcohol-associated pancreatitis figured more prominently than in many European centres. For this reason Ranson (1979) modified his system for use in patients with gallstone pancreatitis and the Glasgow group have also modified their original 9-point systems (Imrie et al, 1978) for this group of patients (Osborne et al, 1981). Recognizing the danger of a proliferation of scoring systems, we in Glasgow attempted to return to a single system for use in acute pancreatitis. In a prospective evaluation of 405 episodes, 8 factors (Table 4) showed a significant association with the outcome and when combined in a scoring system, correctly identified severity in 79% of the attacks (Blamey et al, 1984). Of the 92 patients with three or more positive factors, 39% proved to have severe disease, while only 9% of the 313 episodes judged to be mild on admission ran a complicated course. Schein (1988) has argued strongly for a single scoring system with which to assess all forms of acute surgical disease and has suggested that the APACHE II system (Knaus et al, 1985) deserves study in this context. While agreeing with this sentiment, I believe that for the moment the Glasgow system serves a useful role and goes a long way to meet the aims of a scoring system as outlined above.

TABLE 3
Basis of factor scoring systems to predict the severity of acute pancreatitis

Ranson et al (1974)	Imrie et al (1978)
On admission	
Age > 55 years	
WBC > 16 000/mm³	
Blood glucose > 10 mmol/l	
LDH > 700 IU%	
AST > 250 Sigma Frankel units%	
Within 48 hours	*Within 48 hours*
	Age > 55 years
	WBC > 15 × 10⁹/l
	Blood glucose > 10 mmol/l (no diabetic history)
Blood urea nitrogen rise > 5 mg%	Serum urea > 16 mmol/l (no response to i.v. fluids)
PaO₂ < 8 kPa	PaO₂ < 8 kPa
Serum calcium < 2.0 mmol/l	Serum calcium < 2.0 mmol/l
	Serum albumin < 32 g/l
	LDH > 600 units/l
	AST/ALT > 100 units/l
Haematocrit fall > 10%	
Base deficit > 4 mmol/l	
Fluid sequestration > 6 l	

For either system: severe disease = three or more factors present.
WBC = white blood cell count; LDH = lactic dehydrogenase; AST = asparate aminotransferase; ALT = alanine aminotranferase; PaO₂ = arterial oxygen saturation.

TABLE 4
Significant factors in predicting severity of acute pancreatitis

Factor	Value	No.	Mild (%)	Severe (%)*
Calcium	<2.00	58	62	38
(mmol/l)	>2.00	305	91	9
Urea	>16	13	31	69
(mmol/l)	<16	385	86	14
LDH	>600	70	67	33
(U/l)	<600	165	94	6
Glucose	>10	29	48	52
(mmol/l)	<10	181	74	26
PaO₂	<8	114	75	25
(kPa)	>8	262	89	11
WBC	>15	130	73	27
(×10⁹/l)	<15	237	90	10
Albumin	<32	28	64	36
(g/l)	<32	344	87	13
Age	>55	198	80	20
(years)	<55	207	88	12

LDH = lactic dehydrogenase; PaO₂ = arterial oxygen saturation; WBC = white blood cell count.
* Pancreatitis classified as severe if patient died, underwent surgery because pancreatitis did not settle, or complications became manifest.

Peritoneal lavage

McMahon et al (1980) have advocated peritoneal lavage as a means of identifying severe disease. Pancreatitis is classified as severe if more than 10 ml of free fluid is recovered, if the free fluid has a dark 'prune juice' colour, and if after instillation of 1 l of saline the return fluid is mid-straw colour or darker ('bitter beer' colour). The overall accuracy of prediction is similar to that achieved by the Glasgow system (Corfield et al, 1985b) but lavage has the virtue of immediate availability of the result. In the UK three-centre study of the *therapeutic* value of peritoneal lavage, the Glasgow system proved superior in the assessment of severity of patients with gallstone disease, while *diagnostic* lavage proved superior in those with alcohol-associated acute pancreatitis (Corfield et al, 1985b).

Detection of pancreatic necrosis

As mentioned above, attention has focused recently on the need to distinguish between oedematous and necrotizing pancreatitis. In an attempt to identify patients with necrotic disease and, therefore, a potential need for early surgery, a number of serum markers have been evaluated. C-reactive protein is a non-specific but sensitive index of tissue injury, inflammation, bacterial infection and ischaemia. Elevation of serum levels above 100 mg/l is said by the Ulm group to detect 95% of cases of pancreatic necrosis, the comparable figures for CT scanning and ultrasonography being 85% and 38%, respectively (Buchler et al, 1986). While agreeing with the value of C-reactive protein as a marker of severe and complicated acute pancreatitis, Wilson et al (1989) argue that many patients with severe disease and high C-reactive protein levels can be managed without surgery. It is important to appreciate that necrosis in itself is not an indicator for operation and the Ulm group lay great emphasis on determining whether the necrosis is infected (see below). Other putative serum markers of severe acute pancreatitis and/or necrosis include raised levels of ribonuclease (Warshaw and Lee, 1979), lactic dehydrogenase (Buchler et al, 1986), alpha-1-antitrypsin (McMahon et al, 1984) and fibrinogen (Berry et al, 1982), and a falling level of alpha-2-macroglobulin (McMahon et al, 1984). Depletion of this last marker reflects its consumption during inactivation of circulating proteases and its sensitivity in detecting pancreatic necrosis is estimated to be 85% (Buchler et al, 1986). While all of these markers are of interest, C-reactive protein probably represents the most useful indicator of the likelihood of necrosis and a means of determining the need for intensive radiological and bacteriological investigation.

MANAGEMENT OF ACUTE PANCREATITIS

In many patients, the acute attack appears to be settling by the time the patient reaches hospital and intensive monitoring, resuscitation and treatment are not required. At the other end of the spectrum, the patient with fulminant necrotizing acute pancreatitis requires intensive care from the outset and considerable judgement is required to determine optimal medical care and decide upon the indications for surgery and its timing.

Initial conservative management

The patient is confined to bed, given nothing further by mouth and an intravenous infusion is established. Appropriate pain relief is prescribed; pethidine is traditionally preferred to morphine although when given in equianalgesic doses both agents cause contraction of the sphincter of Oddi. Baseline monitoring consists of hourly pulse and blood pressure recording and 4-hourly temperature determination. Blood is withdrawn to determine serum amylase concentration, full blood count and haemotocrit, arterial pH and blood gas tensions, and the concentration of serum, urea and electrolytes, calcium, albumin, liver function analyses, blood glucose and C-reactive protein. In patients with signs of severe disease the level of monitoring activity is increased without hesitation to include bladder catheterization and measurement of hourly urine output, central venous pressure and pulmonary arterial wedge pressure. A baseline ECG and chest X-ray are obtained looking for pleural effusion, atelectasis and pulmonary oedema. An abdominal plain film should also be obtained, primarily to exclude other causes of the acute abdomen rather than as a means of supporting the diagnosis of acute pancreatitis.

It is generally accepted that elimination of oral intake reduces stimulation of the pancreas and premature return to feeding does carry some risk of reactivating inflammation (Ranson and Spencer, 1977). The value of nasogastric suction is controversial. Review of clinical trials involving a total of 408 patients reveals no benefit but as Ranson (1989) points out many of the patients had alcohol-associated pancreatitis and appeared to have mild disease, given that only five of them died. While not recommending nasogastric intubation routinely, I advocate its use in patients with severe disease, particularly when associated with duodenal ileus and continued vomiting. On theoretical grounds, inhibition of gastric secretion might be expected to reduce the stimulus to pancreatic secretion. In practice, there is no evidence that histamine H_2 receptor antagonists improve outcome and there is evidence that they actually increase the mortality of acute pancreatitis in experimental models (Evander and Ihse, 1979). Anticholinergics have been used in an attempt to inhibit pancreatic secretion but are of no clinical benefit (Cameron et al, 1979) and are not recommended.

A number of potential pancreatic inhibitors have also been evaluated. The list includes glucagon, calcitonin, somatostatin, acetazolamide and 5-fluorouracil but none are of proven benefit for use in routine clinical practice. The same applies to specific and non-specific anti-inflammatory agents such as soya bean trypsin inhibitor, adrenocorticosteroids and prostaglandins and their synthetase inhibitors.

The role of antibiotics in acute pancreatitis is more debatable. In a collective review of three studies involving almost 200 patients, ampicillin was shown not to be of benefit (Ranson, 1989). However, it appears that most of the patients had mild disease associated predominantly with alcohol and only three patients developed abscess formation and one died. Although not part of universal clinical practice, there is a reasonable case for broad spectrum antibiotic administration in gallstone pancreatitis (in which biliary cultures are frequently positive), and in patients deemed to have severe disease (Ranson, 1989).

There has been interest in the use of fresh frozen plasma as a means of supplementing antiprotease activity (Cuschieri et al, 1983) but the value of this approach has not been confirmed by multicentre trial (Leese et al, 1987). In theory, heparin therapy might be of benefit in preventing intravascular coagulation in the pancreas following trypsin activation. In practice, no improvement has been associated with heparin administration in trials involving small numbers of patients but Ranson (1989) argues that a rising platelet count and serum fibrogen level may justify heparin administration (750–1000 units/h monitored by partial thromboplastin time) to reduce the danger of disseminated intravascular coagulation.

Continued cardiorespiratory monitoring is essential for all patients with severe disease. Many of these patients have a high cardiac output and diminished peripheral resistance perhaps reflecting liberation of vasoactive substances as a consequence of pancreatic inflammation. Intravenous infusion of cystalloid solutions coupled with appropriate use of colloid solutions such as albumin is indicated, although as just outlined, there is some debate about whether fresh frozen plasma is desirable if colloid is needed. In cardiocirculatory failure, dopamine or dobutamine infusion may also be required, while respiratory failure as a part of the adult respiratory distress syndrome may require controlled ventilation with oxygen-enriched air to maintain arterial oxygen tension above 8.0 kPa (60 mmHg). Minimal positive end-expiratory pressure is usually recommended if assisted ventilation is required. Urine output should be maintained above 50 ml/h if possible but an output falling consistently below 30 ml/h despite adequate volume replacement and dopamine infusion, coupled with a rising serum creatinine, indicates the need to consider dialysis. In acute pancreatitis, peritoneal dialysis may be particularly appropriate (see below). It cannot be overemphasized that multiorgan failure in these patients is usually associated with infected necrosis, and that survival may ultimately depend upon surgical eradication of necrotic tissue.

In patients with protracted illness, thought must be given early to the provision of nutritional support. There is no justification for the use of parenteral nutrition in *all* patients with acute pancreatitis, indeed the morbidity associated with central venous catheters may far outweigh any potential benefits (Sax et al, 1987). However, in patients with continuing severe illness parenteral nutrition is advisable. If at any time laparotomy is indicated it is our routine practice to insert a tube jejunostomy so that enteral feeding can be used as a long-term alternative to oral or parenteral feeding. In theory, nasoenteric feeding with a fine bore tube offers an alternative means of long-term nutritional support in patients with protracted duodenal ileus; in practice it has not been used widely in patients with acute pancreatitis.

Therapeutic peritoneal lavage

Lavage of the peritoneal cavity offers an attractive prospect of removing pancreatic enzymes and vasoactive substances before they gain entry to the bloodstream. Its value remains controversial despite a large amount of experimental and clinical study. In an early controlled assessment involving 10 patients with severe disease, Ranson et al (1976) found that lavaged patients had less prolonged hyperamylasaemia and that their time in an intensive care unit was halved in comparison to non-lavaged patients; the only death occurred in a non-lavaged patient. In a larger evaluation, *early* mortality was 10% in non-lavaged patients as opposed to only 4% (2 of 48) in those having lavage (Ranson, 1989). Despite this encouraging effect on early mortality, overall mortality was not significantly affected and lavage alone may fail to prevent the late sequelae of pancreatic and peripancreatic necrosis, notably pancreatic abscess.

Four controlled clinical trials of the use of peritoneal lavage also deserve comment. The trial conducted by Stone and Fabian (1980) is impossible to evaluate in that a large number of patients allocated to the non-lavaged group 'crossed over' to receive lavage. In the authors view 'decided improvement' within 24 h was seen in 85% of lavaged patients and only 36% of the control group. For what it is worth, there were eight deaths in the 51 patients (16%) ultimately having lavage as opposed to six deaths in the 19 (32%) non-lavaged patients. In the UK three-centre controlled study, 91 patients with severe disease were identified from 428 evaluated patients with acute pancreatitis. Twelve of the 45 lavaged patients died as opposed to 13 of the 46 control patients and the incidence of major complications was almost identical in the two groups (Mayer et al, 1985). It is however worth mentioning that there was a suggestion of benefit from the lavage in the subgroup of patients with alcohol-associated disease. In a further controlled study involving 39 Swedish patients, Ihse et al (1986) also failed to discern any significant benefit from lavage. Balldin et al (1983) compared the effects of lavage with or without aprotinin; while no significant differences were seen, the three deaths and three cases of abscess formation were all in the group having lavage without aprotinin.

Thus, the position of peritoneal lavage remains uncertain. In the United Kingdom it has not become popular, perhaps as a result of the negative UK study. This is not to say that it is of no value. As will be discussed, lesser sac lavage is an integral part of the successful Ulm regime for the management of necrotizing pancreatitis and it may be of great value in patients with coexisting renal failure. If lavage is to be used without laparotomy, it is safer to insert the catheter by an open approach under local anaesthesia. The peritoneum is exposed through a vertical 5 cm subumbilical incision so that the catheter can be inserted under direct vision, thus minimizing the risk of visceral injury. Approximately 2 l of isotonic lavage fluid are cycled every hour, bearing in mind that the volume may have to be reduced if ventilation is compromised. Given the dextrose content of the dialysate used in many centres, it is also advisable to monitor blood glucose concentration.

Management of gallstone pancreatitis

Detection of gallstones in the early period following an attack of acute pancreatitis may prove difficult. Ultrasonography is frequently employed but it detects only about two-thirds of gallstone pancreatitis patients at this stage (McKay et al, 1982; Neoptolemos et al, 1984). The problem lies in failure to visualize the gallbladder because of the gaseous distension and the fact that the offending stones are often small and in the lower common bile duct, an area not well visualized by ultrasonography. Repeating the ultrasound examination at a later stage is certainly advisable if the initial scan is equivocal. In 99 patients discharged without definition of a cause for their acute pancreatitis, Goodman et al (1985) found that ultrasonography at 6 weeks had a sensitivity of 87% and specificity of 93% in gallstone detection, a performance superior to that of delayed oral cholecystography. However, such delayed investigation still failed to detect gallstones in 13% of the patients from whom stones were eventually recovered by laparotomy or endoscopic papillotomy.

Serum markers and clinical indices have also been used to detect patients with gallstone-associated disease. For example, Mayer and McMahon (1985) showed that transient elevation of serum aspartate aminotransferase above 60 i.u./l was present in 84% of attacks of pancreatitis due to gallstones but in only 15% of those not due to stones. In our own Glasgow experience, five factors (age > 50 years, female sex, and serum alkaline phosphatase, alanine aminotransferase and amylase concentrations) were strongly associated with gallstone pancreatitis (Blamey et al, 1983). In patients with four or five of these factors gallstones were present in 95–100% of cases whereas in those with one or no positive factors gallstones were present in less than 5% of cases. Neoptolemos et al (1984) found that while biochemical tests alone were able to separate only 47% of those with gallstones from those without, combination of biochemical testing and ultrasonography allowed correct diagnosis of 81% of those with gallstone pancreatitis, without any false positive diagnoses.

Given that a patient is deemed to have acute pancreatitis due to gallstones, debate still surrounds the subsequent management. Prior to the availability of endoscopic papillotomy, surgery represented the only means of eradicating gallstones from the duct system. The traditional policy of deferring surgery for some 6 weeks was challenged by the realization that many patients spent much longer awaiting elective surgery (Osborne et al, 1981) and that many had further attacks of pancreatitis while awaiting readmission (Kelly, 1980). Although some have argued that urgent cholecystectomy should be undertaken as soon as possible after admission with acute pancreatitis (Acosta et al, 1980; Stone et al, 1981) this policy has not been adopted widely, perhaps because of the uncertainty of the diagnosis of gallstones as the cause of pancreatitis in some patients. Furthermore, while proponents of urgent biliary surgery emphasize that it relieves biliary and pancreatic obstruction by removing ductal calculi, the counter argument is that many of these stones would pass spontaneously if surgery is deferred, thus obviating the need for choledochotomy and/or duodenotomy, at the time of cholecystectomy.

Many surgeons now adopt a selective policy for patients thought to have gallstone pancreatitis. If the disease is classified as mild on admission or settles rapidly thereafter, biliary surgery can be undertaken safely as a non-urgent procedure during the same hospital admission (Osborne et al, 1981). Surgery under these circumstances should consist of cholecystectomy and operative cholangiography, duct exploration being undertaken only if duct stones are demonstrated radiologically (Osborne et al, 1983). If the patient has severe acute pancreatitis which fails to settle promptly on conservative management, there is now a strong argument for endoscopic papillotomy as an alternative to urgent biliary surgery under potentially dangerous circumstances. In an important prospective trial, the Leicester group (Neoptolemos et al, 1988) divided patients thought to have gallstone pancreatitis into those with mild disease and those with severe disease according to Glasgow criteria. Patients in each group were then randomized to undergo urgent ERCP (with endoscopic papillotomy if appropriate) or conventional treatment. In the patients with mild disease there were no deaths and no significant differences in morbidity. On the other hand in patients with severe disease, conventional treatment carried a significantly higher complication rate (61% versus 24%) and although the difference was not statistically significant, there were five deaths in 28 conventionally managed patients as opposed to one death in the 25 endoscopically managed patients. Although encouraging these results must still be interpreted cautiously. The Leicester experience is based on skilled endoscopic intervention and we still require reassurance that these results can be extrapolated to other hospitals with widely differing standards of endoscopic and surgical management. If gallstone pancreatitis is managed successfully in the acute situation by endoscopic means, the decision regarding the need for subsequent cholecystectomy must depend on the clinical condition of the patients. In the elderly and infirm there may be a strong case for avoiding unnecessary surgery once the prospect of further ductal obstruction has been obviated by papillotomy.

Management of necrotizing pancreatitis

Acute necrotizing pancreatitis constitutes a difficult and controversial problem. As discussed earlier, C-reactive protein is probably the best marker of its presence but the interpretation of results is debated. Mayer et al (1984) used a level of 75 mg/l to predict severity, Buchler et al (1986) report a 95% accuracy in detecting necrosis when levels exceed 100 mg/l, while Wilson et al (1989) suggest a cut-off point of 210 mg/l as an indication of severe pancreatitis (although not necessarily of necrosis). Ultrasonography is generally unhelpful due to the presence of bowel gas and difficulty in differentiating liquid collections from necrotic parenchyma. CT scanning with intravenous contrast enhancement now appears to be the radiological investigation of choice, given that necrotic tissue fails to enhance (Kivisaari et al, 1984). Beger's group have compared contrast enhanced CT, ultrasonography and Ranson's criteria in 77 patients who came subsequently to resection; CT proved superior and identified 90% of the patients with pancreatic necrosis involving more than 50% of the gland and also identified 79% of those with lesser degrees of necrosis (Block et al, 1986).

Given that necrosis is present, bacterial contamination may then become the deciding factor when considering surgery. Bacterial infection is known to occur early in that a quarter of cases became infected within 7 days, and such infection increases mortality in necrotizing pancreatitis from 9% to 38% (Beger et al, 1986). Thus it can now be proposed that C-reactive protein should be used for monitoring purposes, contrast-enhanced CT scanning should be used to detect and determine the extent of necrosis, and percutaneous fine needle aspiration should be used to detect *infected* necrosis. The decision to abandon conservative management in favour of surgery still remains a clinical decision but it may now be argued that a very pressing reason is required not to recommend surgery in patients with infected necrosis. The decision is made more complex by multiorgan failure but in such patients prompt surgical necrosectomy and effective treatment of infection may represent their only hope of survival.

The nature of the surgery in necrotizing acute pancreatitis is still a matter for debate. Formal pancreatic resection is reported recently as having a mortality rate of 33% (Aldridge, 1989) and 22% (Kivilaakso et al, 1984), although the lower mortality rate was achieved in a relatively young, predominantly male patient population with a high preponderance of alcohol-associated pancreatitis. Other workers have stressed the difficulty of differentiating between viable and non-viable pancreas at laparotomy and the long-term sequelae of extensive pancreatic resection cannot be overemphasized (Nordback and Auvinen, 1985).

Recently, there has been a move away from formal pancreatic resection in favour of deferring surgery until the extent of necrosis is better defined so that one removes only necrotic pancreatic and peripancreatic tissue, the procedure being termed necrosectomy. Hollender et al (1986) in a review of the experience of 12 European centres found an average mortality rate of 42% for subtotal pancreatectomy and of 60% for total pancreatectomy, whereas necrosectomy incurred a mortality rate of 37%. In our own Glasgow experience of 21 patients with acute necrotizing pancreatitis, the mortality rate after necrosectomy was 29% (four of 14 patients) whereas following formal pancreatic resection it was 57% (Wilson et al, 1988b). Bradley and Fulenwider (1984) report a 14% mortality in 21 patients treated by necrosectomy and open packing of the lesser sac. In Ulm, Beger et al (1986) report a mortality rate of only 8% in 61 patients treated by necrosectomy followed by lesser sac lavage for a median duration of 21 days.

The outstanding results obtained by Beger's group must be placed in perspective. In the recent review of 744 patients with acute pancreatitis in Ulm, 130 (17%) were classified as having necrotizing pancreatitis and all but 20 of these 130 patients were managed by operative means (Table 2; Beger, 1989). Thus, about 50% of Ulm patients with acute pancreatitis came to necrosectomy, whereas in our own Glasgow experience only 21 (4.6%) of 456 patients came to surgery for acute necrotizing pancreatitis (Wilson et al, 1988b). While it is my subjective view that we require to be more aggressive in our diagnosis and management of necrotizing pancreatitis in the UK, I suspect that an operation rate of 15% in all patients with acute pancreatitis may err too much in the other direction. This said, the achievements of the Ulm group remain extremely impressive and their operative mortality of 8% in necrosectomy patients has yet to be bettered. Beger (1989) lays great stress on the avoidance of formal partial or total duodenopancreatectomy (and the unnecessary removal of healthy tissue/organs), on the merits of blunt digital necrosectomy, and the importance of reconstituting the lesser sac so that continuous through-and-through lavage can be used to wash debris, infected material and biologically active substances from the region.

Management of pancreatic abscess

Pancreatic abscess is a late complication and frequently becomes manifest some 2–6 weeks after the acute attack of pancreatitis appears to have settled. Intestinal bacteria are usually implicated, notably Gram-negative organisms such as E. coli. Abdominal discomfort and pain are common; the pain is experienced in the epigastrium and/or left hypochondrium and may radiate to the back or to the left shoulder. Anorexia, nausea and vomiting are common. Systemic upset in the form of pyrexia, tachycardia and leucocytosis suggests infection and some patients develop septicaemic shock.

General diagnostic measures include full blood count determination and blood culture while ultrasonography is used as a first line localization test. CT scanning is also helpful in confirming the size and location of the collection(s), detecting any retroperitoneal abscesses, and identifying involvement of neighbouring organs such as the spleen and colon. Broad spectrum antibiotics are included in the general resuscitative measures and operation is the preferred method of treatment with institution of free external drainage. Postoperative lavage of the abscess cavity is becoming increasingly popular and the size of the residual cavity can be monitored by sinography. There is a significant risk of inducing intestinal necrosis and fistula formation if rigid drainage tubes are employed and a posterior approach through the bed of the twelfth rib may be preferred for patients with retroperitoneal abscesses. It should be remembered that abscesses are often multiple and that further loculi should be sought radiologically prior to surgery and excluded by a careful search at the time of laparotomy. Further abscesses may form in the postoperative period and vigilance must not be relaxed in case relaparotomy is needed. There is now general agreement that percutaneous drainage techniques, including catheter insertion, frequently fail to deal effectively with pancreatic abscess and should be avoided if possible. Pancreatic abscess remains a dangerous condition and mortality rates until recently ranged from 30% to 70% (Ranson, 1984); given modern diagnosis and management this figure may now have fallen to 10% in specialist centres (Beger, 1989).

Management of pancreatic pseudocyst

Pseudocysts are fluid collections which are frequently rich in pancreatic secretions that have escaped from a duct disrupted by acute inflammation or obstruction. Acute pancreatic and peripancreatic fluid collections frequently resolve spontaneously and are not in themselves an indication for intervention; patients who are stable clinically should be observed for evidence of toxicity or infection but in their absence intervention may still be required if the collection persists for many weeks or increases in size. Ultrasonography or CT scanning can be used to monitor the size of the collection, and in long-standing collections, preoperative ERCP may be valuable to detect evidence of chronic pancreatitis and duct obstruction. The current debate centres on treatment. Conventional internal surgical drainage usually involves draining the cyst into the back wall of the stomach but cyst-duodenostomy or drainage into a Roux loop of jejunum may be necessary, depending on the location of the collection. The complication and recurrence rates should be less than 5% after such surgery (Warshaw and Rattner, 1985). Needle aspiration of the collection under ultrasonographic control carries a recurrence rate of around 75% whereas it is claimed that percutaneous insertion of a catheter for prolonged drainage succeeds in 70–100% of cases (Warshaw, 1989). Endoscopic techniques allowing catheter drainage into the stomach have also been described (Hancke and Henriksen, 1985; Matzinger et al, 1988).

Despite the availability of non-surgical methods it is still our practice to treat persistent or complicated pseudocysts by surgical means unless advanced age and infirmity pose contraindications. Surgery allows free drainage, reduces the risk of abscess formation, avoids the formation of an external fistula and allows exclusion of the presence of a cystic neoplasm (Warshaw, 1989).

Management of pancreatic ascites and fistula

These are relatively rare complications of acute pancreatitis which follow pancreatic duct disruption. An external fistula may form following necrosectomy or after external drainage of an abscess or pseudocyst, while internal fistulae may be created surgically to follow spontaneous drainage into the gut. Less frequently the pancreatic disruption remains free, leading to the formation of pancreatic ascites or a pleural effusion. Patients who develop such fistulae are frequently debilitated by their attack of acute pancreatitis and by fistula complications such as fluid loss, sepsis and bleeding.

In general, spontaneous closure may be expected in patients with low output external fistulae (> 200 ml/day) provided that they receive fluid and electrolyte replacement, nutritional support and continued skin care. Radiological delineation of the fistula is valuable and the surgeon should have a low threshold for intervention to drain any infected intra-abdominal collection(s). High output fistulas frequently require surgery, and fistulography or ERCP is used to define the pathological anatomy and plan resection when conservative management fails. Resection along a line just downstream of the point of duct rupture is the normal treatment in such cases.

Pancreatic ascites is frequently misdiagnosed at presentation and thought to be a manifestation of liver disease. Determination of amylase and protein concentrations in a sample of peritoneal fluid will reveal the correct diagnosis. Ascites is frequently gross and fluid may track upwards into the mediastinum and rupture into the pleural cavity to form an effusion (pancreatico-pleural fistula) or more rarely, into the bronchial tree (pancreatico-bronchial fistula). Protracted conservative treatment (drainage of ascites or pleural fluid and hyperalimentation) exposes the patient to the risk of sepsis and it is now considered unwise to persist with such treatment for more than 2–3 weeks. ERCP is of value in defining the site of duct rupture in such patients. Following duct disruption in the body and tail, pancreatic resection is usually indicated whereas Roux-en-Y cystjejunostomy or pancreatico-jejunostomy may be successful when the lesion is in the head of the gland. If the patient has a pancreatico-pleural fistula there is no need to follow the track to the chest; disruption of the track in the course of pancreatic surgery will prevent further accumulation.

A number of agents have been used over the years to aid closure of a pancreatic fistula or deal with ascites. The list includes atropine, diamox and radiotherapy but interest centres currently on somatostatin and its analogue SMS 201–995 (Ahren et al, 1988).

Pancreatic ascites and fistula are dangerous conditions and in our own experience of 23 patients, five patients succumbed (Fielding et al, 1989).

CONCLUSIONS AND THE WAY FORWARD

Acute pancreatitis remains a common and dangerous problem. While serum amylase determination remains the standard method of diagnosis it has significant shortcomings and serum lipase estimation may supplant it in future. Assessment of severity remains an important basis for management and it is hoped that trypsinogen activation peptides may realize their potential in this context. In gallstone pancreatitis a judicious combination of endoscopic intervention and early surgery seems likely to lower mortality, but it has yet to be demonstrated that endoscopic papillotomy and stone removal will prove safe and effective when used outside specialized centres of excellence. Necrotizing pancreatitis remains a major challenge; it will be important to determine whether the use of markers of necrosis such as C-reactive protein, contrast enhanced CT scanning and needle aspiration to confine infection can be used by other workers to reproduce the results of necrosectomy and lesser sac lavage achieved by the Ulm group (Beger, 1989). There have been useful advances in our understanding and management of acute pancreatitis in the last decade and these should translate into more widespread improvements in outcome for patients developing this disease in future.

REFERENCES

Acosta JM, Pellegrini CA & Skinner DB (1980) Etiology and pathogenesis of acute biliary pancreatitis. *Surgery* **83**: 367.

Ahren B, Tranberg KG & Bengmark S (1988) Treatment of pancreatic fistula with the somatostatin analogue SMS 201–995. *British Journal of Surgery* **75**: 718.

Aldridge MC (1989) Diagnosis of pancreatic necrosis. *British Journal of Surgery* **75**: 99–100.

Balldin G, Borgstrom A, Genell S & Ohlsson K (1983) The effect of peritoneal lavage and aprotinin in the treatment of severe acute pancreatitis. *Research in Experimental Medicine* **183**: 203–312.

Beger HG (1989) Management of pancreatic necrosis and pancreatic abscess. In Carter DC and Warshaw AL (eds) *Pancreatitis*, pp 107–119. Edinburgh: Churchill Livingstone.

Beger HG, Bittner R, Block S & Buchler M (1986) Bacterial contamination of pancreatic necrosis. A prospective clinical study. *Gastroenterology* **91**: 433–438.

Berry AR, Taylor TV & Davies GC (1982) Diagnostic tests and prognostic indicators in acute pancreatitis. *Journal of the Royal College of Surgeons of Edinburgh* **27**: 345–352.

Blamey SL, Osborne DH, Gilmour WH, O'Neill J, Carter DC & Imrie CW (1983) The early identification of patients with gallstone associated pancreatitis using clinical and biochemical factors only. *Annals of Surgery* **198**: 574.

Blamey SL, Imrie CW, O'Neill J, Gilmour WH & Carter DC (1984) Prognostic factors in acute pancreatitis. *Gut* **25**: 1340–1346.

Block S, Maier W, Bittner R, Buchler M, Malfertheiner P & Beger HG (1986) Identification of pancreas necrosis in severe acute pancreatitis: imaging procedures versus clinical staging. *Gut* **27**: 1035–1042.

Bradley HG & Fulenwider JT (1984) Open treatment of pancreatic abscess. *Surgery, Gynecological and Obstetrics* **159**: 509–513.

Buchler M, Malfertheiner P & Beger HG (1986) Correlation of imaging procedures, biochemical parameters, and clinical stage in acute pancreatitis. In Malfertheiner P & Ditschuneit H (eds) *Diagnostic Procedures in Pancreatic Disease*, pp 123–129. Berlin: Springer.

Burkitt DS (1987) The Rapignost-amylase test in acute pancreatitis. *British Journal of Surgery* **22**: 719–724.

Cameron JL, Mehigan D & Zuidema GD (1979) Evaluation of atropine in acute pancreatitis. *Surgery, Gynecology and Obstetrics* **148**: 206–208.

Clavien PA, Burgan S & Moossa AR (1989) Serum enzymes and other laboratory tests in acute pancreatitis. *British Journal of Surgery* **76**: 1234–1243.

Corfield AP, Cooper MJ & Williamson RCN (1985a) Acute pancreatitis: a lethal disease of increasing incidence. *Gut* **26**: 724–729.

Corfield AP, Cooper MJ & Williamson RCN (1985b) Prediction of severity in acute pancreatitis: a prospective comparison of three prognostic indices. *Lancet* **ii**: 403–406.

Cuschieri A, Wood RAB, Cumming JRG, Meehan SE & Mackie CR (1983) The treatment of acute pancreatitis with fresh frozen plasma. *British Journal of Surgery* **70**: 710–712.

Dickson AP & Imrie CW (1984) The incidence and prognosis of the body wall ecchymosis in acute pancreatitis. *Surgery, Gynecology and Obstetrics* **159**: 343–347.

Evander A & Ihse I (1979) Influence of cimetidine on acute experimental pancreatitis. *Danish Medical Bulletin* **26**: 13.

Fielding GA, McLatchie GR, Wilson C, Imrie CW & Carter DC (1989) Acute pancreatitis and pancreatic fistula formation. *British Journal of Surgery* **76**: 1126–1128.

Garden OJ, Dominiczak MH, Shenkin A & Carter DC (1985) The diagnosis of acute pancreatitis in the presence of hyperlipaemia. *Scottish Medical Journal* **30**: 235–236.

Goodman AJ, Neoptolemos JP, Carr-Locke DL, Finlay DBL & Fossard DP (1985) Detection of gallstones after acute pancreatitis. *Gut* **26**: 125.

Gudgeon AM, Heath DI, Hurley P. et al (1990) Trypsinogen activation peptides assay in the early prediction of severity of acute pancreatitis. *Lancet* **i**: 4–8.

Hancke S & Henriksen FW (1985) Percutaneous pancreatic cytogastrostomy guided by ultrasound scanning and gastroscopy. *British Journal of Surgery* **72**: 916–917.

Hollender LF, Meyer C & Keller D (1986) Planned operations for necrotizing pancreatitis: the continental experience. In Howard JM, Jordon GI & Reber HA (eds) *Surgical Diseases of the Pancreas*, pp 450–460. Philadelphia: Lea and Febiger.

Ihse I, Evander A, Gustafson I & Holmberg JT (1986) Influence of peritoneal lavage on objective prognostic signs in acute pancreatitis: the effect of hyoalbuminaemia. *Current Medical Research Opinion* **4**: 101–116.

Imrie CW, Benjamin IS & Ferguson JC (1978) A single centre double-blind trial of Trasylol therapy in primary acute pancreatitis. *British Journal of Surgery* **65**: 337–341.

Kelly TR (1980) Gallstone pancreatitis: the timing of surgery. *Surgery* **88**: 345–350.

Kivilaakso E, Lempinen M, Makelainen A, Nikki P & Schroder T (1984) Pancreatic resection versus peritoneal lavage for acute fulminant pancreatitis. *British Journal of Surgery* **199**: 426–431.

Kivisaari L, Somer K, Stranderskjold-Nordenstam CG, Schroder T, Kivilaakson E & Lempinen M (1984) A new method for the diagnosis of acute hemorrhage-necrotizing pancreatitis using contrast-enhanced CT. *Gastrointestinal Radiology* **9**: 27–30.

Knaus WA, Draper EA, Wagner DP & Zimmerman JE (1985) APACHE II: A severity of disease classification system. *Critical Care Medicine* **13**: 818–829.

Leese T, Holliday M, Heath D, Hall AW & Bell PRF (1987) Multicentre clinical trial of low volume fresh frozen plasma therapy in acute pancreatitis. *British Journal of Surgery* **74**: 906–911.

McKay AJ, Imrie CW, O'Neill J & Duncan JG (1982) Is an early ultrasound scan of value in acute pancreatitis? *British Journal of Surgery* **69**: 369–371.

McMahon JM, Playforth JM & Pickford IR (1980) A comparative study of methods for the prediction of severity of attacks of acute pancreatitis. *British Journal of Surgery* 67: 22–25.

McMahon JM, Bowen M, Mayer AD & Cooper EH (1984) Relationship of alpha-macroglobulin and other antiproteases to the clinical features of acute pancreatitis. *American Journal of Surgery* 147: 164–70.

Matzinger FRK, Ho CS & Yee AC (1988) Pancreatic pseudocysts drained through a percuntaneous transgastric approach: further experience. *Radiology* 167: 431–434.

Mayer AD & McMahon MJ (1985) Biochemical identification of patients with gallstones associated with acute pancreatitis: aims, indications and timing. *Annals of the Royal College of Surgeons of Edinburgh* 201: 68.

Mayer AD, McMahon MJ, Bowen M & Cooper EH (1984) C-reactive protein: an aid to assessment and monitoring in acute pancreatitis. *Journal of Clinical Pathology* 37: 207–211.

Mayer AD, McMahon MD & Corfield AP (1985) A randomised trial of peritoneal lavage for the treatment of severe acute pancreatitis. *New England Journal of Medicine* 312: 399–404.

Moller-Petersen JK, Klaerbe M, Dali T & Toth T (1986) Immunochemical qualitative latex agglutination test for pancreatic lipase. *Clinical Chemistry* 31: 1207–1210.

Moossa AR (1984) Diagnostic tests and procedures in acute pancreatitis. *New England Journal of Medicine* 311: 639–643.

Neoptolemos JP, Hall AW, Finlay DBL, Berry JM, Carr-Locke DL & Fossard DP (1984) The urgent diagnosis of gallstones in acute pancreatitis: a prospective study of three methods. *British Journal of Surgery* 71: 230.

Neoptolemos JP, Carr-Locke DL, London NJ, Bailey IA, James D & Fossard DP (1988) Controlled trials or urgent endoscopic retrograde cholangiopancreatography and endoscopic sphincterotomy versus conservative treatment for acute pancreatitis due to gallstones. *Lancet* 10: 980–983.

Nordback IH & Auvinen OA (1985) Long-term results after pancreas resection for acute necrotizing pancreatitis. *British Journal of Surgery* 72: 687–689.

Osborne DH, Imrie CW & Carter DC (1981) Biliary surgery in the same admission for gallstone-associated acute pancreatitis. *British Journal of Surgery* 68, 758–761.

Osborne DH, Harris NWS, Gilmour H & Carter DC (1983) Operative cholangiography in gallstone associated acute pancreatitis. *Journal of Royal College of Surgeons of Edinburgh* 28: 96.

Ranson JHC (1979) The timing of biliary surgery in acute pancreatitis. *Annals of Surgery* 189: 654–663.

Ranson JHC (1984) Acute pancreatitis: Pathogenesis, outcome and treatment. In *Clinics in Gastroenterology*, pp 804–843. Philadelphia: Saunders.

Ranson HC (1989) Medical management of acute pancreatitis. In Carter DC & Warshaw AL (eds) *Pancreatitis*, pp 44–57. Edinburgh: Churchill Livingstone.

Ranson HC & Pasternack BS (1977) Statistical methods for quantifying the severity of clinical acute pancreatitis. *Journal of Surgical Research* 22: 77–79.

Ranson HC & Spencer FC (1977) Prevention, diagnosis and treatment of pancreatic abscess. *Surgery* 82: 99–106.

Ranson JHC, Rifkind KM, Moses DF, Flink SD, Eng K & Spencer FC (1974) Prognostic signs and the role of the operative management in acute pancreatitis. *Surgery, Gynecology and Obstetrics* 139: 69–81.

Ranson JHC, Rifkind KM & Turner JW (1976) Prognostic signs and non-operative peritoneal lavage in acute pancreatitis. *Surgery, Gynecology and Obstetrics* 142: 209–219.

Sax HC, Warner BW & Talamini MA (1987) Early total parenteral nutrition in acute pancreatitis: lack of beneficial effects. *American Journal of Surgery* 153: 117–124.

Schein H (1988) Acute surgical disease and scoring systems in daily surgical practice. *British Journal of Surgery* 75: 731–732.

Stone HH & Fabian TC (1980) Peritoneal dialysis in the treatment of acute alcoholic pancreatitis. *Surgery, Gynecology and Obstetrics* 150: 878–882.

Stone HH, Fabian WH & Dunlop WE (1981) Gallstone pancreatitis. Biliary tract pathology in relation to time of operation. *Annals of Surgery* **194**: 305–312.

Thompson HJ, Obekpa PO, Smith AN & Brydon WG (1987) Diagnosis of acute pancreatitis: a proposed sequence of biochemical investigations. *Scandinavian Journal of Gastroenterology* **22**, 719–724.

Warshaw AL (1989) Pancreatic cysts and pseudocysts: new rules for a new game. *British Journal of Surgery* **76**: 533–534.

Warshaw AL & Lee KH (1979) Serum ribonuclease evaluations and pancreatic necrosis in acute pancreatitis. *Surgery* **86**, 227–234.

Warshaw AL & Rattner DW (1985) Timing of surgical drainage for pancreatic pseudocyst. Clinical and chemical criteria. *Annals of Surgery* **202**, 720–724.

Weaver DW, Bouwman DL, Walt AJ, Clink D, Resto A & Stephany J (1982) A correlation between clinical pancreatitis and isoenzyme patterns of amylase. *Surgery* **92**: 576–580.

Wilson C, Imrie CW & Carter DC (1988a) Fatal acute pancreatitis *Gut* **29**: 782–788.

Wilson C, McArdle CS, Carter DC & Imrie CW (1988b) Surgical treatment of acute necrotizing pancreatitis. *British Journal of Surgery* **75**: 1119–1123.

Wilson C, Heads A, Shenkin A & Imrie CW (1989) C-reactive protein, antiproteases and complement factors as objective markers of severity in acute pancreatitis. *British Journal of Surgery* **76**: 177–181.

8

ACUTE INTESTINAL ISCHAEMIA

Adrian Marston

INTRODUCTION

The main route of blood supply to the intestine is the superior mesenteric artery (SMA), occlusion of which is rapidly fatal. However, because there is an abundant collateral blood supply via the coeliac axis above, and the inferior mesenteric artery below, vascular accidents occur less frequently in the intestine than in the heart, brain, kidney or limbs. None the less the incidence is on the increase and in a community of 250 000 one would expect one case of acute gut ischaemia each month (Wilson et al, 1987) so that this is one of the commoner vascular emergencies encountered by a general surgeon. It is frustrating to recognize that progress in this area has been so slow that mortality has remained at 70–100% since 1930 (Clavien et al, 1987; Wilson et al, 1987). It was observed over 50 years ago (Hibbard et al, 1933) that 'The difficulty in arriving at an early diagnosis undoubtedly accounts for the high mortality. The delay in diagnosis is often unavoidable due to the lack of definite symptoms, even though the damage to the intestinal tract is severe.' It is often said that an aggressive diagnostic and therapeutic approach offers the only hope of reducing the morbidity and death rate of the condition, but this is not easily achieved because in the early stages the clinical features are vague and non-specific, and routine laboratory data and radiographs are unhelpful.

CAUSATION

It is customary to consider the aetiology of acute intestinal ischaemia in terms of the following:

(1) Mesenteric arterial embolus: (a) from the left heart (arrhythmia or recent endocardial infarct) (Baue and Austen, 1963; Kairolvoma et al, 1977); (b) from the great vessels (detachment of an atheromatous plaque) (Kairolvoma et al, 1977); (c) paradoxical embolus (rare).

(2) Mesenteric arterial thrombosis: (a) from atheroma; (b) due to clotting disorder (Wilson et al, 1987); (c) traumatic or iatrogenic (Lucas et al, 1981).

(3) Mesenteric venous thrombosis: (a) due to clotting disorder (e.g. antithrombin III deficiency) (Umpleby, 1987); (b) secondary to a tumour; (c) complicating portal hypertension schistosomiasis or splenectomy (Anayi and Al Nasiri, 1987; Umpleby, 1987); (d) resulting from peritoneal infection; (e) associated with pregnancy or oral contraceptives (Cavin et al, 1982).

(4) Non-occlusive infarction: (a) complicating cardiac failure (Polansky et al, 1964); (b) associated with diuretics or digitalis toxicity (Bynum and Hanley, 1982); (c) as part of an Arthus or Schwartzmann phenomenon; (d) secondary to vasoconstrictive bacterial toxins (e.g. clostridial exotoxin) (Murrel et al, 1966; Lauon and Price, 1987); (e) manifestation of inflammatory arteritis or Burgers disease (Deitch and Sikkema, 1981); (f) from unexplained causes.

However, this classification is oversimplified. Mesenteric embolus is nowadays uncommon, and few infarctions are due to this cause. Acute thrombosis certainly occurs, although in one-third of patients perishing from gut necrosis there is no vascular occlusion to be seen at autopsy (Ottinger and Austen, 1967). Moreover, stenoses, plaques, and even complete occlusions of the mesenteric vessels can be found post-mortem in individuals who have had no alimentary symptoms during life (Croft et al, 1981) so that the relationship between the vascular and the intestinal lesions is uncertain. There is circumstantial evidence, however (Marston, 1962), that partial obstruction of the visceral arteries may lead to an infarction if for some reason the pressure across the lesion is reduced.

Recent evidence suggests that reduction in blood flow to the mucosa of the gastrointestinal tract occurs in a wide variety of clinical situations, including major vascular surgery (Bergquist et al, 1986), sepsis (Dahn et al, 1987) and cardiogenic and haemorrhagic shock (Fiddian-Green and Grantz, 1984; Rutherford et al, 1976). In the absence of mechanical arterial occlusion, the underlying mechanism is almost certainly vasoconstriction in the arterioles in response to circulating or locally released pressor amines, or to release of vasopressin, which has a greater effect on splanchnic than on systemic vessels (Bailey et al, 1986). In a young and healthy individual with a resilient splanchnic circulation these may not prove crucial, but in a patient whose vessels are less adaptable and in whom other organ systems may be impaired, a vicious circle may be initiated, leading to a catastrophic series of life-threatening events (Figure 1).

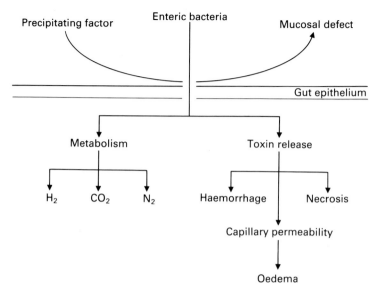

FIGURE I   The metabolic consequences of acute intestinal ischaemia.

ACUTE ISCHAEMIA OF THE SMALL INTESTINE

Clinical features

Acute intestinal ischaemia, however caused, presents with abdominal pain which is usually periumbilical, but is sometimes felt in the right upper quadrant or right iliac fossa. An early event is intense peristaltic activity and gut emptying. Vomiting and loose stools frequently follow. Bloody diarrhoea is usually not evident until several hours later in the course of the disease, when mucosal infarction has begun. The majority of patients with mesenteric emboli are in the sixth or seventh decades and give a history of cardiac arrhythmia or recent myocardial infarction. A history of previous embolism to the brain, extremities or viscera can be elicited in 25–40% of these patients (Bergan and Yao, 1981).

Physical findings are few in the early stages. Pain out of proportion to the objective signs is an important clue to the presence of ischaemia.

Peritoneal irritation signals the onset of full-thickness bowel necrosis, and carries a grave prognosis.

Early in the course of the disease vital signs, including temperature, are normal. With progressive ischaemia, the circulating volume contracts as fluid is lost into the intestinal lumen, the bowel wall and the peritoneal cavity, leading to signs of hypovolaemia. The temperature, if elevated, is usually below $38°C$. Laboratory findings in acute ischaemia are initially unremarkable, with the exception of leucocytosis. Leucocyte counts in excess of 20 000 are common. Raised serum levels of tissue enzymes such as amylase, alkaline phosphatase, lactic dehydrogenase and creatine phosphokinase occur frequently, but are non-specific and unhelpful (Wilson et al, 1987). Metabolic acidosis is a later finding and suggests bowel necrosis (Jamieson et al, 1982). Early reports indicating that hyperphosphataemia (Jamieson et al, 1982) might be a useful pointer to infarction have not been confirmed.

Thus, the overriding impression in the early stages is of a patient who appears sicker and in more pain than would be suggested by the physical examination. This deceptively mild clinical picture lasts from a few hours to 1 or 2 days. As necrosis proceeds outward to the serosa there is a peritonitic reaction and the clinical state becomes that of a desperate illness with distension, ileus, exquisite tenderness and a characteristic odour on the breath. Pain and distension interfere with respiratory movements, resulting in anxiety, restlessness, air hunger and cyanosis. Urine output falls off as dehydration proceeds, and lowered tissue perfusion and metabolic acidosis contribute to the shock-like picture. Eventually the patient succumbs to multiorgan and multisystem failure.

Radiographic changes

The plain radiograph in the earliest stages is normal, or may show an empty bowel. Later, a non-specific picture of distended small gut loops develops, difficult to distinguish from the changes found in peritonitis or early mechanical obstruction. Thickening of the bowel wall (Frimann-Dahl, 1960) has been reported, but again is not a constant or reliable feature.

The presence of gas bubbles in the mesenteric or portal veins (see Figure 2) was previously regarded as a terminal finding (Stewart, 1963). However, there have

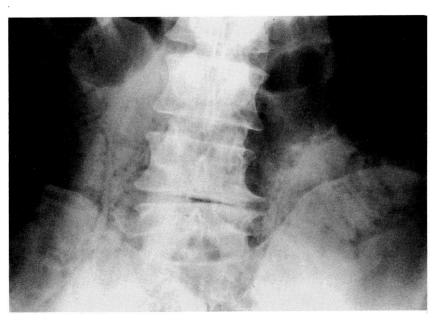

FIGURE 2 Gas bubbles in the portal circulation.

been reports of patients surviving revascularization who had gas in the portal vein preoperatively (Kranendonk et al, 1983).

If intestinal ischaemia is suspected, the surgeon must decide whether to perform an immediate exploratory laparotomy or to carry out a preliminary arteriogram. Obvious peritonitis points clearly to an immediate operation. However, arteriography may be a useful diagnostic step in those patients who have equivocal signs and are haemodynically stable. A retrograde study via the femoral artery can be performed safely in most patients, provided that they are not allergic to the contrast medium, are well hydrated and have adequate renal function (Koehler and Kressel, 1978). Films must be exposed in anteroposterior and lateral projections, to demonstrate all three visceral arteries. If there is clear evidence of an embolus (see Figure 3) the surgeon can embark confidently on a laparotomy with a view to embolectomy and revascularization of the gut.

However the position is not so simple, and many surgeons would oppose the routine use of aortography on the following grounds.

(1) It delays definitive treatment of the lesion.

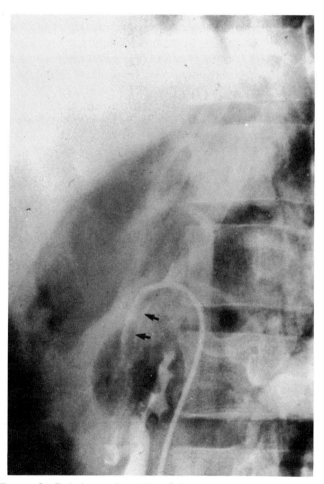

FIGURE 3 Embolus at the origin of the superior mesenteric artery.

(2) A normal arteriogram does not exclude ischaemia, because as many as one-third of cases are 'non-occlusive' in nature (Ottinger and Austen, 1967).

(3) Conversely, the radiographic finding of an occluded or stenosed SMA does not necessarily imply that this is the cause of the patient's pain. Such lesions are quite frequent, and are often asymptomatic and of no haemodynamic significance (Croft et al, 1981).

Management

Resuscitation and support

Threatened death of the intestine involves loss of body fluids, the effects of bacterial invasion, and the absorption of toxic factors into the portal (and, later, systemic) circulations. Therapy is, therefore, directed against all these processes.

The loss is initially of water, electrolytes and protein. This results in a rise in haematocrit with a fall in circulating volume, leading to impaired flow both in the gut wall itself and in the rest of the body. Replacement is planned by serial measurements of the haematocrit, central venous or wedged pulmonary arterial pressure, and urine output. Depending on the patient's known cardiac status and reserve, liberal quantities of balanced saline, colloid or protein solutions are given, until the haematocrit falls to below 45 and the central venous pressure rises to 5–10 cm saline.

Bacterial invasion and toxaemia clearly demand the use of antibiotics. Whilst animal studies have shown that pretreatment with such agents mitigates the effects of intestinal ischaemia, in the clinical context it is difficult to ensure that the antibiotic in fact reaches the site of the damage. Blood is taken for culture (it is almost always sterile), and the chosen drug is then given intravenously. This will usually be an aminoglycoside, such as gentamicin, together with metronidazole to combat anaerobic organisms. The dose given will depend on the weight of the patient, the urine output, and the serum level of the drug. There is recent evidence that polymyxin B may have a specific protective effect against mucosal ischaemia and endotoxaemia (Ingoldby, 1980).

Heparin is given in order to prevent extension of thrombus in the mesenteric vessels and gut wall and, perhaps more importantly, to counteract disseminated intravascular coagulation. Full heparinization is achieved by the immediate intravenous injection of 20 000 IU supplemented by 90 000–60 000 IU in 24 h by continuous infusion. This therapy may need to be interrupted during surgery.

Metabolic acidosis is brought about by the combination of low tissue perfusion, haemoconcentration, and absorption of the products of tissue necrosis. To this is added a respiratory component due to interference with respiratory movement and increased blood viscosity, with intrapulmonary sludging. Measurements of pCO_2 and arterial pH will guide the amount of intravenous saline and bicarbonate therapy required. Given reasonably normal pulmonary and renal function, however, restoration of the circulating blood volume will do much to restore correct acid–base equilibrium.

Laboratory evidence suggests that the use of α-blocking agents (phenoxybenzamine), β-stimulators (isoprenaline), and inotropic agents (dopamine and glucagon) increases flow in the mesenteric circuit and helps to preserve viability. There is little clinical information, and it is doubtful if, in the presence of a mesenteric vascular occlusion or massive shutdown of the minute vessels, any such drug can penetrate to the gut wall. Additionally, the fall in arterial pressure that these agents (particularly phenoxybenzamine) bring about may steal blood from the splanchnic circuit, and prove difficult to control. By contrast, the use of vasoconstrictor agents, such as metaraminol or noradrenaline, is obviously contraindicated.

The intestinal mucosa is uniquely rich in the enzyme xanthine dehydrogenase, and the noxious role of oxygen-derived free radicals such as superoxide (O_2^-) and reactive oxygen metabolites such as peroxide (H_2O_2) and hydroxyl ($\cdot OH$) which are generated in hypoxic states when this enzyme converts to xanthine oxidase (Granger et al, 1981; Parks and Granger, 1983) has been intensively studied. This particularly applies to the phase of reperfusion, when mucosal injury is exacerbated. Experimentally, it is known that ischaemic damage can be mitigated by the use of superoxide dismutase (SOD) (Dalsing et al, 1983) which 'scavenges' O_2, by catalase, which reduces H_2O_2 (Turner et al, 1984) and by dimethyl sulfoxide (DMSO) which scavenges $\cdot OH$ (Marston, 1986). It would seem logical to apply such therapy clinically, but so far there are no reports of this. Another possibly useful agent in the preservation of threatened intestine is allopurinol, which blocks xanthine oxidase and scavenges $\cdot OH$ (Moorehouse et al, 1987).

The use of massive doses of corticosteroids, popular in the 1970s, would not now find general acceptance.

Digitalis and other cardiac glycosides constrict the mesenteric vessels and hence are a possible cause of intestinal necrosis (Polansky et al, 1964; Bynum and Hanley, 1982). Their cautious use may none the less be justified in the control of fast atrial fibrillation, as in this circumstance the effect will be to raise cardiac output and increase intestinal blood flow.

The place of interventional radiology

Some authors have advocated an 'aggressive' management, using preoperative arteriography and selective injections into the SMA of vasodilators, such as papaverine (Boley et al, 1981), phenoxybenzamine (Athanasoulis et al, 1975), or prostaglandin E1 (Clark and Gallant, 1984). These agents have been claimed to be of value in overcoming vasospasm in non-occlusive infarction, but of course this assertion is difficult to sustain in patients who recover without operative proof of the diagnosis, and vasospasm (Banks et al, 1985; Bulkley et al, 1987) is a more complex matter than an angiographic appearance. There is evidence, furthermore, that such therapy may be harmful by selective stealing of blood from less well-perfused areas of the gut (Chou and Kvietys, 1981).

If clot can be demonstrated within the mesenteric system, lysis may be possible with streptokinase (Flickinger et al, 1983). A catheter is placed in the SMA immediately proximal to the occlusion and streptokinase infused. The arteriogram is repeated in 1–3 h and if there is no resolution, the concentration is increased. Should the patient's abdominal condition deteriorate, the procedure is terminated and a laparotomy performed. The few preliminary reports have been encouraging, but streptokinase therapy has many associated problems, including anaphylaxis, febrile reactions and bleeding. Possibly the newer agents such as urokinase, recombinant tissue plasminogen activator (rTPA) (Robin et al, 1988) or anisoylated plasminogen streptokinase activator complex (APSAC) will prove to have an application here. Clinical reports are awaited.

Operative management

Once the diagnosis has been established and the metabolic defects corrected or brought under control, the decision regarding surgery is made. Bearing in mind that complete infarction of the midgut is always lethal, exploration should be carried out if there is the remotest hope of success.

Under light anaesthesia with two intravenous lines in place, tracheal intubation and muscular relaxation, the abdomen is opened through a long midline or paramedian incision, and the diagnosis confirmed. The situation is usually immediately obvious, because of the characteristic 'musty' smell of ischaemic bowel.

In early cases the small intestine may appear healthy. On close inspection there is loss of the normal glistening appearance of the serosa, and palpation of the mesenteric vascular arcades reveals absent pulsation. With advanced ischaemia, the bowel appears oedematous and blue, and eventually green or black. Frank perforation is unusual.

The distribution of ischaemia is a useful indicator of the site of arterial obstruction. Thrombosis of the SMA occurs at the origin and produces ischaemia throughout the midgut from the ligament of Treitz to the splenic flexure of the colon. Emboli usually lodge at, or distal to, the origin of the middle colic artery, thereby sparing the proximal jejunum. Small emboli migrate peripherally to produce segmental damage.

Once the peritoneal cavity is entered the extent of damage to the bowel is usually quite obvious and a choice must be made between the following options.

(1) To close the abdomen with no further action. This used to be common practice, but now is only adopted if the entire alimentary tract is dead in a patient already very sick from other causes.

(2) To revascularize the gut. The decision to attack the arterial lesion will depend on the state of the bowel, the fitness of the patient and the experience of the operator. Reperfused ischaemic bowel imposes a very heavy physiological load on the patient, and the origin of the SMA is an unfamiliar and difficult area for most surgeons.

(3) To resect the damaged bowel and exteriorize the end. For the less experienced surgeon, this may well be the wisest choice. The availability of simple techniques of parenteral nutrition has transformed the management of these patients.

Revascularizing the bowel The proximal SMA is exposed by retracting the transverse colon upwards and drawing down the small bowel mesentery (Figure 4). The ligament of Treitz is incised and the fourth part of the duodenum and upper jejunum thoroughly mobilized. If an embolus is present, palpation along the root of the mesentery in front of the duodenum and below the pancreas will reveal a pulse proximal to the embolus, and the distal vessels are soft and normal. Proximal and distal control of the SMA is obtained by encircling the artery with

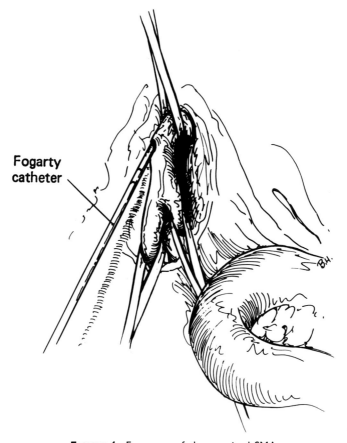

Fogarty catheter

FIGURE 4   Exposure of the proximal SMA.

silicone rubber loops. Following systemic heparinization, the artery is occluded and opened transversely. Catheter embolectomy is performed, taking care to avoid overinflating the balloon, which can result in arterial rupture or intimal injury (Figure 5). After proximal and distal embolectomy is completed, the arterial bed is flushed with 30–40 ml of heparinized saline and the arteriotomy closed with a fine vascular suture.

Once adequate arterial flow has been established and if possible documented by completion arteriography, the bowel must be carefully inspected in order to determine the need for resection. A 20–30 min period of observation will often reveal adequate perfusion of segments initially thought to be non-viable.

Intra-operative assessment of intestinal viability remains an unsolved clinical problem. Most surgeons still rely on clinical judgement on deciding whether to resect non-viable bowel. The criteria usually employed for viability are the return of colour and pulsation and the resumption of peristalsis in the injured segment. Several techniques designed to determine the presence of adequate perfusion of gut wall including electromyography (Schamaun, 1967), pH recordings (Katz et al, 1974) and fluorescein injections (Carter et al, 1984) have been tried, advocated and abandoned. Probably the most useful current adjunct to clinical judgement is the use of the Doppler laser ultrasonic probe (Cooperman et al, 1979; Shah and

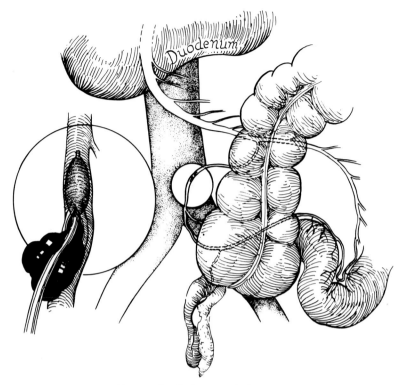

FIGURE 5 Catheter embolectomy.

Anderson, 1981). Non-viable segments must of course be resected, but primary anastomosis is not advised; it is much safer to bring out the ends. Extensive and multiple areas of non-viability are an indication for enterectomy (see below).

To correct a thrombosis of the SMA a reconstructive procedure is required. The mesenteric vessels are approached by exposing the aorta at the level of the renal arteries. Extensive thromboendarterectomy of the mid-aortic region, including the origins of the visceral vessels, has been advocated (Brittain and Early, 1963). However, bypass grafting from the infrarenal aorta to the mesenteric vessels just distal to their origin is easier to carry out and more reliable (Bergan and Yao, 1981) (see Figure 6). In the presence of advanced ischaemia autologous saphenous vein is the preferred graft material. Careful alignment of the graft from the aorta to the superior mesenteric or coeliac arteries is required to prevent kinking. Before completing the bypass, a balloon catheter is passed to ensure patency of the distal arterial tree.

Such a direct attack on the origin of the SMA for emergency revascularization of the gut involves a dissection which is difficult and prolonged, especially in an obese patient. Access is hampered by the portal vein, the neck of the pancreas with its many small veins, and the thick lymphatic tissues in the root of the mesentery. However, success can occasionally be achieved by this means, and in a thin patient it may be worth attempting.

An alternative approach is illustrated in Figure 7, which utilizes the ileocolic artery. The common iliac arteries are cleared and controlled with snares and atraumatic clamps, in order to prevent dislodgement of thrombus into the legs.

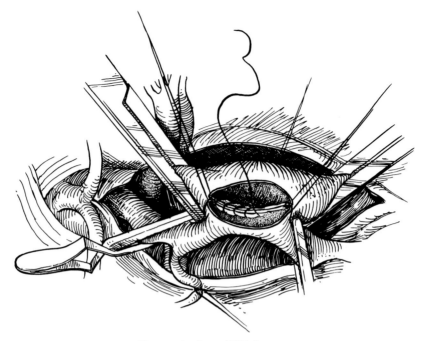

FIGURE 6 Aorta/SMA bypass.

The ileocolic artery is then dissected proximally until a reasonable diameter (3–4 mm) has been attained, and is controlled with tapes. The vessel is easily found in the caecal mesentery, and is usually of adequate calibre. A 1 cm arteriotomy is made in this vessel, and a size 4F embolectomy catheter is gently worked into the aorta, and repeatedly drawn back, so as to retrieve as much occlusive material as possible. As the occlusion is extracted the ileocolic artery progressively dilates. When all possible thrombus has been withdrawn, the mesentery is milked back to clear the distal vessels, the SMA is flushed from the aorta and the catheter passed again. The iliac arteries are checked, and if any debris is felt to have accumulated within them this is removed through short longitudinal incision.

If at this point the SMA picks up pulsation and the bowel becomes pink and is obviously revascularized, the incision in the ileocolic artery is closed, or (if the pattern of collateral appears to make this safe) the vessel is simply ligated. If, however, doubt remains as to restoration of blood supply and it is felt that the origin occlusion has not been completely relieved, the bowel must be revascularized in another way. It is quite a simple matter to make a short (1.5 cm) arteriotomy in the common iliac artery and to carry out a side-to-side anastomosis between this vessel and the already opened ileocolic, using two running sutures of 4/0 or 5/0 material. When clamps are finally removed, the bowel is revascularized in a retrograde fashion, the blood passing up the ileocolic artery into the SMA and hence to the arcades.

Following revascularization of the gut, any obviously non-viable area is resected, and the ends brought out at a suitable point on the abdominal wall, avoiding tension. Any subsequent ischaemia is then immediately apparent, and can be dealt with appropriately.

The patient is returned to the intensive care unit with central intravenous lines, tracheal intubation, urethral catheter, gastrostomy and appropriate drains in place. Fluid replacement, antibiotics and inotropic agents are continued.

Previously (Shaw and Rutledge, 1957) it was advocated that, regardless of the clinical state, any patient who had undergone a revascularization of the gut should be returned to the operating room the following day, because it is difficult to assess success at the first operation. Since surgeons have learned to avoid primary anastomoses, such revisions are seldom required.

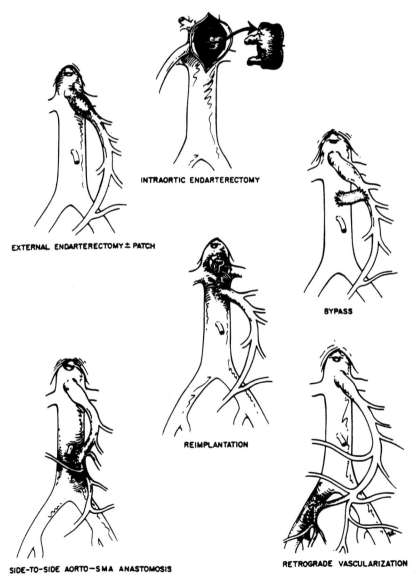

FIGURE 7 Techniques for reconstruction of the intestinal circulation.

Resection of bowel Despite all that has been said above, the fact remains that the most frequent situation which the emergency surgeon encounters is not that of recoverable ischaemia, but of a major infarction of the mid-gut loop (Figure 8). The patient's abdomen will have been opened on a diagnosis of unexplained peritonitis, and the infarction then discovered. Not so very long ago many surgeons would have accepted this as a death sentence, but the advent of effective parenteral nutrition has revolutionized our approach to the management of massive ischaemia. Clearly, a visceral infarction in an elderly individual with multiple system disease is not often a remediable event, but, given that the patient is in other ways recoverable, then it is worthwhile to resect large lengths of dead bowel (thus eliminating the source of the metabolic problem) and to exteriorize the ends in a convenient position. It is nowadays quite simple to replace the massive losses which occur from the high level fistula thus created. Loss of large lengths of bowel leads to gastric hypersecretion, and parenteral H_2 blockers are routinely given. Following 2–3 weeks parenteral feeding, intestinal continuity can be restored in a reasonably healthy individual. The capacity of the small bowel mucosa to regenerate was quite unappreciated before the advent of parenteral support, because at that time all such patients died. For the surgeon inexperienced in reconstruction of the visceral arteries (and surely this must be the majority) it is far safer to resect the gut rather than to attempt to revascularize it. Many of these patients will eventually maintain themselves on oral feeding, though an unlucky few will require lifelong parenteral nutrition. The detailed management of the 'short bowel syndrome' lies outside the scope of this chapter.

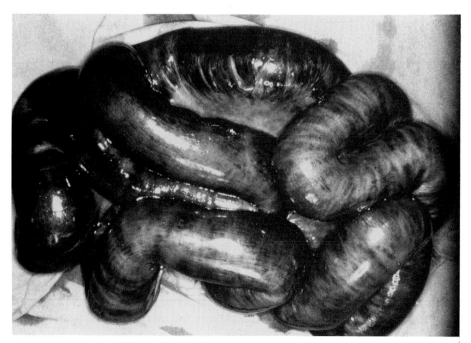

FIGURE 8   Total infarction of the midgut loop.

MESENTERIC VENOUS THROMBOSIS

Mesenteric venous thrombosis accounts for less than 10% of cases of intestinal ischaemia. The main causes are described on page 143 and include portal vein thrombosis (Anayi and Al Nasiri, 1987; Umpleby, 1987), distal thrombosis due to oral contraceptives (Cavin et al, 1982), hypercoagulable states (Horsbrugh, 1976; Khodadadi et al, 1980) and neoplasia. Trauma is another important cause, which will be clear from the history and may arise from stab or gunshot wounds, or surgical mishap. Many cases, however, do no fit into these categories and are unexplained (Berry and Bougas, 1950).

Clinical presentation

Mesenteric venous thrombosis tends to be insidious in onset. The duration of symptoms prior to presentation or diagnosis is much longer with venous than with arterial occlusion. Vague abdominal pains, distension, change in bowel habit (usually diarrhoea and often with blood), nausea and mild fever are common. Abdominal tenderness, hyperactive bowel sounds and leucocytosis are often present. The features of an acute abdomen appear late. The most common acute presentation is that of cramping epigastric or periumbilical pain with nausea, vomiting and diarrhoea. Physical examination usually reveals generalized tenderness and distension. Evidence of hypovolaemia may also be present. Signs of peritoneal irritation and shock suggest bowel infarction and carry a poor prognosis. Leucocytosis and hyperamylasaemia are common.

Diagnosis

Plain X-ray of the abdomen usually shows features of small bowel obstruction with dilated loops and air fluid levels. Whether angiography is clinically indicated here is subject to the same criteria as are discussed in relation to arterial occlusion. The features include: (1) reflux of contrast into the aorta; (2) spasm of the SMA and its branches; (3) opacification of a few distal arterial branches; (4) prolongation of the arterial phase beyond 40 s; (5) non-opacification of the SMV within 40 s; (6) opacification of the thickened bowel walls; (7) visible contrast within the bowel lumen. In practice, the condition is most often discovered when the abdomen has already been opened.

Operative management

The first step in the operation is quickly to exclude arterial occlusion as described above. Because in mesenteric venous thrombosis the infarction is often limited and segmental, a short bowel syndrome is less likely to occur than after treatment of arterial occlusion. Any infarcted bowel is resected. Thrombectomy of the superior mesenteric vein has been described. The vessel can be approached in three ways from the right side of the root to the mesentery of the small bowel.

(1) The right colon is mobilized extensively from right to left until all the right lumbar gutter structures are exposed and the SMV is visualized as it crosses the third part of the duodenum.

(2) The lesser peritoneal sac is opened by detaching the greater omentum from the transverse colon and following the middle colic vessels until the middle colic vein dips underneath the neck of the pancreas to join the SMV.

(3) Using a Kocher manoeuvre, the supraduodenal portion of the portal vein can be exposed behind the hepatic artery and the common bile duct, and thrombectomy can be performed through the portal vein using balloon catheters.

All three approaches may be necessary in order to ensure adequate clearance. The patient is maintained on full heparinization, and later on oral anticoagulants which are continued for life.

ISCHAEMIA OF THE COLON

Hindgut ischaemia is a less common clinical problem but is easier to diagnose. The clinical syndromes produced are well delineated and often simulate those of more common non-vascular lesions of the colon, with clear evidence of the site of the lesion and the need for surgical intervention. Acute hindgut ischaemia differs from small bowel ischaemia in that it can often be treated successfully using well-established general surgical principles without having to resort to an arterial reconstruction (Marston et al, 1966).

The commonest cause of IMA occlusion is arteriosclerosis. Some cases follow ligation of the IMA during operations on the distal aorta. There are also reported associations with rheumatoid arthritis, the contraceptive pill and phaeochromocytoma (Cotton and Thomas, 1971; Marcuson and Farman, 1971; Rosati and Augur, 1971; Cavin et al, 1982).

The most frequent sites for acute colon ischaemia are at the splenic flexure and the rectosigmoid junction (Marston et al, 1966; Reeders et al, 1984). Anatomical defects in the marginal artery have been described angiographically. Whether these defects are the result of congenital maldevelopment or of occlusion by an arteriosclerotic process is not always certain.

Major infarction of the hindgut is about one-tenth as common as small bowel gangrene and presents with severe peripheral circulatory failure, sepsis and obvious clinical features of generalized peritonitis' and rectal bleeding. The exact cause of the abdominal catastrophe is often only recognized at laparotomy or at autopsy. It may follow aortic thrombosis or aortic surgery, and has also been reported following unrelated non-vascular operations, including haemor-rhoidectomy, vagotomy and pyloroplasty, ureteric transplantation and above knee amputation. It is postulated that an episode of low cardiac output from heart failure is the underlying aetiology, even though the IMA may still be patent. Thus, the equivalent of 'non-occlusive' bowel ischaemia may be more common in the colon than is generally recognized (Bailey et al, 1986). Evidence in support of this is that colon necrosis occurs only in about 1% of cases following ligation of the IMA during resection of abdominal aortic aneurysms. Much, of course, depends on the state of the collateral pathways from the SMA and internal iliac and middle colic arteries. In the presence of advanced disease of the SMA and coeliac axis, the IMA forms the main visceral blood supply and its ligation may cause ischaemia which extends beyond the distal colon.

Acute necrotizing colitis

Acute necrotizing colitis can occur from many causes (neonatal disease is a special case which will not be discussed here) and is now recognized as a complication of colonic obstruction (Teasdale and Mortensen, 1983). The increased intraluminal pressure diminishes blood flow through the colon wall even in the absence of major vessel occlusion. Ischaemia confined initially to the mucosa may begin a train of events which allows resident bacteria, especially clostridia, to become lethally invasive. The changes observed at laparotomy have ranged from mucosal necrosis to frank gangrene of the colon proximal to the obstructing lesion. Gram stains of resected colon have demonstrated Gram-positive bacilli invading the mucosa and submucosa.

Treatment

This follows the lines described above. When the colon is involved, it is obviously even more important to avoid primary anastomosis, and to exteriorize the ends of the compromized bowel. In many patients both the small and the large bowel are involved, and the extent of the lesion is only identified at laparotomy.

CONCLUSIONS AND THE WAY FORWARD
(Marston et al, 1989)

Acute intestinal ischaemia remains a challenging problem, and in spite of increased understanding of the pathophysiology and of better methods of critical care, the results of treatment have scarcely improved. Early diagnosis is essential before the gut has undergone full thickness necrosis. Following correction of the metabolic deficits, operation is almost always necessary, when the choice must be made between revascularization and resection. Although complete vascularization of blood supply is the ideal to be aimed at, it may be wiser and safer to settle for resection in the doubtful case, bearing in mind the methods now available for nourishing a patient with inadequate small bowel function. The place of aortography is still undecided, and in spite of some encouraging results of intra-arterial therapy for early ischaemia, these methods have not gained wide acceptance.

REFERENCES

Anayi S & Al Nasiri N (1987) Acute mesenteric ischaemia caused by *Schistosoma mansoni* infection. *British Medical Journal* **294**: 1197.

Athanasoulis CA, Wittenberg J, Berenstein J & Williams LF (1975) Vasodilatory drugs in the management of non-occlusive bowel ischaemia. *Gastroenterology* **68**: 146–150.

Bailey RW, Bulkley GB, Hamilton SR et al (1986) Pathogenesis of non-occlusive ischemic colitis. *Annals of Surgery* **203**: 590–599.

Banks RO, Gellern RH, Zimmer MJ, Bulkley GB, Hughes SL & Granger DN (1985) Vasoactive agents in the control of the mesenteric circulation. *Federation Proceedings* **40**: 12.

Baue AE & Austen GW (1963) Superior mesenteric artery embolism. *Surgery, Gynecology and Obstetrics* **116**: 474–477.

Bergan JJ & Yao JS (1981) Acute intestinal ischemia. In Rutherford P (ed.) *Vascular Surgery*, 2nd edn, pp. 948–963. Philadelphia: WB Saunders.

Bergquist D, Bowater S, Erikkson I, Lannerstad O & Jakolanden R (1986) Small intestinal necrosis after aorto-iliac reconstruction. *British Journal of Surgery* **73**: 28–30.

Berry FB & Bougas JA (1950) Agnogenic venous mesenteric thrombosis. *Annals of Surgery* **132**: 450–474.

Boley SJ, Feinstein FR, Sammartano R, Brandt LJ & Sprayregen S (1981) New concept in the management of emboli of the superior mesenteric artery. *Surgery, Gynecology and Obstetrics* **153**: 561–569.

Brittain RS & Early TK (1963) Emergency thromboendarterectomy of the superior mesenteric artery. *Annals of Surgery* **158**: 138–143.

Bulkley GB, Hammond VH & Mains GB (1987) Mesenteric infarction and the pathophysiology of intestinal ischemia. In Bergan JJ & Yao JST (eds) *Vascular Surgical Emergencies*. New York: Grune and Stratton.

Bynum TE & Hanley HG (1982) Effect of digitalis on estimated splanchnic blood flow. *Journal of Clinical Medicine* **99**: 84–91.

Carter M, Fantini G, Sammartano R, Mitsudo S, Silverman D & Boley SJ (1984) Qualitative and quantitative fluorescein fluorescence for determining intestinal viability. *American Journal of Surgery* **147**: 117–125.

Cavin R, Boumghar M, Loosli H & Saegesser F (1982) Les accidents digestifs aigus des contraceptifs oraux. *Chirurgie* **108**: 64–74.

Chou CC & Kvietys PR (1981) Physiological and pharmacological alterations in gastrointestinal blood flow. In Granger DN & Bulkley GB (eds) *Measurement of Blood Flow—Application to the Splanchnic Circulation*, pp 477–509. Baltimore: Williams & Wilkins.

Clark AZ & Gallant TE (1984) Acute mesenteric ischemia. *American Journal of Roentgenology* **142**: 555–562.

Clavien PA, Muller C & Harder F (1987) Treatment of mesenteric infarction. *British Journal of Surgery* **74**: 500–503.

Cooperman M, Martin EW, Keith LM & Carey LC (1979) Use of Doppler ultrasound in intestinal surgery. *American Journal of Surgery* **138**: 850–859.

Cotton PB & Thomas ML (1971) Ischaemic colitis and the contraceptive pill. *British Medical Journal* **3**: 27–29.

Croft RJ, Menon GP & Marston A (1981) Does intestinal angina exist? A critical study of obstructed visceral arteries. *British Journal of Surgery* **68**: 316–318.

Dahn MS, Lange P, Lobdel K, Hans B, Jacobs LA & Mitchell RA (1987) Splanchnic and total body oxygen concentration differences in septic and injured patients. *Surgery* **101**: 69–80.

Dalsing MC, Grosfeld JA, Shiffler MA et al (1983) Superoxide dismutase: a cellular protective enzyme in bowel ischemia. *Journal of Surgical Research* **34**: 589–596.

Deitch EA & Sikkema WW (1981) Intestinal manifestations of Burger's Disease. *American Surgeon* **47**: 326–328.

Fiddian-Green RG & Gantz M (1984) Hypotension, hypoxia and arterial acidosis in ICU patients. *Circulatory Shock* **21**: 326.

Flickinger EG, Johnsrude IS, Ogburn NL, Weaver MD & Pories WJ (1983) Local streptokinase infusion for superior mesenteric thromboembolism. *American Journal of Roentgenology* **140**: 771–772.

Frimann-Dahl J (1960) *Roentgen Examination in Acute Abdominal Disease*. Oxford: Blackwell.

Granger DN, Rutili G & McCord JM (1981) Superoxide radicals in feline intestinal ischemia. *Gastroenterology* **81**: 22–29.

Hibbard JS, Swenson PC & Levin AG (1933) Roentgenology of experimental mesenteric vascular occlusion. *Archives of Surgery* **26**: 20–26.

Horsbrugh AG (1976) Occlusion of the mesenteric veins. In Hadfield J & Hobsley M (eds) *Current Surgical Practice*, Vol. 1. London: Edward Arnold.

Ingoldby CJH (1980) The value of polymyxin B in endotoxaemia due to experimental obstructive jaundice and mesenteric ischaemia. *British Journal of Surgery* **67**: 565–567.

Jamieson WG, Marchuk S, Rowson J & Durand J (1982) The early diagnosis of massive acute intestinal ischaemia. *British Journal of Surgery* **69 (supplement)**: S52–S53.

Kairolvoma MI, Karkola P, Heikinnen E et al (1977) Mesenteric infarction. *American Journal of Surgery* **133**: 188–193.

Katz S, Wahab A, Murray W & Williams L (1974) New parameters of viability in ischemic bowel disease. *American Journal of Surgery* **127**: 136–141.

Khodadadi J, Rozencwajg J, Nacach N, Schmidt B & Feuchtwanger MM (1980) Mesenteric vein thrombosis. *Archives of Surgery* **115**: 315–317.

Koehler RE & Kressel HY (1978) Arteriographic examination in suspected small bowel ischemia. *Digestive Diseases* **23**: 853–861.

Kranendonk SE, Bruining HA & van Urk H (1983) Survival after portal venous gas due to mesenteric vascular occlusion. *British Journal of Surgery* **70**: 183–184.

Lauon HE & Price AB (1987) Pseudomembranous colitis: presence of clostridial toxin. *Lancet* **2**: 1312–1314.

Lucas AE, Richardson JD, Flint LM & Polk HC (1981) Traumatic injury to the proximal superior mesenteric artery. *American Surgeon* **193**: 30–34.

Marcuson RW & Farman JA (1971) Ischaemic disease of the colon. *Proceedings of the Royal Society of Medicine* **64**: 1080–1083.

Marston A (1962) The bowel in shock. *Lancet* **2**: 365–370.

Marston A (1986) *Vascular Disease of the GI Tract*. London: Edward Arnold.

Marston A, Pheils MT, Thomas ML & Morson BC (1966) Ischaemic colitis. *Gut* **7**: 1–10.

Marston A, Bulkley GB, Fiddian-Green RG & Hagland U (1989) *Splanchnic Ischaemia and Multiple Organ Failure*. London: Edward Arnold.

Moorehouse PC, Gronveld M, Halliwell B, Quinlan JG & Gutteridge JMC (1987) Allopurinol and oxypurinol are hydroxyl radical scavengers. *FEBS Letters* **213**: 23–26.

Murrel TGC, Roth L, Egerton J, Samuels J & Walker PD (1966) Pig-bel: enteritis necroticans. *Lancet* **1**: 217–222.

Ottinger LW & Austen WG (1967) A study of 136 patients with mesenteric infarction. *Surgery, Gynecology and Obstetrics* **124**: 251–261.

Parks DA & Granger DN (1983) Ischemia induced microvascular changes: role of xanthine oxidase and hydroxyl radicals. *American Journal of Physiology* **245**: G285–G289.

Polansky BJ, Berger RL & Byrne JJ (1964) Massive nonocclusive intestinal infarction associated with digitalis toxicity. *Circulation* **30 (supplement)**: 141–145.

Reeders JWAJ, Tytgat GNJ, Rosenbusch G & Gratama S (1984) *Ischaemic Colitis*. The Hague: Martinus Nijhoff.

Robin P, Gruel Y, Lang M et al (1988) Complete thrombolysis of mesenteric vein occlusion with rTPA. *Lancet* **1**: 1391.

Rosati LA & Augur NA (1971) Ischemic enterocolitis in pheochromocytoma. *Gastroenterology* **60**: 581–583.

Rutherford RB, Ballis JV, Trow RS & Graves GM (1976) Comparison of regional blood-flow changes at equivalent stages of endotoxin and hemorrhagic shock. *Journal of Trauma* **16**: 886–897.

Schamaun M (1967) Electromyography to determine viability of injured small bowel segments. *Surgery* **62**: 899–909.

Shah S & Anderson C (1981) Prediction of small bowel viability using Doppler ultrasound. *American Surgeon* **194**: 97–99.

Shaw RS & Rutledge RH (1957) Superior mesenteric embolectomy in the treatment of massive mesenteric infarction. *New England Journal of Medicine* **157**: 595–600.

Stewart JOR (1963) Portal gas embolism, a prognostic sign in mesenteric vascular occlusion. *British Medical Journal* **1**: 1328.

Teasdale C & Mortensen NJMcC (1983) Acute necrotizing colitis and obstruction. *British Journal of Surgery* **70**: 44–47.

Turner DF, Crapo D et al (1984) Protection against toxicity of intravenous infusion of liposome encapsulated catalase and superoxide dimutase. *Journal of Clinical Investigation* **73**: 87–95.

Umpleby HC (1987) Thrombosis of the superior mesenteric vein. *British Journal of Surgery* **74**: 694–696.

Wilson C, Gupta R, Gilmour DG & Imrie CW (1987) Acute superior mesenteric ischaemia. *British Journal of Surgery* **74**: 279–281.

9

ACUTE INFLAMMATORY BOWEL DISEASE ASSESSMENT AND MEDICAL MANAGEMENT

D. J. Gertner and J. E. Lennard-Jones

INTRODUCTION

Acute ulcerative colitis is a serious and potentially life-threatening condition. Crohn's disease tends to be more chronic and may affect any part of the gastrointestinal tract. For the purposes of this chapter, the two conditions are discussed together under the heading of colitis, but Crohn's disease is considered separately when other areas of the gastrointestinal tract are described.

MANAGEMENT OF COLITIS

Clinical features

The first attack of ulcerative colitis usually occurs in young adults below the age of 40 but can occur at any age. Crohn's disease also presents early in life, but has a bimodal incidence with a secondary peak later in life when it is rather more common in females.

The onset of colitis is usually insidious, with rectal bleeding and mild bowel looseness. However, an acute presentation may be characterized by diarrhoea, with the passage of frequent liquid stools by day and night. The passage of liquid stools usually indicates an extensive colitis; formed stools with the passage of blood and pus per rectum suggests a distal proctosigmoiditis. Blood and mucus seen with the stool is more likely to indicate ulcerative than Crohn's colitis.

Abdominal pain, which may take the form of a constant dull ache or attacks of colic, is variable and may be absent even with profuse bloody diarrhoea. Patients may experience general malaise, weakness, rapid weight loss and fever.

Examination of the patient should include assessment of the state of hydration, the presence of fever, tachycardia and anaemia. The pharynx may reveal aphthous ulcers or sometimes monilia infection. Abdominal tenderness may be localized to the left iliac fossa in distal colitis, or be generalized with extensive disease.

Abdominal pain with evidence of peritonism suggests severe inflammation, perhaps with incipient toxic megacolon. Abdominal distension is a late sign of megacolon and the diagnosis should be made at an earlier stage whenever possible.

Anal lesions such as florid tags, perianal fistulae and abscesses are much more common in Crohn's disease. Sigmoidoscopy is mandatory in the evaluation of undiagnosed acute bloody diarrhoea. Expected appearances in acute severe colitis include an inflamed haemorrhagic mucosa with a purulent exudate. Discrete ulcers separated by areas of normal mucosa are typical of Crohn's disease but can occur in infective colitis.

Differential diagnosis

Specific causes of colitis include infections, which may be antibiotic associated, ischaemia and irradiation (see Table 1). Ulcerative colitis, Crohn's disease, collagenous and microscopic colitis are all of unknown cause.

The distinction between non-specific colitis and infective colitis may prove difficult especially in the acute stage. The absence of blood associated with the diarrhoea is more likely to indicate an infective cause, though blood can be seen with severe infections. Bacterial causes include *Salmonella* sp., *Shigella* sp., *Campylobacter jejuni* and *Yersinia* sp. *Campylobacter* enteritis is often a particularly painful condition, but generally the infective forms of colitis are clinically indistinguishable. Recently, a toxigenic form of *Escherichia coli* (*E. coli* 0157) has been implicated in sporadic outbreaks of severe haemorrhagic colitis of short duration (Symonds, 1988).

Immunodeficient patients, for example those with HIV disease or after chemotherapy, are prone to unusual colonic infections, particularly cytomegalovirus and atypical mycobacteria.

TABLE I
Differential diagnosis of acute colitis

Inflammatory bowel disease
Ulcerative colitis
Crohn's colitis
Infective
(1) Immunocompetent
    (a) Bacterial: *Salmonella, Shigella*
                    Campylobacter,
                    Yersinia
    (b) Parasitic: Amoebiasis
                 Schistosomiasis
    (c) Antibiotic associated: *Clostridium difficile*
(2) Immunodeficient: cytomegalovirus,
                    atypical mycobacteria
Ischaemic colitis
Radiation colitis
Miscellaneous
Collagenous colitis
Microscopic colitis

A careful history should include recent drug treatment, foreign travel, possible contaminated food and contact with people having similar symptoms. It is also important to take a sexual history and enquire about previous blood transfusions, with HIV disease in mind.

The diagnosis of most infective forms of colitis relies on positive stool cultures. The diagnostic yield is improved if three separate fresh samples are sent to the microbiology laboratory.

Amoebic colitis may be diagnosed by the presence of motile parasites in a hot stool sample or cysts on routine microscopy. The parasites may also be seen on histological examination of a rectal biopsy. Serological tests may alert the clinician to the possibility of amoebiasis, although they are often negative in non-invasive disease.

Clostridium difficile has been implicated as the organism responsible for antibiotic-associated colitis. It does not always produce the classical pseudomembrane seen at sigmoidoscopy to be covering the rectal mucosa. Culture of the organism and the presence of toxin in the stool indicate clinically significant infection. Many patients with ulcerative colitis who have been treated with antibiotics or sulphasalazine have evidence of *Clostridium difficile* on stool culture but its significance is doubtful (Greenfield et al, 1983).

Some non-steroidal anti-inflammatory drugs may cause a colitis which returns to normal when the drug is stopped.

Other conditions important in the differential diagnosis of acute bloody diarrhoea include ischaemic colitis (usually a localized area at the splenic flexure visualized at colonoscopy and/or barium enema) and radiation enteritis in patients with a history of previous pelvic or abdominal radiotherapy. Rectal bleeding in the absence of diarrhoea and associated with a normal sigmoidoscopy is not due to ulcerative colitis, but may rarely be associated with localized Crohn's disease in the sigmoid colon. Haemorrhoids, colonic neoplasia, diverticular disease and angiodysplasia are likely diagnoses. Collagenous colitis, a poorly understood histologically diagnosed condition, does not usually present acutely.

Early investigation of suspected inflammatory colitis

Patients presenting with a first attack of colitis will require more extensive investigations than those with a known diagnosis of non-specific inflammatory bowel disease. Even in the latter, it is important to re-examine the stools for pathogens as coincidental infection occurs. The important early investigations are summarized in Table 2.

Diagnostic

The diagnosis of colitis relies upon histological confirmation and exclusion of infective causes. Rigid sigmoidoscopy is a rapidly available procedure and should be part of the examination of the patient with undiagnosed bloody diarrhoea. Typical features have already been described. A rectal biopsy sent for histological assessment is mandatory in undiagnosed colitis but not necessary in patients with a recurrence of known inflammatory colitis.

Three fresh stool samples should be sent for microbiological assessment. The

TABLE 2
Investigation of suspected colitis

Haematology/chemical pathology
General condition
    Haemoglobin, urea and electrolytes
Inflammatory indices
    White cell count, platelets, C-reactive protein, albumin
Nutritional state
    Albumin

Microbiology
Stool microscopy and cultere (*C. difficale* toxin)
Blood cultures, serology (*Yersinia*)

Endoscopy
Sigmoidoscopy

Radiology
Plain abdominal radiograph, unprepared barium enema

Histology
Rectal biopsy

---

request should include bacterial culture and sensitivity, microscopy for ova, cysts and parasites and a test for *Clostridium difficile* toxin.

Assessment of colon

Delineating the extent of the disease is important in the assessment of the patient and the subsequent decision-making process. A plain abdominal X-ray at presentation may define the extent of colonic inflammation. Typical appearances in severe colitis include a lack of faecal residue and an abnormal mucosal outline, in the most severe cases with soft tissue shadows projecting into the gas-filled colon ('mucosal islands'; Bartram, 1976) (see Figure 1). Colonic dilatation is apparent from the air-filled colon, the upper limit of normal being 6 cm. 'Toxic megacolon' should be diagnosed only if there is both dilatation and an abnormal mucosal pattern (Jones and Chapman, 1969). (Note: the colonic diameter may be falsely exaggerated following sigmoidoscopy with air insufflation).

A barium enema without preparation of the colon and taking only three or four films is more likely to accurately delineate the disease extent, but is precluded immediately after a rectal biopsy. Performed gently, this examination does not usually upset the patient. The radiographs will show loss of haustration, areas of ulceration and granularity and commonly a tubular appearance in the affected region (Thomas, 1979) (Figure 2). Discontinuous areas of inflammation seen on a barium enema suggest Crohn's disease rather than ulcerative colitis although rectal sparing may be seen in any patient using topical therapy.

Colonoscopy during an acute severe attack of colitis is usually contraindicated because of the risk of disease exacerbation or even colonic perforation.

Blood tests

A full blood count may demonstrate anaemia (normocytic, normochromic if

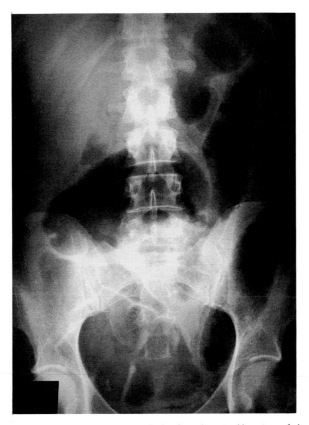

FIGURE I   Plain abdominal X-ray showing mucosal islands and toxic dilatation of the transverse colon.

acute and microcytic, hypochromic if chronic), neutrophil leucocytosis and thrombocytosis. Biochemical screening will indicate the degree of uraemia if the patient is dehydrated and possible associated electrolyte imbalance (hypokalaemia and hyponatraemia) which require correction. A low serum albumin is a useful indicator of disease activity and nutritional status. The C-reactive protein or orosomucoid are markers of inflammation and one of these acute phase reactants can be used to monitor the progress of the disease particularly in Crohn's colitis.

Assessment of severity

The severity of an acute attack of ulcerative or Crohn's colitis depends on the following factors: (1) the extent of the inflammation; (2) the depth of the mucosal ulceration; (3) the systemic response; (4) the metabolic depletion; (5) the age and physique of the patient.

Inflammation confined to the rectum and sigmoid colon rarely causes severe illness. When the whole or a substantial proportion of the colon is involved, the attack is likely to be more severe with some systemic upset. Even though much of the colon is inflamed the illness can still be mild if ulceration is absent or superficial, but deep ulceration, especially if the deep muscle layer is exposed over

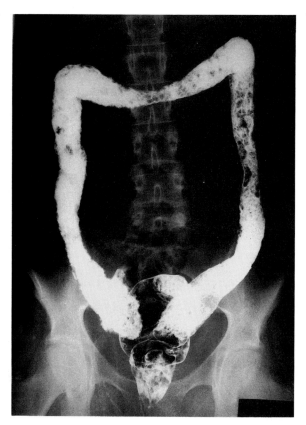

FIGURE 2   Instant barium enema showing a total colitis.

a large area, causes severe illness (Buckell et al, 1980). Systemic manifestations of colitis such as erythema nodosum, arthritis or pyoderma do not bear a direct relation to the extent and severity of the mucosal inflammation, but they are more common when the disease is extensive. Depletion of protein with a low serum albumin, loss of muscle bulk and loss of body weight is a common feature of severe colitis. Colitis in the elderly tends to be a more dangerous illness than in younger patients and the postoperative mortality after colectomy for acute disease is greater.

Attempts have been made to categorize patients with active colitis into mild, moderate and severe groups based on the clinical features and laboratory findings (Truelove and Witts, 1955). Such divisions may be arbitrary but can be useful in determining the level of medical intervention required. Factors involved in the assessment of severity are illustrated in Table 3.

Patients do not necessarily fit neatly into a particular category. For example some patients may have severe bloody diarrhoea with little constitutional upset or evidence of abnormal laboratory indices. In one retrospective study (Lennard-Jones et al, 1975) four features were found to have the greatest predictive value in determining the outcome of an attack of acute colitis: (1) maximum daily body temperature; (2) maximum daily pulse rate; (3) bowel frequency; (4) serum albumin.

TABLE 3
Severity of the attack of colitis

	Mild	Moderate	Severe
Local features			
(a) Stools/24 h	<4	4–6	>6
(b) Blood	Small	Moderate	Copious
(c) Abdominal tenderness	Absent	Slight	Peritonism
Constitutional upset			
Fever } Tachycardia	Absent	Mild	Severe
Nutritional state	Normal	Mildly undernourished	Cachectic
Laboratory			
(a) Inflammatory response WBC Platelets ESR CRP	Normal	Mildly elevated	Significantly elevated
(b) Evidence of loss Haemoglobin Albumin Electrolytes	Normal	Mildly depleted	Significantly depleted

Intensive medical treatment

Patients with a severe attack of colitis require admission to hospital. They may
need replacement of deficient fluids and in some cases nutritional support as well
as intensive drug therapy. The use of nutrition as a primary therapy has not been
established for ulcerative colitis but may be beneficial in Crohn's colitis.

Nutritional replacement

Dehydration and electrolyte imbalances should be corrected with intravenous
fluids and a blood transfusion may be necessary to correct anaemia. Profound
hypoalbuminaemia may be treated with infusions of human albumin, but these
are expensive, scarce and unlikely to provide long-term improvement. Deficiencies
of blood, fluid and electrolytes may be rapidly corrected, but replacing lost body
tissue is a much slower process. Nutritional support to treat malnutrition is
described below in the management of acute Crohn's disease.

Nutrition as primary therapy

It is now becoming apparent that Crohn's disease responds differently to
nutritional therapy compared with ulcerative colitis. In two controlled studies,
bowel rest with parenteral nutrition was ineffective in the management of acute
ulcerative colitis (Dickinson et al, 1980; McIntyre et al, 1986). This contrasts with
the evidence in Crohn's disease, colonic or small bowel, which suggests that

bowel rest with parenteral nutrition or elemental diets significantly reduces inflammation (see fuller discussion below).

We therefore occasionally use an elemental diet (E028, Scientific Hospital Supplies) for the treatment of acute Crohn's colitis. We do not advocate the use of parenteral nutrition or an elemental diet as a primary treatment to reduce inflammation in acute ulcerative colitis.

Drugs

Corticosteroids

Severe attacks. The primary aim in the treatment of severe acute colitis is to reduce mortality. The mainstay of specific therapy remains corticosteroids, first used more than 30 years ago (Truelove and Witts, 1955). Several questions pertaining to corticosteroid therapy remain controversial:

(1) *Which steroid preparation to use?* Corticotrophin (ACTH) and hydrocortisone in equivalent dose have a similar therapeutic effect in acute colitis. Both mortality and the need for colectomy are reduced by the use of these agents (Truelove and Witts, 1959). Corticotrophin may have a reduced effect in patients previously treated with corticosteroids (due to adrenal gland suppression) (Myers et al, 1983) and most clinicians do not use this treatment. Intravenous hydrocortisone is as effective as corticotrophin (Myers et al, 1983) but tends to cause sodium and water retention. For this reason prednisolone, which has fewer mineralocorticoid effects, is commonly used.

(2) *How long to treat for?* The problem of how long to persist with intensive medical therapy is controversial. Early surgical intervention undoubtedly reduces the mortality of severe acute colitis. A balance has to be struck between an adequate period of medical treatment to permit possible response and unduly prolonged therapy that jeopardizes the outcome of surgery should it become necessary. Truelove and Jewell (1974) advocated a strict 5 day period of intravenous steroid therapy after which, if there was no decisive improvement, surgery was advised. A Scandinavian study suggested an increase in the proportion of patients attaining remission with treatment prolonged beyond 5 days (Jarnerot et al, 1985). Another report suggested that treatment prolonged for more than 10 days did not seem to give any advantage (Meyers and Janowitz, 1985).

(3) *What dose and route of administration?* Intravenous administration is widely held to give better therapeutic results than an equivalent oral dose. Equivalent intravenous doses by bolus injection or infusion produce higher plasma prednisolone levels than by oral ingestion in acute colitis (Berghouse et al, 1982). Intravenous steroids are therefore preferred for severe attacks.

Truelove and Jewell (1974) advocated 60 mg prednisolone daily (as the 21-phosphate) in divided doses by intravenous infusion and this regimen has been widely practised. There are no controlled trials comparing bolus injections with a constant infusion or indeed comparing different doses. High-dose therapy with methyl prednisolone, daily for 3 days, did not improve the therapeutic result (Ireland et al, 1988).

Suggested regimen. For severe attacks, a 5 day intravenous course of methylprednisolone 48 mg/day in three divided doses is initiated (see Table 4). (Prednisolone 21-phosphate used previously in the equivalent dose of 60 mg is no longer available as an intravenous preparation.)

The majority of patients responding to this regime do so promptly and dramatically. A few patients may make little progress during the 5 days of intensive therapy. Most clinicians would advocate surgical intervention for these patients at this stage, or earlier if their condition deteriorates. If there is some, but not clear-cut, improvement, we adopt a flexible approach but would not delay operation for longer than about 10 days. It is important to emphasize the importance of a combined medical and surgical evaluation at all stages for these very sick patients.

If a less potent drug regime has been used as a first step, then it is reasonable to substitute an intravenous corticosteroid if there is no response to the initial treatment.

High dose corticosteroid therapy may increase the complication rate (perforation and haemorrhage) of peptic ulceration and as undiagnosed peptic ulcer is one of the, albeit infrequent, causes of death in acute severe colitis, we prescribe an H_2-receptor blocker (cimetidine or ranitidine) by mouth.

Mild/moderate attacks

Oral therapy. The patient with a less severe exacerbation of colitis who presents with an exacerbation may not require hospital admission and intensive therapy. If the patient is not constitutionally ill and can tolerate oral medication, prednisolone 40 mg/day is given by mouth and the situation reviewed as an out-patient.

Topical therapy. Some patients with active colitis whether moderate or severe suffer unduly with symptoms of urgency and frequency due to rectal inflammation. This group as well as those with less extensive but nevertheless

TABLE 4
Regime for intensive therapy of colitis

(1) Intravenous infusion if necessary for:
    (a) Fluid and electrolyte replacement
    (b) Blood transfusion
(2) Methylprednisolone 16 mg tds i.v. ($+H_2$ blocker if there is a history of peptic ulcer or dyspepsia, or routinely)
(3) Sulphasalazine 1 g tds or 5-ASA 1.2 g tds by mouth, if well tolerated
(4) Enemata for acute distal or left-sided disease if relevant:
    (a) Prednisolone-21-phosphate 20 mg in 100 ml water; or
    (b) 5-ASA enema

active disease may benefit from topical therapy. The rationale for using a topical preparation is that a high concentration of the active drug is brought into contact for an adequate time with the whole area of inflamed mucosa.

Conventional prednisolone phosphate or hydrocortisone enemas are significantly absorbed and may cause adrenal suppression and steroid side effects. Equally effective steroid preparations are now becoming available which are poorly absorbed (McIntyre et al, 1985) or metabolized so rapidly that side effects are limited (e.g. prednisolone metasulphobenzoate).

In adults a retention enema of 100 ml always reaches the sigmoid colon, but the proximal spread varies greatly. If extensive colitis is to be treated topically, then it is important to know that the enema penetrates far enough into the colon. This can be judged from an abdominal radiograph performed at an interval after administration of the enema with a little barium (Swarbrick et al, 1974).

Many patients are unable to retain corticosteroid retention enemas. In this circumstance, a foam preparation has the advantage that it can be retained more easily than a fluid enema, but studies show that the extent of penetration is limited to the rectum and sigmoid colon (Farthing et al, 1979). Administration of a fluid retention enema via a rectal drip may be an alternative to the usual method in the presence of severe rectal urgency. A suppository can be used for disease confined to the rectum.

Sulphasalazine and related compounds Sulphasalazine, a compound of 5-aminosalicylic acid (5-ASA) linked to sulphapyridine (SP) by an azo bond, has been shown by controlled trial to benefit patients with mild active colitis. In the context of severe acute colitis it may be used as an adjuvant to steroid therapy. The maximum dose usually used is 4 g in divided doses but side effects are fairly common and most of them are dose dependent. Dyspepsia may be alleviated by using enteric coated tablets.

Some of the side effects of sulphasalazine (fatigue, nausea, abdominal pain) may exacerbate the symptoms of acute colitis and its value in severe attacks is not proven. With severe diarrhoea and rapid transit or with co-administration of antibiotics the bacterial splitting of sulphasalazine into the active moiety 5-ASA may be impaired and drug efficacy reduced. Sulphasalazine tends to act more slowly than corticosteroids and for all these reasons is often not used in severe acute colitis, though it is useful in moderate/mild attacks.

A number of orally active preparations of 5-ASA (olsalazine (Dipentum), mesalazine (Asacol, Pentasa) are now available. Although these preparations appear to be as efficacious as sulphasalazine with fewer side effects, their value in severe acute colitis is unproven, but two trials have shown benefit in moderate/mild colitis (Riley et al, 1988; Rachmilevitz et al, 1989).

Topical preparations of sulphasalazine or 5-ASA, either as a retention enema or suppository, can be beneficial in acute distal colitis.

Antibiotics The use of antibiotics is controversial. Neither metronidazole (Chapman et al, 1986) nor vancomycin (Dickinson et al, 1985) had any significant impact on remission rates in acute colitis. Broad spectrum antibiotics have been tested but at present there is no conclusive evidence of benefit although a recent report suggests that tobramycin may be efficacious (Burke et al, 1987).

There is a good indication for giving antibiotics prophylactically when an operation is undertaken for acute colitis in order to reduce the risk of infective postoperative complications.

Antidiarrhoeal agents Antidiarrhoeal agents reduce stool frequency and might be anticipated to offer significant syptomatic relief. In fact, a controlled trial has shown little benefit from diphenoxylate in acute colitis (Engbaek et al, 1975). Those patients with inflammation confined to the left side of the colon may accumulate hard stools in the normal right side of the colon (Lennard-Jones et al, 1962), a situation which can be aggravated by anti-diarrhoeal drugs. We prescribe codeine phosphate and/or loperamide very rarely in colitis, though these drugs are useful in other types of diarrhoea.

Indications for surgery

About two-thirds of patients with severe acute attacks of colitis respond well, but up to 30% of patients will require surgical intervention (Truelove and Jewell, 1974; Truelove et al, 1978). In general, patients with Crohn's colitis seem to require urgent surgical treatment less frequently than those with ulcerative colitis (Mortensen et al, 1984).

Patients with severe attacks of colitis should be kept under careful clinical observation by physician and surgeon working closely together. The plain abdominal X-ray may be repeated daily if there is a suspicion that toxic megacolon is developing. Worrying clinical features during therapy include onset of fever, tachycardia, abdominal distension or tenderness. If a patient deteriorates despite intensive therapy, or a toxic megacolon or colonic perforation is suspected, urgent surgery is indicated. Surgery is also indicated if there is no response to intravenous steroids over 5–7 days. A few patients improve slowly and incompletely. For them, continued medical treatment is often justified. A total colectomy, ileostomy and retention of the rectum with mucous fistula is the safest procedure and preserves the long-term surgical options.

Subsequent medical treatment for those who respond to therapy

After 5 days of intensive intravenous therapy, oral prednisolone (60 mg/day) is substituted. The steroid dosage is gradually reduced, usually over the subsequent 4–6 weeks and sulphasalazine (1 g bd to tds) or 5-ASA (400–800 mg tds) given in maintenance doses. Azathioprine (2 mg/kg/day) may be a useful adjunct for the occasional patient in whom disease activity persists with steroid dependence.

Complications of colitis and their treatment

Toxic megacolon

The most severe complication (see Table 5) of colitis is toxic megacolon, which is more common in ulcerative than Crohn's colitis. The presence of extensive deep ulceration denudes the colonic lining and damages the underlying muscle (Buckell et al, 1980). The colon is then liable to dilate, and may perforate spontaneously or

Table 5
Complications of acute inflammatory bowel disease

(a) Colitis
    Toxic megacolon
    Colonic perforation
    Colonic haemorrhage
    Enteric superinfection
    Acute anal lesions
(b) Small bowel disease (Crohn's)
    Intestinal obstruction
    Abscess and septicaemia
    Fistulae (internal and external)
    Haemorrhage
    Anorectal lesions
    Ileostomy dysfunction
(c) Manifestations of IBD outside the gastrointestinal tract
    Skin: erythema nodosum, pyoderma gangrenosum
    Eyes: iritis
    Joints: monoarthritis, ankylosing spondylitis
    Liver: sclerosing cholangitis

rupture during surgical removal. Toxic megacolon is potentially lethal and even following prompt surgery death may occur from intra-abdominal sepsis or related complications. Colonic dilatation is usually associated with extensive colitis, often a first attack, but may complicate left-sided disease (Kisloff and Adkins, 1981) and may also occur in bacterial and pseudomembranous colitis.

Risk factors A number of factors have been suggested in the pathogenesis of this complication including various pharmacological agents such as narcotic analgesics, anticholinergics and antidiarrhoeal drugs. A barium enema or colonoscopy may be associated with apparent worsening of acute colitis, perhaps related as much to the preparation of the colon as to the procedure itself.

Clinical features The patient is always ill but there may be no localizing symptoms or physical signs. The onset of pain, which is usually diffuse and constant, or a change in the nature of pre-existing pain may herald a toxic megacolon. Fever and/or tachycardia are common but not invariable; a change in the mental state may occasionally occur in the most severe cases. Abdominal examination may reveal signs of peritonism; distension with increase in abdominal girth is a late sign.

Investigations The plain abdominal radiograph is the only reliable means of diagnosing this condition and is mandatory in all patients with severe acute colitis. Dilatation may be recognized from an abnormal gas shadow anywhere in the colon depending on the patient's position. The transverse colon is most often seen to be dilated (> 6 cm) because the radiograph is taken supine and this part of the colon is uppermost. Dilatation is associated with a loss of haustration, an irregular edge at the junction of the air and soft tissue shadows and, in the most severe cases, the presence of mucosal islands (see Figure 1).
  Abnormal laboratory investigations usually associated with this condition include a neutrophil leucocytosis, anaemia, and hypoproteinaemia.

Treatment Because this condition is potentially lethal, the crucial decision is when to intervene surgically. A patient with a toxic megacolon should be evaluated by both a physician and a surgeon. A decision to operate is usually made at the onset of this problem, but under some circumstances it may be reasonable to persist with a trial of intensive medical therapy for a period of 24–48 h. This approach relies on meticulous monitoring of the patient's condition and regular medical review. Most clinicians advocate nil by mouth and nasogastric suction, and a few use a tube passed per rectum with the aim of relieving colonic pressure.

Outcome In Britain, toxic megacolon is generally treated by colectomy, and in most centres the mortality is now low. In the United States medical treatment is more often undertaken. In a retrospective series from America, 79% of 75 cases of toxic megacolon presenting in a 20 year period were treated surgically with a 16% mortality rate. Factors increasing mortality included age (those under 40 carry a much better prognosis), female sex, transfer from another hospital and most importantly preoperative colonic perforation (Greenstein et al, 1985).

Colonic perforation

Colonic perforation may occur freely into the peritoneal cavity, the site may be sealed off by omentum, or it may be retroperitoneal when the colon becomes adherent to neighbouring structures or an abscess develops. Free perforation occurs more commonly in ulcerative than in Crohn's colitis. It may occur as a sequel to toxic megacolon or unexpectedly in its absence. The sigmoid colon is the most vulnerable site. Perforation appears to occur more often during the first attack of colitis (Edwards and Truelove, 1964). Corticosteroids have been implicated in the development of colonic perforation but this has not been borne out by retrospective studies (Edwards and Truelove, 1964). It is said that corticosteroids may mask the physical signs of perforation but, in fact, colonic perforation can be almost painless in patients not taking drugs.

Diagnosis of colonic perforation is easy if the patient manifests the sudden onset of an 'acute abdomen' with signs of peritonitis. In many cases, the patient has significant pre-existent abdominal pain and changes in the physical signs may be subtle. Abrupt onset of tachycardia or fever may alert the attending clinician to a perforation. Perforation into the peritoneal cavity may be confirmed by a prompt abdominal radiograph, either upright or in the lateral decubitus position, which demonstrates the presence of free gas.

Treatment Prompt surgical intervention offers the best chance of survival with this complication.

Colonic haemorrhage

Profuse colonic bleeding rarely complicates colitis. In ulcerative colitis the bleeding is often diffuse but in Crohn's colitis it is likely to be localized to a site of deep penetrating ulceration. Occasionally, major haemorrhage in ulcerative colitis can be from the rectum and this may be a contraindication to the operation of colectomy leaving a rectal stump.

The patient's haemodynamic state should be stabilized with blood and clotting factors as necessary. It may be possible to assess the colon and localize the haemorrhage by colonoscopy if an acute colitis is not present. If profuse bleeding persists, an emergency colectomy is unavoidable.

Acute anal lesions

Anorectal lesions are common in Crohn's disease, occurring in up to 80% of patients, but may also complicate ulcerative colitis. Only the acute lesions are discussed here.

Anal fissure This is often asymptomatic in Crohn's disease but may cause exquisite local pain during or after defaecation in ulcerative colitics. A fissure can be seen as an ulcer or linear split at the anal verge. A topical steroid cream or ointment may be of some benefit when introduced into the anal canal regularly by a gloved finger.

Perianal abscesses Perianal abscesses occur in up to one-quarter of patients with Crohn's disease and in less than 10% with ulcerative colitis. An abscess usually presents as a very painful swelling related to the anus. Clinically it appears as an area of induration, swelling and redness and it may be fluctuant. These lesions may drain spontaneously but surgical drainage is usually needed. Early drainage of an abscess may avoid fistula formation. Systemic antibiotics including anaerobic cover (ampicillin and metronidazole) are usually given but should not delay surgical drainage.

Enteric infections

Enteric infections, such as *Salmonella* or *Campylobacter*, may apparently trigger a first attack of colitis or complicate pre-existing colitis. It is advisable to culture the stool if a patient with known inflammatory bowel disease develops a severe relapse because a coincidental infection may be present. If a pathogen is present in the stool and the colitis is moderate to severe, experience suggests that both antibacterial and corticosteroid therapies are needed (Dronfield et al, 1974). We treat *Clostridium difficile* only if the toxin is detectable in the stool (metronidazole 400 mg tds or vancomycin 125 mg qds by mouth).

Extra-intestinal manifestations

Several extra-intestinal manifestations of acute inflammatory bowel disease may occur. Target organs include skin (erythema nodosum and pyoderma gangrenosum), eyes (episcleritis or iritis), joints (arthritis) and the liver (see Table 5). In general, these associated disorders other than sclerosing cholangitis respond to treatment of the colitis. Patients with eye inflammation may require local steroid eye drops. Sclerosing cholangitis may be occasionally complicated by acute cholangitis with fever and jaundice; antibacterial treatment is then required.

Colitis in pregnancy

Colitis has no effect on fertility or childbirth and the outcome of pregnancy is the same as that for the general population (Willoughby and Truelove, 1980). Active disease at conception produces a slightly less favourable outcome for the baby. Very severe attacks may precipitate premature labour and stillbirth and the outcome for the fetus of urgent surgical treatment for the mother is very poor (Anderson et al, 1987). The risks of prescribing corticosteroids in pregnancy are minimal and are far outweighed by the risks of uncontrolled colitis. Colitis in pregnancy may be treated conventionally with standard doses of prednisolone and sulphasalazine or mesalazine with no documented deleterious effects on the fetus or unborn child (Mogadam et al, 1981). Sulphasalazine may also be prescribed without harm for breast-feeding mothers in the puerperium.

MANAGEMENT OF ACUTE CROHN'S DISEASE

Clinical features

Classical ileocolic Crohn's disease accounts for some 40% of cases; the management of patients with mainly or entirely (30%) colonic disease has already been discussed. Disease limited to the small bowel occurs in some 30% of patients, most of whom have involvement of the distal ileum. Jejuno-ileitis is rare and gastroduodenal involvement extremely uncommon. The symptomatology, investigations and therapy may vary with disease location.

The characteristic pathological lesion in Crohn's disease is the deep penetrating ulcer. The disease is often discontinuous along the length and around the circumference of the gut, unlike the uniformity and continuity of colonic inflammation in ulcerative colitis.

If the ulcerating mucosal lesion penetrates through the bowel wall, an abscess (if the breach is localized) or fistula (if an adjacent viscus or nearby skin is involved) will develop. Drainage of an abscess, while essential, may lead to fistula formation. Healing by fibrosis characterizes this condition and predisposes to stricture formation with obstruction. Hence Crohn's disease is often a 'complicated' condition which requires treatment of the underlying inflammatory process (usually by means of 'medical' therapy) and the accompanying complications by surgery.

A number of clinical features are common in acute Crohn's disease wherever it may occur in the gut. Patients often give a history of anorexia, nausea and occasionally vomiting. Fever and sweats indicate active disease. Diarrhoea is very common, but the bowel habit may be infrequent if bowel obstruction is present. A typical patient with active Crohn's disease will be underweight, anaemic and febrile. A resting tachycardia may be present even without dehydration or significant blood loss.

Ileocolic Crohn's disease

Patients with acute ileocolitis usually have abdominal pain, localized to the right iliac fossa. If there is narrowing of the terminal ileum, the patient may experience obstructive symptoms, typically colicky pain which is usually related to eating. There is usually localized right iliac fossa tenderness and occasionally peritonism.

There may be a right iliac fossa mass and this should alert the clinician to the possibility of a complicating abscess (see below).

Acute jejuno-ileitis

Involvement of the proximal small bowel is often extensive, causing a protein-losing enteropathy and malabsorption. Patients may present with abdominal pain, usually colicky, diarrhoea, which may be frankly steatorrhoeic, and oedema due to hypoalbuminaemia. Stricturing disease may cause upper intestinal obstruction with postprandial pain, distension, vomiting and resultant electrolyte and acid–base disturbance.

Differential diagnosis

Acute Crohn's disease may present with very similar features to acute appendicitis and many patients are discovered to have Crohn's disease at appendicectomy (see Table 6). Specific forms of terminal ileitis with enlarged lympth nodes are due to *Yersinia pseudotuberculosis* or *Yersinia enterocolitica*. Non-specific mesenteric lymphadenitis may also present with right iliac fossa pain, fever and diarrhoea. Other important specific infections involving the small bowel include *Campylobacter jejuni* and *Salmonella* sp., both of which may cause diarrhoea with abdominal pain and fever. Ulcerative jejunitis and small bowel lymphoma are very rare.

A mass in the right iliac fossa may be a feature of ileocaecal tuberculosis, more common in the Third World and not necessarily associated with active pulmonary disease. Fungal conditions such as actinomycosis and histoplasmosis are rare but a caecal carcinoma should always be suspected in the older patient with a mass in the right iliac fossa (See Table 6).

Early investigation of acute Crohn's disease

The laboratory investigations are similar to those in acute colitis (see Table 2). Radiological studies of the small bowel define the presence and extent of disease. A plain abdominal radiograph is indicated if there is suspected intestinal obstruction and will show dilated small bowel loops. Typical features on a barium follow-through include cobblestoning of the mucosa, ulcers, which may be aphthous or deep, fissuring and luminal narrowing (see Figure 3). Endoscopy with biopsy for histological evaluation is helpful if there is disease in the terminal ileum or upper small bowel. Stool culture for *Campylobacter*, *Yersinia* and other pathogens is important in acute enteritis.

Intensive medical therapy

The patient with severe acute Crohn's disease may require hospitalization and intensive medical therapy. Constitutional problems of anaemia, dehydration and electrolyte disturbance should be managed in the same way as described for

TABLE 6
Differential diagnosis of
acute Crohn's disease

Acute enteritis
Acute appendicitis
Mesenteric lymphadenitis
Enteric infections
   Campylobacter jejuni
   Yersinia sp.
Ulcerative jejunitis
Small bowel lymphoma

Right iliac fossa mass
Ileocaecal tuberculosis
Actinomycosis
Histoplasmosis
Caecal carcinoma

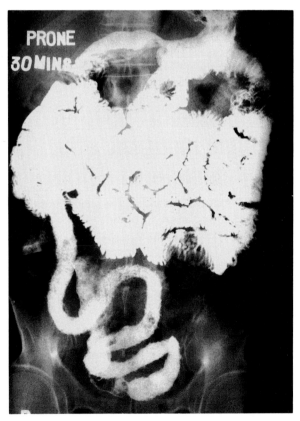

FIGURE 3 Barium follow-through showing extensive ileal Crohn's disease with deep penetrating ulcers and loss of fold pattern.

ulcerative colitis. Nutritional deficiencies and sepsis (localized and systemic) are much more common than in ulcerative colitis and these warrant special attention (*vide infra*).

Role of diet and parenteral nutrition

The use of nutrition in inflammatory bowel disease may be supportive or as a primary therapy to reduce inflammation or improve symptoms. Nutritional measures could reduce inflammation by altering the body's response, by altering the contents of the gut or by removing nutrients from the gut lumen.

Nutrition as a primary therapy

Liquid/low-residue diet to improve symptoms. Patients with obstructive symptoms due to stricturing disease may improve dramatically by taking a low-residue or even liquid diet. A regime of small frequent meals often improves symptoms and enables an increased calorific intake.

Supplemented nutrition. A cross-over study comparing a 2 month period on a normal diet with a similar period on a diet supplemented with a polymeric liquid drink demonstrated not only significant weight gain, increased mid-arm circumference and plasma albumin but also an increased T-cell lymphocyte count and reduced serum orosomucoid (Harries et al, 1983). These findings suggest both an improved nutritional state and an anti-inflammatory effect. It seems possible that improved nutritional status enhances immunological function in some way.

Bowel rest and parenteral nutrition. The possibility that total parenteral nutrition (TPN) could be beneficial in active inflammatory bowel disease was first suggested in the late 1960s. In a recent uncontrolled study, short-term nutritional therapy (TPN given for a mean period of 25 days) improved the majority of 100 patients with complicated acute Crohn's disease. Obstructive symptoms disappeared in 75% of patients with small bowel obstruction, an abdominal mass subsided in 82%, a fistula closed in 62% and active disease remitted in 89% (Ostro et al, 1985).

The beneficial effect of TPN had been attributed to 'resting the bowel'. However, recent carefully controlled studies have shown that the therapeutic benefit of a normal or chemically defined diet supplemented with parenteral nutrition is not significantly different from parenteral nutrition without any nutrients by mouth (Lochs et al, 1983; Greenberg et al, 1988). Furthermore, enteral nutrition with a defined formula diet appears to be as efficacious as parenteral nutrition in inducing disease remission.

Elemental diets. Enteral feeding with an elemental diet is as effective as prednisolone in first attacks of active Crohn's disease (O'Morain et al, 1984; Sanderson et al, 1987). The efficacy of an elemental diet could be due to its 'hypoallergenic' nature. Similar beneficial effects with polymeric, whole-protein diets have been described (Greenberg et al, 1988; Giaffar et al, 1989; Park et al, 1989) suggesting that these liquid diets may be acting by some other means, possibly by altering the bacterial flora.

Exclusion diets. Although food intolerance producing a variety of abdominal symptoms occurs more frequently in patients with Crohn's disease than controls, the use of exclusion diets (Jones et al, 1985) as a primary therapy for acute disease is not yet generally accepted. Most patients spontaneously exclude those dietary items which offend, and there does not appear to be a diet which benefits every patient. The foods which seem to cause symptoms most commonly are dairy and wheat products.

Current policy. In terms of primary therapy, a 1 month trial with a chemically defined elemental diet (E028, Scientific Hospital Supplies) as the sole nutritional intake can be advised as an alternative to corticosteroids for patients with acute Crohn's disease, providing the enteral route of administration is possible. This diet is not very palatable and restriction of dietary intake to such a liquid for several weeks is demanding for a patient. The diet can be made as palatable as possible by sipping it as a chilled drink with ice. For those who cannot tolerate it as a drink, a nasogastric tube feed is often acceptable.

Parenteral nutrition is not usually justified as a primary treatment because of its cost and liability to dangerous complications. However, its use can be considered in exceptional circumstances.

Nutrition as support

Patients with severe disease may be malnourished due to a variety of causes (Table 7). Significant malnutrition leads to weakness, apathy, depression and possibly an increased incidence of infection and impaired wound healing. Acutely ill patients with both ulcerative colitis and Crohn's disease benefit from nutritional support if their nutritional status is suboptimal.

The nutritional state should be part of the initial and ongoing assessment of every patient. Important factors to consider are the dietary intake during the recent past, excessive losses from the gut, actual weight as compared with usual weight, and a general impression of deficient muscle bulk and subcutaneous fat.

How to intervene? The simplest and often most successful intervention is to encourage the patient to eat larger amounts of ordinary food. If this is not sufficient, enteral or parenteral supplementation is required. A high calorie liquid supplement should ideally be palatable, have a high nutrient density, empty easily from the stomach and not cause diarrhoea. Many commercially available liquid formulas are suitable and most are low in fat, yield about 1 kcal/ml and contain appropriate minerals and vitamins.

TABLE 7
Causes of malnutrition in inflammatory bowel disease

Inadequate intake
Anorexia, nausea and vomiting, avoidance
Increased requirements
Fever, stress, growth, inflammation, repletion of stores
Decreased absorption
Resection, bypass, inflammation, stagnant loop
Excessive losses
Diarrhoea, protein-losing enteropathy, fistulae
Miscellaneous
Metabolic effects of inflammation

Ill patients may not be able to increase their calorific intake by drinking an adequate volume of a liquid supplement because of early satiety. A constant or overnight drip feed by means of a fine-bore nasogastric tube may overcome this problem.

The parenteral route for nutritional supplementation should be reserved for patients who are acutely ill with intestinal failure. It is expensive, requires careful supervision preferably by a 'nutrition team' and has a higher morbidity rate than other methods of support. Nevertheless in selected patients, it may be essential and life saving: (1) patients with excessive gastrointestinal losses in whom oral intake is less than output, including high output enterocutaneous fistulae and the short bowel syndrome; (2) patients with gastrointestinal obstruction or ileus; (3) patients with severe malabsorption due to extensive mucosal disease.

The nutritional requirements are well established and these may be modified according to individual needs. Some patients may only require parenteral replacement of fluid and electrolytes.

Specific nutritional deficiencies Large losses from the small intestine, especially in patients with a short gut, may cause sodium deficiency and hypomagnesaemia. The average concentration of sodium in small bowel effluent is about 100 mmol/l. Negative sodium balance leads to dehydration, postural hypotension and pre-renal uraemia. Magnesium deficiency may present with frank tetany or even generalized convulsions, but more often with a complaint of cramps and paraesthesiae. Trousseau and Chvostek's signs will be positive with significant magnesium deficiency. A serum magnesium of less than 0.5 mmol/l often requires intravenous replacement using magnesium sulphate 12–24 mmol over 24 h. With a low serum magnesium, there is often hypocalcaemia and hypokalaemia; magnesium supplementation often corrects all these abnormalities.

Drug therapy

Pharmacological therapy of Crohn's disease is hampered by the lack of a curative agent and the fact that evaluation of drug therapy is complicated by the unpredictability of the disease. There is both a significant spontaneous remission rate and placebo response. Several agents are available for use and some are now established as being effective for the treatment of active disease.

Corticosteroids

As with ulcerative colitis, the mainstay of treatment remains a corticosteroid drug. Two large-scale controlled, prospective double-blind studies have confirmed the benefit of corticosteroid therapy in active Crohn's disease. In the American National Cooperative Crohns Disease Study (NCCDS) (Summers et al, 1979) 85 patients received prednisone in doses determined by their disease activity (0.25–0.75 mg/kg) for 17 weeks; 60% achieved remission compared with 30% in the placebo-treated group. The extra-intestinal manifestations and perianal disease were both unresponsive. The European Cooperative Crohns Disease Study (ECCDS) demonstrated the efficacy of 6-methyl prednisolone (80% in remission at 100 days), initially at 48 mg/day and tapered to 12 mg/day over 6 weeks for disease in all sites compared with placebo (15% in remission at 100 days) (Malchow et al, 1984).

Which agent and dose? Just as in the therapy of ulcerative colitis, the questions over which agent, dosage and route of administration to use is unresolved. Most patients, even with very active disease, do not require intravenous therapy. We favour prednisolone, initially as a single daily oral dose of 40 mg and then tapered on a weekly basis depending on the patient's response. If the patient is unable to take oral medication or is constitutionally very ill, intravenous methyl-prednisolone 48 mg daily in three divided doses may be given and an oral preparation substituted after 5–7 days. Caution in prescribing corticosteroids is indicated if there is obvious sepsis or an abdominal mass. Broad spectrum antibiotic cover including a drug active against anaerobes should be given in these circumstances (see below).

Sulphasalazine and 5-ASA

Several studies including the American and European collaborative trials have suggested some, albeit modest, improvement with sulphasalazine in active Crohn's disease. This is most obvious for colonic disease, less pronounced for ileocaecal disease and absent for small bowel disease alone. This is not surprising in view of the mode of action of sulphasalazine which relies on colonic bacterial splitting to yield the active moiety of 5-ASA.

5-ASA (mesalazine) preparations formulated to be released along the length of the small intestine (Pentasa) or in the distal small intestine (Claversal or Asacol) have recently become available. These are attractive agents for the treatment of acute small bowel or ileocaecal disease but evidence of drug efficacy from controlled studies is not yet available. It seems reasonable to advise Pentasa (1 g tds) for active extensive small bowel disease, and Claversal or Asacol for ileocaecal disease. Sulphasalazine, olsalazine (Dipentum), Claversal or Asacol can be used for active colonic disease.

Antibiotics

The use of broad spectrum antibacterial agents is attractive for several reasons. Bacterial toxins and metabolites may play a role in the pathogenesis of Crohn's disease. Measures to modify gut flora, reduce the antigenic load and presence of enteroadhesive bacteria may be beneficial. Unfortunately, despite several favourable uncontrolled studies, there is no controlled study showing evidence of benefit. At present the use of broad spectrum antibiotics in active Crohn's disease should be limited to patients in whom there is evidence of secondary bacterial invasion of tissue to produce an inflammatory mass or abscess. In a Swedish randomized double-blind study metronidazole (800 mg/day) was found to be as efficacious as sulphasalazine (3 g/day) in active Crohn's colitis (Ursing et al, 1982). As sulphasalazine produces only a modest improvement in Crohn's colitis, it follows that metronidazole is also only moderately effective. Potential side effects include peripheral neuropathy, metallic taste and glossitis; they are unusual at a dose of 800 mg/day. Metronidazole is of no proven benefit in small bowel Crohn's disease.

Anti-mycobacterial antibiotics have been advocated since *Mycobacterium paratuberculosis* has been isolated from a few patients with Crohn's disease and there is the possibility that mycobacteria may be involved in the pathogenesis of the disease. Double therapies have been tried in controlled studies without demonstrable benefit and quadruple drug regimes have now been advocated. There is no controlled evidence that these regimes are effective and any beneficial effect could be due to a non-specific antibiotic action rather than anti-mycobacterial action. These agents commonly produce side effects and we do not prescribe them at present.

Immunosuppressive agents

Several studies have shown that azathioprine or its metabolite 6-mercaptopurine (6MP) may be beneficial in chronic active disease and have a steroid sparing effect (O'Donoghue et al, 1978; Present et al, 1980). Use of these agents is however limited by their potential toxicity. Neutropaenia, particularly likely to occur in those patients with an inherited deficiency of the methyl-transferase enzyme (about one in 300) (Lennard et al, 1989), is life threatening but reversible. Pancreatitis, another potentially serious complication, is also important but reversible. The other important consideration in the use of these drugs is their slow onset of action. Benefit is usually only seen after 2–3 months of therapy. This really precludes their use in acute disease but they should still be considered as an adjunct for steroid-dependent patients.

Cyclosporin is currently being evaluated and appears to act rapidly. It may turn out to be a useful treatment given for a short period in acute disease but further data are needed before its general use can be considered (Brynskov et al, 1989; Sachar, 1989).

Symptomatic relief

Patients with active Crohn's disease are often severely incapacitated by pain and diarrhoea. Effective analgesia is important but as far as possible avoiding drug dependence. Antidiarrhoeal agents (loperamide 2–4 mg tds or codeine phosphate 30–60 mg tds) may provide symptomatic relief and the latter has a minor analgesic effect.

Complications of acute Crohn's disease and their management

The complications of acute Crohn's disease are summarized in Table 5.

Intestinal obstruction

Patients with Crohn's disease may present with intestinal obstruction due to a variety of causes. Strictures may be the end result of healing by fibrosis ('mechanical') or, alternatively, actively inflamed bowel may be oedematous with luminal narrowing ('inflammatory'). Usually intestinal narrowing is due to a combination of mechanical and inflammatory factors. Sometimes, patients who have had previous surgery develop adhesions which may cause bowel obstruction. The symptomatology depends on the site, degree and extent of narrowing of bowel and consistency of the intestinal content. Significant strictures cause bowel obstruction which may present acutely (rare) or subacutely. Abdominal colic and distension, vomiting and constipation may be precipitated by poorly digested foods (e.g. nuts and orange pith) causing so-called bolus colic. Colonic strictures may well be asymptomatic especially if the stool is loose or semi-formed.

Vomiting is an early symptom of gastric outlet obstruction due to gastroduodenal Crohn's disease and this may cause rapid electrolyte disturbance with alkalosis, hyponatraemia and dehydration. Small bowel obstruction is much more likely to be distal than proximal as a consequence of terminal ileal disease.

Radiological investigation will usually define the site and extent of narrowing. A plain abdominal radiograph in the erect position may confirm the presence of intestinal obstruction. A barium small bowel X-ray is the preferred study in small bowel obstruction but is contraindicated in complete obstruction. Colonoscopy with brush cytology and biopsy of the strictured area is the definitive investigation for colonic strictures.

Therapy of small bowel obstruction depends on the cause. If active disease is present on the basis of disease assessment clinically and using laboratory indices (raised C-reactive protein, low albumin and haemoglobin), then a trial of medical therapy, usually with a corticosteroid is warranted. If the obstruction is felt to be due to a 'mechanical' stricture in the absence of active disease, then medical therapy is most unlikely to be helpful and surgical resection is indicated. In practice, most patients fall into the grey area and have a combination of active disease and mechanical obstruction.

Intra-abdominal abscess

Intra-abdominal abscesses may arise spontaneously or in a postsurgical situation due to an anastomotic leak or infected haematoma (within 2 months of surgery).

Abscesses present with pain (either new or a change in preexisting pain), fever, and often a palpable mass. An ileopsoas abscess classically causes spasm of the muscle with fixed flexion of the (usually right) hip (Burul et al, 1980).

Laboratory investigations are non-specific but a neutrophil leucocytosis is characteristic. Very often the serum albumin is low. Blood cultures may be positive if the abscess causes bacteraemia. Ultrasonography is the most accessible investigation to delineate the problem. In difficult cases, computerized tomography provides more accurate anatomical visualization. Radioisotope-labelled leucocytes may help in localizing an abscess but this facility is not generally available.

Intra-abdominal or intrapelvic abscesses usually require surgical drainage but sometimes percutaneous drainage under ultrasound control is possible, thus avoiding surgery (Casola et al, 1987). Drainage of an abscess may be followed by development of an enterocutaneous fistula.

Fistulas

Enterovesical fistulas Enterovesical fistulas are more common in males and usually associated with long-standing disease. They can be asymptomatic but generally present with pneumaturia, recurrent cystitis and occasionally faecaluria. Barium studies of the colon or small bowel or intravenous urography may define the fistula; cystoscopy may be of further help. These fistulas usually require surgical repair and localized intestinal resection, though vesicocolic fistulas can sometimes be controlled for long periods with azathioprine (Glass et al, 1985).

Enterocutaneous fistulas Enterocutaneous fistulas usually complicate surgically treated Crohn's disease. They present with a leak of bowel content through a defect in the abdominal wall and overlying skin. Fistulography will confirm a connection with the intestine and define the anatomy. Postoperative fistulas may heal with bowel rest and parenteral nutrition for a 4–6 week period. Those due to underlying active disease usually require resection of the diseased segment of gut.

Enteroenteral fistulas Enteroenteral fistulas are often asymptomatic and found incidentally on barium studies. Connections may occur between adjacent loops of small bowel, small bowel and colon and adherent loops of colon (Glass et al, 1985) (Figure 4). Bacterial contamination of the upper small intestine due to an enterocolonic fistula can lead to malabsorption. If the fistula contributes to ill health, surgery is usually necessary to disconnect the adjacent loops and resect the involved bowel. Nutritional support may be indicated for those patients with significant malabsorption.

Very rarely, fistulating Crohn's disease may involve the joints presenting as an acute septic arthritis (Shreeve et al, 1982).

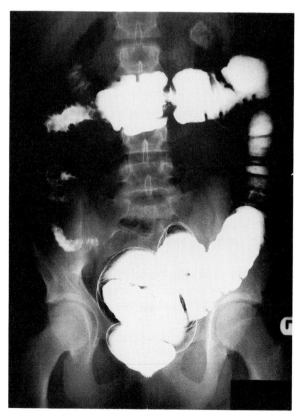

FIGURE 4 Barium enema showing an ileotransverse anastomosis with ulceration of the distal ileum and a duodenocolic fistula.

Haemorrhage

Upper gastrointestinal haemorrhage may complicate gastroduodenal or jejunal disease in a small proportion of cases. Patients present with melaena; haematemesis is unusual. It is mandatory to perform upper gastrointestinal panendoscopy if haemorrhage is suspected. This may reveal an unsuspected peptic ulcer or demonstrate involvement of the upper gastrointestinal tract with Crohn's disease. Terminal ileal disease with bleeding may be visualized at colonoscopy but often a small bowel source of bleeding remains obscure after 'top and tail' endoscopy. If the rate of bleeding is greater than 0.5 ml/min, mesenteric angiography may help to localize the site.

Disorders of the clotting cascade may complicate Crohn's disease if there is significant malabsorption of vitamin K and also if the haemorrhage is prolonged. A full clotting screen is essential prior to transfusion as replacement of clotting factors (with fresh frozen plasma) may be necessary.

Definitive management of massive colonic or upper gastrointestinal bleeding involves resection of the involved segment of gut. The surgeon will want to limit the resection and should be provided with as much information as possible regarding the site of bleeding and the extent of local inflammation.

Anorectal lesions

Anorectal lesions are common in Crohn's disease, occurring in up to 80% of patients. They may predate gastrointestinal symptoms by some years. They are more commonly associated with colonic disease than with small bowel disease. The treatment of anal fissure and perianal abscess has been described above.

Perianal fistula A perianal fistula may occur *de novo* or more commonly complicate an abscess. Fistulas are often multiple and complex in Crohn's disease. They present as a discharging hole close to or distant from the anus. These lesions often produce fewer symptoms than their appearance suggests. Pain is rarely a problem unless drainage becomes obstructed and the most common complaint is of a messy discharge requiring the use of a pad. Surgery is generally limited to laying open low fistulas or ensuring free drainage in high fistulas.

Rectovaginal fistulas A rectovaginal fistula is due to extension of an abscess in the rectovaginal septum. It usually presents with a painless foul discharge per vagina. This may be accompanied by faeces and flatus. Sigmoidoscopy and speculum examination may define the connection, which is often at the level of the anorectal junction, but sometimes a barium enema examination is required.

Treatment of these fistulas may not be necessary if, as is often the case, the problem is well tolerated. Symptoms may be minimal as long as the stools are solid, but become troublesome if liquid diarrhoea develops. Metronidazole, 800 mg/day, may reduce pain and discharge. Surgical correction is sometimes attempted usually with a diverting colostomy. In severe cases, the fistula may be an indication for rectal excision.

For recurrent or resistant perianal disease, metronidazole has been shown to suppress the inflammation but this tends to recur when the drug is stopped (Bernstein et al, 1980). The use of immunosuppressives in this context remains controversial. An elemental diet may improve intestinal absorption, reduce diarrhoea and disease activity and speed healing of perianal disease.

High stomal output

Patients with an ileostomy may become unwell due to an abnormally high stomal output. This may be due to recurrent disease, infectious enteritis, subacute bowel obstruction, or occult sepsis (for example a pelvic abscess). Salt (ileostomy effluent contains approximately 100 mmol Na/l) and water are rapidly lost and the patient quickly dehydrates. Hypotension and oliguria are typical features and the urine will contain less than 10 mmol Na if the kidneys are working normally. Increasing the water intake by mouth exacerbates the high output and leads to severe loss. Some patients may maintain fluid balance by taking 1–1.5 l of a glucose–electrolyte solution (NaCl 90 mM, glucose 100 mM) by mouth over 24 h. Intravenous saline replacement is indicated in those with a persistent negative fluid balance.

Crohn's disease and pregnancy

Patients with active disease at conception tend to continue with active disease during pregnancy and this group has a high rate of spontaneous abortion. (Khosla et al, 1984). As for colitis in pregnancy, corticosteroids, sulphasalazine or mesalazine may be given in conventional doses.

CONCLUSIONS AND THE WAY FORWARD

Acute ulcerative colitis remains a serious and potentially life-threatening problem, but improvements in medical therapy and prompt surgical intervention for non-responders have contributed to a considerable reduction in mortality. Crohn's disease presents in a variety of ways and tends to be less acute. The possible development of orally active poorly absorbed steroid preparations is an exciting advance which may significantly reduce the side effects of traditional therapy. A better understanding of the inflammatory process and identification of the chemical mediators is likely to yield novel and more specific anti-inflammatory drugs.

Until these advances are realized, or other special treatment becomes available, we must concentrate on prompt diagnosis, close patient supervision and liaison between physicians and surgeons to minimize the morbidity and mortality of inflammatory bowel disease.

REFERENCES

Anderson JB, Turner GM & Williamson RCN (1987) Fulminant ulcerative colitis in late pregnancy and the puerperium. *Journal of the Royal Society of Medicine* **80**: 492–494.

Bartram CI (1976) Plain abdominal X-ray in acute colitis. *Proceedings of the Royal Society of Medicine* **69**: 617–618.

Berghouse LM, Elliott PR, Lennard-Jones JE et al (1982) Plasma prednisolone levels during intravenous therapy in acute colitis. *Gut* **23**: 980–983.

Bernstein LH, Frank MS, Brandt LJ & Boley SJ (1980) Healing of perineal Crohn's disease with metronidazole. *Gastroenterology* **79**: 357–365.

Brynskov J et al (1989) A placebo-controlled, double-blind, randomized trial of cyclosporine therapy in active chronic Crohn's disease. *New England Journal of Medicine* **321**: 845–850.

Buckell NA, Williams GT, Bartram CI & Lennard-Jones JE (1980) Depth of ulceration in acute colitis. Correlation with outcome and clinical and radiological features. *Gastroenterology* **79**: 19–25.

Burke DA, Axon ATR, Clayden SA, Dixon MF & Lacey RW (1990) The efficacy of tobramycin in the treatment of ulcerative colitis. *Alimentary Pharmacology and Therapeutics* **4**: 123–129.

Burul CJ, Ritchie JK, Hawley PR & Todd IP (1980) Psoas abscess: a complication of Crohn's disease. *British Journal of Surgery* **67**: 355–356.

Casola G, van Sonnenberg E, Neff CC, Saba RM, Withers C & Emarine CW (1987) Abscesses in Crohn's disease: percutaneous drainage. *Radiology* **163**: 19–22.

Chapman RW, Selby WS & Jewell DP (1986) Controlled trial of intravenous metronidazole as an adjunct to corticosteroids in severe ulcerative colitis. *Gut* **27**: 1210–1212.

Dickinson RJ, Ashton MG, Axon ATR, Smith RC, Yeung CK & Hill GL (1980) Controlled trial of intravenous hyperalimentation and total bowel rest as an adjunct to routine therapy of acute colitis. *Gastroenterology* **79**: 1199–1204.

Dickinson RJ, O'Connor HJ, Pinder I, Hamilton I, Johnston D & Axon ATR (1985) Double-blind controlled trial of oral vancomycin as adjunctive treatment in acute exacerbations of idiopathic colitis. *Gut* **26**: 1380–1384.

Dronfield MW, Fletcher J & Langman MJ (1974) Coincident salmonella infection in ulcerative colitis. Problems of recognition and management. *British Medical Journal* **1**: 99–100.

Edwards FC & Truelove SC (1964) The course and prognosis of ulcerative colitis. Part 3: Complications. *Gut* **5**: 15–22.

Engbaek J, Ersboll J, Faurby V, Binder V & Riis P (1975) The constipating effect of diphenoxylate in ulcerative colitis. *Scandinavian Journal of Gastroenterology* **10**: 695–698.

Farthing MJG, Rutland MD & Clark ML (1979) Retrograde spread of hydrocortisone containing foam given intrarectally in ulcerative colitis. *British Medical Journal* **2**: 822–824.

Giaffar MH, North G & Holdsworth CD (1989) Controlled trial or polymeric elemental diet in the treatment of active Crohn's disease. *Gut* **30**: A1515.

Glass RE, Ritchie JK, Lennard-Jones JE, Hawley PR & Todd IP (1985) Internal fistulas in Crohn's disease. *Diseases of the Colon and Rectum* **28**: 557–561.

Greenberg GR, Fleming CR, Jeejeebhoy KN, Rosenberg IH, Sales D & Tremaine WJ (1988) Controlled trial of bowel rest and nutritional support in the management of Crohn's disease. *Gut* **29**: 1309–1315.

Greenfield C, Aguilar Ramirez JR, Pounder RE, Williams T, Danvers M, Marper SR & Noone P (1983) Clostridium difficile and inflammatory bowel disease. *Gut* **24**: 713–717.

Greenstein AJ, Sachar DB, Gibas A, Schrag D, Heimann T, Janowitz HD & Aufses AH (1985) Outcome of toxic dilatation in ulcerative and Crohn's colitis. *Journal of Clinical Gastroenterology* **7**: 137–144.

Harries AD, Danis V, Heatley RV, Jones LA, Fifield R, Newcombe RG & Rhodes J (1983) Controlled trial of supplemented oral nutrition in Crohn's disease. *Lancet* **i**: 887–890.

Ireland A, Rosenberg W & Jewell DP (1988) High dose methylprednisolone in the treatment of active ulcerative colitis. *Gut* **29**: A1466.

Jarnerot G, Rolny P & Sandberg-Gertzen H (1985) Intensive intravenous treatment of ulcerative colitis. *Gastroenterology* **89**: 1005–1013.

Jones JH & Chapman M (1969) Definition of megacolon in colitis. *Gut* **10**: 562–564.

Jones VA, Workman E, Freeman AH, Dickinson RJ, Wilson AJ & Hunter JO (1985) Crohn's disease: maintenance of remission by diet. *Lancet* **2**: 177–180.

Khosla R, Willoughby CP & Jewell DP (1984) Crohn's disease and pregnancy. *Gut* **25**: 52–56.

Kisloff B & Adkins JC (1981) Toxic megacolon developing in a patient with long standing distal ulcerative colitis. *American Journal of Gastroenterology* **75**: 451–453.

Lennard L, Van Loon JA & Weinshilboum RM (1989) Pharmacogenetics of acute azathioprine toxicity: Relationship to thiopurine methyltransferase genetic polymorphism. *Clinical Pharmacology and Therapeutics* **46**: 149–154.

Lennard-Jones JE, Langman MJS & Avery-Jones F (1962) Faecal stasis in proctocolitis. *Gut* **3**: 301–305.

Lennard-Jones JE, Ritchie JK, Hilder W & Spicer CC (1975) Assessment of severity in colitis: A preliminary study. *Gut* **16**: 579–584.

Lochs H, Meryn S, Marosi L, Ferenci P & Hortnagel H (1983) Has total bowel rest a beneficial effect in the treatment of Crohn's disease? *Clinical Nutrition* **2**: 61–64.

Malchow H, Ewe K, Brandes JW, Goebell H, Elms H, Sommer H, Jesdinsky H (1984) European Co-operative Crohn's Disease Study (ECCDS): results of drug treatment. *Gastroenterology* **86**: 249–266.

McIntyre PB, Macrae FA, Berghouse L, English J & Lennard-Jones JE (1985) Therapeutic benefits from a poorly absorbed prednisolone enema in distal colitis. *Gut* **26**: 822–824.

McIntyre PB, Powell-Tuck J, Wood SR, Lennard-Jones JE, Lerebours E, Hecketsweiler P, Galmiche JP & Colin R (1986) Controlled trial of bowel rest in the treatment of severe acute colitis. *Gut* **27**: 481–485.

Meyers S & Janowitz HD (1985) Systemic corticosteroid therapy of ulcerative colitis. *Gastroenterology* **89**: 1189–1190.

Meyers S, Sachar DB, Goldberg JD & Janowitz HD (1983) Corticotropin versus hydrocortisone in the intravenous treatment of ulcerative colitis. *Gastroenterology* **85**: 351–357.

Mogadam M, Dobbins WO, Korelitz BI & Ahmed SW (1981) Pregnancy in inflammatory bowel disease: effect of sulfasalazine and corticosteroids on fetal outcome. *Gastroenterology* **80**: 72–78.

Mortensen NJ McC, Ritchie JK, Hawley PR, Todd IP & Lennard-Jones JE (1984) Surgery for acute Crohn's colitis; results and long-term follow up. *British Journal of Surgery* **71**: 783–784.

O'Donoghue DP, Dawson AM, Powell-Tuck J, Bown RL & Lennard-Jones JE (1978) Double-blind withdrawal trial of azathioprine as maintenance treatment for Crohn's disease. *Lancet* **2**: 955–957.

O'Moráin C, Segal AW & Levi AJ (1984) Elemental diet as primary therapy of acute Crohn's disease: a controlled trial. *British Medical Journal* **288**: 1859–1862.

Ostro MJ, Greenberg GR & Jeejeebhoy KN (1985). Total parenteral nutrition and complete bowel rest in the management of Crohn's disease. *Journal of Parenteral and Enteral Nutrition* **9**: 280–287.

Park RHR, Galloway A, Danesh BJZ & Russell RI (1989) Double-blind trial comparing elemental and polymeric diet as primary treatment for active Crohn's disease. *Gut* **30**: 1453.

Present DH, Korelitz BI, Wisch N, Glass JL, Sachar DB & Pasternak BS (1980) Treatment of Crohn's disease with 6-mercaptopurine: a long-term randomised double-blind study. *New England Journal of Medicine* **302**: 981–987.

Rachmilevitz D et al (1989) Coated mesalazine (5-aminosalicylic acid) versus sulphasalazine in the treatment of active ulcerative colitis: a randomised trial. *British Medical Journal* **298**: 82–86.

Riley SA, Mani I, Goodman MJ, Herd ME, Dutt S & Turnberg LA (1988) Comparison of delayed release 5-aminosalicylic acid (mesalazine) and sulphasalazine in the treatment of mild to moderate ulcerative colitis relapse. *Gut* **29**: 669–674.

Sachar DB (1989) Cyclosporine treatment for inflammatory bowel disease: a step backward or a leap forward? *New England Journal of Medicine* **321**: 894–896.

Sanderson IR, Udeen S, Davies PSW, Savage MO & Walker-Smith JA (1987) Remission induced by an elemental diet in small bowel Crohn's disease. *Archives of Disease in Childhood* **62**: 123–127.

Shreeve DR, Ormerod LP & Dunbar EM (1982) Crohn's disease with fistulae involving joints. *Journal of the Royal Society of Medicine* **75**: 946–948.

Summers RW, Switz DM, Sessions JT jr., Becktel JM, Best WR, Kern F Jr & Singleton JW (1979) National Co-operative Crohn's Disease Study: results of drug treatment. *Gastroenterology* **77**: 847–869.

Swarbrick ET, Loose H & Lennard-Jones JE (1974) Enema volume as an important factor in successful topical corticosteroid treatment of colitis. *Journal of the Royal Society of Medicine* **67**: 23–24.

Symonds J (1988) Haemorrhagic colitis and Escherichia coli 0157—a pathogen unmasked. *British Medical Journal* **296**: 875–876.

Thomas BM (1979) The instant enema in inflammatory disease of the colon. *Clinical Radiology* **22**: 434–442.

Truelove SC & Jewell DP (1974) Intensive intravenous regimen for severe attacks of ulcerative colitis. *Lancet* **i**: 1067–1070.

Truelove SC & Witts LJ (1955) Cortisone in ulcerative colitis. Report on therapeutic trial. *British Medical Journal* **2**: 1041–1048.

Truelove SC & Witts LJ (1959) Cortisone and corticotropin in ulcerative colitis. *British Medical Journal* **1**: 387–394.

Truelove SC, Lee EG, Willoughby CP & Kettlewell MGW (1978) Further experience in the treatment of severe attacks of ulcerative colitis. *Lancet* **ii**: 1086–1088.

Ursing B et al (1982) A comparative study of metronidazole and sulfasalazine for active Crohn's disease: The cooperative Crohn's disease study in Sweden. 2. Result. *Gastroenterology* **83**: 550–562.

Willoughby CP & Truelove SC (1980) Ulcerative colitis and pregnancy. *Gut* **21**: 469–474.

10

THE PLACE OF SURGERY IN ACUTE INFLAMMATORY BOWEL DISEASE

J. Alexander-Williams and A. Allan

In patients with a first attack of acute colitis and with no previous symptoms, it may be unclear whether the patient is suffering from ulcerative or Crohn's colitis. However, because the management of these two conditions is similar they can be conveniently described together in the first part of the chapter.

THE PLACE OF SURGERY IN SEVERE ACUTE COLITIS

The characteristics of patients presenting with severe acute colitis

Severe acute colitis is the most common indication for urgent surgery in patients with inflammatory bowel disease. Nevertheless, a district general hospital admits only about three patients with acute colitis each year as emergencies (Buckell and Lennard-Jones, 1979). This relative rarity of a potentially lethal disease may increase the hazard to the patient because of unfamiliarity of the medical team with the condition. Buckell and Lennard-Jones (1979) have shown that patients with acute colitis presenting to physicians at district general hospitals are more likely to be suffering from a first attack of the condition and, when compared with patients presenting at specialist gastrointestinal units, are less likely to have a firm diagnosis of their illness before admission. So the 'generalist' may be faced with a more difficult diagnostic problem than the 'specialist'.

Although it is often impossible to be sure whether severe acute colitis in a particular individual is due to ulcerative or Crohn's colitis there are usually some differences in presentation. Compared with patients with ulcerative colitis, those with severe acute Crohn's colitis usually have a shorter history and less diarrhoea, present more frequently with anal lesions, have lower serum albumin levels, higher temperatures and more profound weight loss.

Colonic dilatation was found to occur in 12% of 187 patients admitted with severe acute colitis (Buckell and Lennard-Jones, 1979). This complication was seen on plain X-rays usually by the end of the second day following admission. When colonic dilatation was first recognized radiologically the clinical features had no consistent pattern and, because clinical signs do not predict colonic dilatation, general practitioners should be encouraged to refer for X-ray any patient with relapse of colitis or persistent severe unexplained diarrhoea. In Buckell and Lennard-Jones' series the response rate to intensive medical treatment was approximately 80%. However, seven patients died, two during medical treatment and five after urgent operation. This gave an overall mortality of 4.5% for patients with a severe attack of ulcerative colitis and a mortality of 8.3% for those with a severe attack of Crohn's colitis (Buckell and Lennard-Jones, 1979).

Intensive medical treatment for severe acute colitis

On admission to hospital many patients with acute colitis are severely ill. In these patients, urgent resuscitation must be combined with an attempt to diagnose the nature of the colitis as accurately as possible. Infective colitides must be excluded by culture of stools for enteropathic bacteria including *Campylobacter* spp. and *Clostridium difficile*. There should also be an examination of a hot stool for ova, cysts and parasites. Rigid sigmoidoscopy is a convenient way to obtain faeces for culture, to confirm the presence of proctitis and take a rectal biopsy for histological examination. Plain X-ray of the abdomen is essential to exclude colonic dilatation and, in ill patients, should be repeated every 24 h.

Patients with severe acute colitis are usually fluid depleted and may have multiple nutritional deficiencies as a result of anorexia as well as intestinal blood and protein loss. It is common to find that patients have severe hypokalaemia, and hypoalbuminaemia. Anaemia is common and is usually caused by a combination of blood loss and bone marrow depression.

Medical treatment consists of specific drug therapy for the colitis, therapy to improve the general condition of the patient and nutritional support.

Intravenous steroids are useful in the treatment of acute colitis. In one study 80% of patients with severe acute colitis responded to steroids within 5 days (Buckell and Lennard-Jones, 1979). In other studies both prednisolone 60 mg daily or hydrocortisone 300 mg daily were associated with remission in 60% of cases; a further 15% of cases improved on this regimen, but 25% remained in a severe condition (Truelove et al, 1978; Truelove, 1988).

If the patient can retain it, hydrocortisone acetate foam can be given by rectal infusion at a dose of 125 mg twice daily. Intravenous fluid is given to correct fluid and electrolyte deficiencies and, where necessary, albumin solutions to restore imbalances in oncotic pressures and whole blood if there is severe anaemia. Regular monitoring of serum electrolyte levels ensures that abnormalities are corrected to the normal ranges; this is particularly important should urgent operation become necessary.

There is no evidence from controlled studies to support the use of antibiotics in the treatment of acute colitis; in particular metronidazole has been shown to confer no advantage (Chapman et al, 1986). However, if the differential diagnosis includes pseudomembranous colitis there might be an indication to use oral metronidazole or vancomycin. Antidiarrhoeal drugs should be avoided during the acute attack, because they may precipitate toxic megacolon.

Nutritional support is important for patients with severe acute colitis, especially if the patient is to be in optimal condition for major surgery. Although a controlled trial of intravenous hyperalimentation and total bowel rest has shown no advantage in the final outcome of patients with acute colitis, those receiving intravenous hyperalimentation preserved their nutritional status compared with a mean loss of 7.3% of body protein mass in the control group (Dickinson et al, 1980). Enteral nutrition is well tolerated in patients with acute colitis; although small bowel transit is increased, both fat and sugars are absorbed normally. Provided there are no signs of colonic dilatation enteral nutrition is safe in patients with acute colitis and has been shown to be associated with a rise in serum albumin levels (Rao et al, 1987).

Prediction of success of medical management

Lennard-Jones et al (1975) found that at the end of the first 24 h in hospital, if the stool frequency of the patient was less than eight and the maximum temperature was 38°C or less there was a high probability that the patient would respond to medical treatment. However, patients with a higher stool frequency and a temperature greater than 38°C had an 80% chance of failing to respond to medical treatment and of needing surgical treatment.

The optimal timing of operation for severe acute colitis

Operation is indicated in patients with severe acute colitis if the patient continues to deteriorate despite the treatment programme outlined above. Patients who do not improve significantly after 5 days treatment should also be considered for operation.

Patients with severe acute attacks of ulcerative colitis managed by intensive medical means for more than 12 days have been compared with patients similarly managed for a maximum of 8 days. In the patients treated for at least 12 days, 52% went into spontaneous remission and this is not significantly different from the patients managed medically for less than 8 days. Furthermore, in the patients treated for less than 8 days the medical mortality was 0.7% and the operative mortality was 7% compared with a medical mortality of 4.8% and operative mortality of 20% in those treated for longer. Therefore there is a strong case for operating on patients with severe acute colitis after 5–8 days of medical treatment, because by prolonging medical treatment for another week few extra remissions were achieved and the associated mortality rose sharply with prolonged medical treatment (Goligher et al, 1970). The policy of advocating early operation in patients who do not respond to medical treatment was further supported by a series of patients studied by Truelove and Marks (1981). They reported no mortality in patients initially treated medically and resorting to surgery if there was no marked improvement within the first 5 days.

We normally recommend operation in patients who do not respond to intensive medical treatment within 5 days as well as in patients with radiological signs of progressive colonic dilatation. In addition, patients who deteriorate suddenly, especially with a sudden rise in pulse rate, are considered for urgent surgical intervention because such deterioration may herald a colonic perforation; it may be hazardous to await local physical signs (de Dombal et al, 1965).

Some patients respond sufficiently to avoid urgent operation during the first week of treatment but remain without complete remission, the so-called 'smouldering' case. In such 'smouldering' cases azathioprine has been tried but the response was disappointing (Jewell and Truelove, 1974). We believe that it is important to avoid prolonged medical treatment in the 'smouldering' case beyond a point where nutritional parameters such as serum albumin can be made optimal. In practice we aim to operate on those patients who have not resolved completely within 1 month of the onset of their attack.

Which operative procedure for patients with severe acute colitis?

Twenty years ago, the operation most widely favoured for the treatment of patients with severe acute colitis was a one stage proctocolectomy and ileostomy (Goligher et al, 1970; Binder et al, 1975). Ileostomy and subtotal colectomy with preservation of the rectal stump was reserved for either the very ill or those with some rectal sparing. In the ill patients the disadvantages of leaving the diseased rectum were outweighed by avoiding the trauma associated with rectal excision and in patients with rectal sparing subsequent restoration of continuity was a possibility.

Flatmark et al (1975) have shown no significant difference in mortality or morbidity between the results of one stage total proctocolectomy and total colectomy with preservation of the rectal stump. During the last 15 years there has been a steady swing away from proctocolectomy towards total colectomy with preservation of a rectal stump. There are good reasons for this change in policy. Many patients who require an emergency operation do so during an early phase of the disease, sometimes as a culmination of the first severe attack. Such patients will be unprepared psychologically for the prospect of living with a permanent ileostomy. The retention of the rectal stump leaves a possibility of restoration of continuity at a later stage, either as an ileoanal pouch procedure or as an ileorectal anastomosis. The potential benefit from staging the operation is that the patient can be restored to health before the major restorative operation, with an improved nutritional status and a decreased steroid intake. Furthermore, the excised colon can be examined histologically and this may reduce the risk of constructing a pouch in a patient with Crohn's disease.

Recent evidence has confirmed that morbidity and mortality rates are reduced by retention of the rectal stump, probably by reducing the blood loss associated with rectal excision. In a series of 176 patients treated for severe acute ulcerative colitis at St Mark's Hospital between 1963 and 1986, 62 had a panproctocolectomy and seven died (an operative mortality of 11%), whereas 111 had a total colectomy and iloestomy and four died (an operative mortality of 4%) (Hawley, 1988). We have used colectomy with immediate ileorectal anastomosis with good results but recognize the risk of anastomotic dehiscence even when the anastomosis is covered with a loop ileostomy. We would not recommend the procedure to inexperienced or trainee surgeons.

Some surgeons who are particularly experienced with ileoanal pouch procedures have used the operation in patients with severe acute colitis with satisfactory results. We do not advocate this, because our patients are generally nutritionally depleted and immunocompromised. In the last 20 years we have not used ileostomy and decompression of the distal colon as recommended by Turnbull et al (1970), although we recognize that others have used it with good results (Fazio, 1980).

Perioperative management

We start a combination of intravenous antibiotics such as cefuroxime (1.5 g) and metronidazole (0.5 g) at induction of anaesthesia and continue this treatment for 5 days following operation (Hares et al, 1982). Anti-embolism stockings are fitted before operation (Allan et al, 1983). We prefer to avoid the use of prophylactic subcutaneous heparin in patients with inflammatory bowel disease. Intravenous hydrocortisone (100 mg) is given as steroid cover during and immediately after operation.

Operation

The patient is placed supine with a small balloon catheter in the bladder and a large one in the rectum. The ileostomy site may be trephined before the midline incision is made so that all layers of the anterior abdominal wall are correctly orientated. However, we usually simply mark its site by a scratch until the operative plan is confirmed.

The colon is mobilized with care, from caecal pole to rectosigmoid junction. Particular care should be taken in mobilizing the splenic flexure and in cases of difficulty the midline incision is extended or a lateral subcostal T-shaped extension made. Areas of colon stuck to omentum or parietal peritoneum should be mobilized with a patch of adherent tissue to avoid opening a sealed perforation. The ileocaecal junction can be neatly divided and closed by applying the GIA cutting and stapling instrument, which removes the risk of soilage associated with clamp slippage. All ligatures to vessels should be absorbable. It is convenient to place the mobilized colon into a plastic isolation bag. The dissection of the mesorectum proceeds sufficiently for the divided distal sigmoid colon to be brought out to the anterior abdominal wall without tension.

The distal sigmoid or rectal mucosa can be sutured to the skin margin at the lower end of the midline wound to form a mucus fistula, or the stump, already closed by staples, is sutured to the lower end of the anterior rectus sheath. The surgeon must take care if the stump is friable; the sutures may cut out of the serosa with subsequent stump retraction into the abdomen. An alternative way of closing the rectal stump with more secure fixation is to use the blade of a crushing Zachary–Cope clamp which is left attached to the patient at skin level. It separates, or is removed, on the seventh or eighth day after operation.

If there has been no perforation or soiling, the peritoneal cavity can be closed without drainage. We use large-bite continuous polydioxanone to close the midline incision in one layer. The skin is closed loosely with a few interrupted nylon sutures except over the mucous fistula, or stapled stump, where it is left open.

Colonic dilatation

Progressive colonic dilatation is an absolute indication for urgent surgery in patients with severe acute colitis. The diameter of the gas-filled dilated colon is said to be about 8 cm (Jones and Chapman, 1969). However, many authorities consider that a diameter of greater than 5 cm is a cause for concern, particularly if air contrast X-rays indicate ulceration penetrating the muscle layer (Buckel et al, 1980) (Figure 1). In this complication the colonic muscle fibres become pale, swollen and surrounded by inflammatory exudate. Damage to smooth muscle cells leads to a loss of intestinal motility over such a length of colon that the proximal bowel is unable to project its contents through the paralysed segment (Sampson and Walker, 1961). Clinical signs bear little relationship to the severity of colonic

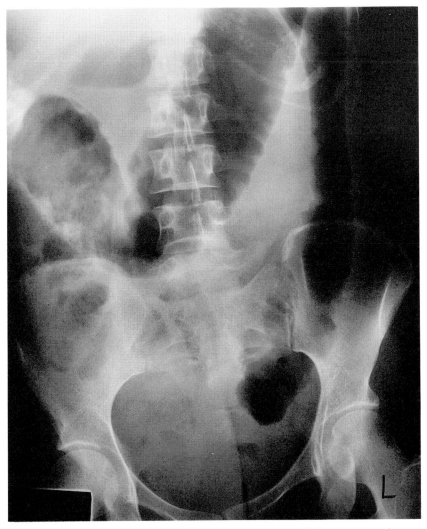

FIGURE I   Plain X-ray of the abdomen showing faecal distension of the caecum and a transverse diameter of the transverse colon of 5 cm.

dilatation and, if this complication is to be detected before perforation occurs, a daily plain abdominal film is necessary. When the patient has had frequent bowel motions, the number becomes strikingly reduced as dilatation increases. In an ill patient, complete cessation of the passage of faeces or flatus is a serious sign.

All patients with colonic dilatation should have urgent resuscitation followed by early operation. Resuscitation should not take longer than 6 h because of the risk of colonic perforation, which may increase the postoperative mortality to as high as 50% (Binder et al, 1974). Although 'less than colectomy' was advocated by Turnbull et al (1970, 1971) who performed a loop ileostomy and a 'blow-hole' decompressing colostomy, this is a technique that has not found favour in our centre and today is rarely used except at the Cleveland Clinic where it was originated and where they still have referred a few seriously ill patients with neglected megacolon (Fazio, 1980). In our centre we always aim to undertake surgical treatment before the patient has become too ill to preclude total colectomy. Total colectomy and ileostomy and a distal mucous fistula is our preferred operation for toxic megacolon. In some of our patients in whom the histological diagnosis has proved to be Crohn's colitis we have been able to perform a secondary ileorectal reconstruction and in many patients in whom the diagnosis has been confirmed as ulcerative colitis we have been able to perform a secondary proctectomy, preserving the anus and restoring continuity with an ileal anal pouch. The results of prolonged medical treatment for toxic dilatation of the colon are extremely poor. Grant and Dozois (1984) reported that, even in patients responding to medical treatment within 48 h, 58% had an unsatisfactory long-term outcome. Youth did not confer any benefit to the outcome of medical treatment and patients with toxic dilatation of the colon secondary to Crohn's colitis did as badly as patients with dilatation secondary to ulcerative colitis (Grant and Dozois, 1984).

In patients with colonic Crohn's disease free perforation of the colon is uncommon; it was 3% in the series of Bundred and colleagues (1985) and has not occurred in our own unreported series. Colonic dilatation is said to occur only in patients already known to have colonic Crohn's disease and who are on steroids (Orda et al, 1982).

Bleeding

Although chronic blood loss and anaemia are common in inflammatory bowel disease, it is relatively uncommon to have continued acute bleeding as the principal indication for emergency surgical intervention either in Crohn's disease or in ulcerative colitis. In the Amsterdam series of 228 patients who had surgical treatment for Crohn's disease, there were only two in whom bleeding was the indication for operation and both of these were due to colonic disease (van Coevorden, 1989). In our own series of 900 operations there have been only four in whom continued bleeding has been the principal indication for surgical intervention; in three of these the bleeding was from the colon. In ulcerative colitis bleeding is usually a subsidiary factor but the continued need for blood transfusion often precipitates the decision to operate. In earlier decades we used to be concerned that patients might continue to bleed from the rectum if we performed an emergency total colectomy and left the rectum *in situ*. However, in the last 20 years we have not been forced to reoperate because of continued bleeding from a retained rectal stump following emergency total colectomy for ulcerative colitis.

Severe acute ulcerative colitis and pregnancy

Although women with ulcerative colitis often become pregnant, fulminant colitis requiring operation is rare during pregnancy. Nevertheless four such patients who needed emergency colectomy during pregnancy or in the puerperium have been reported (Anderson et al, 1987). Three had inactive colitis at conception whilst the fourth had active disease during early pregnancy. Three needed subtotal colectomy and ileostomy for toxic dilatation during the third trimester or within 5 days of delivery. The fourth underwent proctocolectomy following delivery for severe intractable colitis. There were no maternal deaths but two babies were stillborn, the third was delivered at term without complication and one survived delivery at 33 weeks. In the last case, the β-sympathomimetic agent ritodrine was given to prevent premature labour following emergency resection of a toxic megacolon. It is interesting to note the social morbidity of these unfortunate patients; three of the four women separated from their partners although two remarried (Anderson et al, 1987).

EMERGENCY OPERATION FOR SMALL BOWEL CROHN'S DISEASE

Indications

Urgent surgical treatment is usually not required for small bowel Crohn's disease. There is usually time to evaluate, plan and choose the time of operation. The crises indicating urgent surgical intervention in Crohn's disease include peritonitis, septicaemia, obstruction and bleeding. Free perforation and exsanguinating bleeding are rare (Bundred et al, 1985); obstructive symptoms normally subside on rest, rehydration and medication whereas septicaemia needs antibiotics and initial resuscitation before operation. However, there are times of relative urgency, often because the exacerbation has been neglected by the patient or physician until a crisis such as septicaemia occurs. Recently there has been interest in the hypothesis that certain patients with Crohn's disease may be at increased risk of requiring surgery because they suffer from a more aggressive form of the disease. Greenstein et al (1988) studied 770 patients with Crohn's disease and subdivided them into 375 in whom operations were carried out for 'perforating' disease, including acute free perforations, subacute perforations with abscess and chronic perforations with fistula. In this study, if any perforating indication was present, the case was classified as 'perforating' regardless of the coexistence of additional 'non-perforating' indications. Of the 375 patients operated on for 'perforating' indications, 128 required a second operation a mean of 4.7 years later, and 73% of these were for another 'perforating' indication. In contrast, those with 'non-perforating' Crohn's disease who required a second operation did so a mean of 8.8 years later, with perforation as the indication in only 29%. Further support to this hypothesis is provided by the recent retrospective review of our patients. The reoperation rates following resections for Crohn's disease of the small bowel showed two peaks of incidence at 40 and 110 months. The early peak was composed almost exclusively of patients noted to have widespread disease at their initial operative procedure, whereas the major component of the late peak was from patients with less extensive disease (Sayfan et al, 1989). Observations such as these suggest that there may be an aggressive form of the disease, which shows a greater propensity to require recurrent operations.

Abscess

The commonest indication for urgent operation in patients with Crohn's disease of the small bowel is to drain an intra-abdominal abscess. Although the site of the sepsis is sometimes obvious, it may be difficult to locate even with the help of ultrasound, CT or radiolabelled leucocyte scanning (Saverymuttu et al, 1986). The abscess, once detected and located, requires open or percutaneous drainage. Although non-operative drainage is an attractive option it often fails, particularly when the abscess is extensive with tracks leading beyond the abdomen into the thigh, buttock or perineum. In such patients adequate drainage is difficult to achieve and it is often necessary to operate to remove the affected bowel from which the abscess originates. In many patients we have found extraperitoneal connections with abscesses, such as psoas abscesses, that have evaded preoperative detection by scanning. Simple drainage of abscesses is almost invariably followed by a fistula so that, if laparotomy has to be performed for an abscess, it is best also to resect the affected gut.

Patients with an acute abscess secondary to Crohn's disease may be severely ill, with septicaemia and fluid depletion. Initial treatment includes intravenous fluid and antibiotics. It should be possible to control the septicaemia within 12–24 h of admission. The precise timing of surgery to drain an abscess will depend upon the site of the abscess and on the response of the patient to intensive resuscitation. It may be a simple matter to drain a large palpable subcutaneous collection in the anterior abdominal wall of even a severely ill patient but a complex abscess deep in the pelvis may not become apparent until the patient is adequately resuscitated and can then be investigated more extensively with ultrasound or CT scanning.

Immediate treatment of fistula for patients with Crohn's disease

It is always advisable to avoid a major operation on ill patients as they are often immunocompromised from prolonged malnutrition, steroid therapy and immunosuppressive drugs. Furthermore, blood transfusion may be needed, which further compromises the immune response (Tartter et al, 1988). It is not surprising therefore that the postoperative complication rate is high. Heimann et al (1985) reported 130 patients needing early operation, usually for septic complications of their Crohn's disease, 30% of whom had at least one serious postoperative complication. Our own experience is similar; therefore where possible, we try simple drainage first with urgent measures to improve the patient's nutrition, and delay definitive laparotomy and resection for from 2 to 12 weeks. Total parenteral nutrition is rarely required and then rarely for more than 2 weeks. Although there is uncontrolled evidence to suggest that preoperative intravenous feeding will improve the patients nutritional status and decrease the risk of complications (Gouma et al, 1988) we only use it as a preliminary to restarting alimentary feeding and not as a substitute for timely surgical intervention.

The use of loop or split ileostomy in sick patients with a severe acute exacerbation of ileocaecal Crohn's disease

On opening the abdomen the surgeon may be faced with a large oedematous mass of lower small bowel, the serosa of which bleeds freely as soon as an attempt is made to separate one bowel loop from another. In this situation a surgeon who is inexperienced in the management of inflammatory bowel disease may feel that it is not safe to attempt to free the loops of bowel forming the mass and that a safer alternative is to carry out a defunctioning ileostomy immediately above the mass. This procedure will often produce a rapid clinical improvement (Harper et al, 1983; Zelas and Jagelman, 1980), and a defunctioning operation with continued steroid and antibiotic therapy will restore the patient to good nutritional status. The acute inflammation of the Crohn's lesion is reduced prior to a definitive procedure, which can then be undertaken in safer circumstances. The definitive procedure should not be long delayed as there may be further complications and sepsis arising from the defunctioned disease.

We find that with increasing experience in the management of complicated Crohn's disease we now rarely need to use this two stage approach but usually resect the inflammatory mass at the first operation, creating an end ileostomy and mucous fistula for later reconnection.

CONCLUSIONS AND THE WAY FORWARD

Until about 20 years ago surgical intervention for acute complications in inflammatory bowel disease was fraught with dangers, and was attended by many complications and a risk of death. Although the potential for complications is still great today we have now sufficient knowledge about the indications and timing of operations and the accompanying safety precautions so that we may bring the vast majority of patients safely through their acute complications.

In patients with acute colitis the difficulties in making a precise distinction between Crohn's disease and ulcerative colitis give the strongest support for the policy of staged surgical intervention; first ridding the patient of the acute diseased bowel and second trying to restore intestinal continuity with preservation of sphincter function. Although there are clear-cut rules that govern the indications and timing of surgical intervention, their precise interpretation still exercises the niceties of clinical judgement. The message that we wish to impart is not to delay operation until treatable complications become dangerously complicated. Now that ileal reservoir-to-anus pouches have become perfected technically there is no need to feel that early surgical intervention for acute colitis is condemning the patient unnecessarily to a lifetime of an end ileostomy.

For all acute complications of colitis the preferred surgical management is a total colectomy, end ileostomy and mucous fistula of the distal bowel. The distal defunctioned bowel rarely gives serious complications and once the patient has recovered for about 6 months we consider advising proctectomy and ileoanal pouch for ulcerative colitis or an ileorectal anastomosis for Crohn's colitis.

The principal factors that have improved the safety of surgical intervention are the recognition of the importance of adequate nutrition and a healthy body defence response. Nowadays patients can usually be improved and made better able to withstand surgical reintervention.

Emergency surgical intervention in small bowel Crohn's disease is managed with the application of the same principles as already outlined. Seriously ill patients should have minimal initial intervention to allow them to be made fit for early definitive operations. Abscesses should be drained and septicaemia treated; the patients are then rapidly renourished so that they may have safe surgical intervention to overcome the primary complication of bowel stenosis.

In the future it is easy to foresee some gradual refinements of present successful measures, such as the better localization and drainage of local sepsis, the better control of sepsis with antimicrobial agents, the better, safer and speedier correction of malnutrition. It is also easy to forecast a gradual improvement in the safety and efficient function of ileal reservoir-to-anus pouches in patients with ulcerative colitis. We would like to forecast a general improvement in the collaboration between physician and surgeon in the management of inflammatory bowel disease. We would like to believe that the lessons we have learned in our own centre about the closest possible collaboration between physician and surgeon and the absence of rivalry and a struggle for patient control are being widely applied.

It is rather more difficult to forecast 'breakthrough' discoveries because, by definition, they are unexpected. We cannot see any clear indication of the expected major breakthrough in the understanding of the pathogenesis and therefore potential prevention of ulcerative colitis or Crohn's disease but, surely, some day these riddles will be solved. Until they are, good medical and surgical collaboration will mean that most patients with inflammatory bowel disease will be able to be kept at work, able to enjoy life and have confidence in the future.

REFERENCES

Allan A, Williams JT, Bolton JP & Le Quesne LP (1983) The use of graduated compression stockings in the prevention of postoperative deep vein thrombosis. *British Journal of Surgery* **70**: 172–174.
Anderson JB, Turner GB & Williamson RCN (1987) Fulminating ulcerative colitis in late pregnancy and the puerperium. *Journal of the Royal Society of Medicine* **80**: 492–494.
Binder SC, Patterson JF & Glotzer DJ (1974) Toxic megacolon in ulcerative colitis. *Gastroenterology* **66**: 909–915.

Binder SC, Miller HH & Deterling RA (1975) Emergency and urgent operations for ulcerative colitis. *Archives of Surgery* **110**: 284–289.

Buckell NA & Lennard-Jones JE (1979) How District Hospitals see acute colitis. *Lancet* **1**: 1226–1229.

Buckel MA, Williams GT, Bartram CI et al (1980) Depth of ulceration in acute colitis. *Gastroenterology* **79**: 19–25.

Bundred NJ, Dixon JM, Lumsden AB, Gilmour HB & Davis GC (1985) Free perforation in Crohn's disease. *Diseases of the Colon and Rectum* **28**: 35–37.

Chapman RW, Selby WAS & Jewell DP (1986) Controlled trial of intravenous metronidazole as an adjunct to corticosteroids in severe ulcerative colitis. *Gut* **27**: 1210–1211.

de Dombal FT, Watts J, Watkinson G & Goligher JC (1965) Intraperitoneal perforation of the colon in ulcerative colitis. *Proceedings of the Royal Society of Medicine* **58**: 713–714.

Dickinson RJ, Ashton MG, Axon ATR, Smith RC, Young CK & Hill G (1980) Controlled trial of intravenous hyperalimentation and total bowel rest as an adjunct to the continued therapy of acute colitis. *Gastroenterology* **79**: 1199–1204.

Fazio VW (1980) Toxic megacolon in ulcerative colitis and Crohn's colitis. *Clinical Gastroenterology* **9(2)**: 389.

Flatmark A, Fietheim B & Gjone E (1975) Early colectomy in severe ulcerative colitis. *Scandinavian Journal of Gastroenterology* **10**: 427–429.

Goligher JC, Hoffman DC & de Dombal FT (1970) Surgical treatment of severe attacks of ulcerative colitis with special reference to the advantages of early operation. *British Medical Journal* **4**: 703–706.

Gouma DJ, Maarten Fum M, Rouflart M & Soeters PB (1988) Preoperative total parenteral nutrition (T.P.N.) in severe Crohn's disease. *Surgery* **103**: 648–651.

Grant CS & Dozois RR (1984) Toxic megacolon: ultimate fate of patients after successful medical management. *American Journal of Surgery* **147**: 106–109.

Greenstein AJ, Lachman P, Sachar DB, Springhorn J, Heumann T, Janowitz HD & Aufses AH (1988) Perforating and non-perforating indications for repeated operations in Crohn's disease: evidence for two clinical forms. *Gut* **29**: 588–592.

Hares MM, Bently S, Allan RN, Burdon DW & Keighley MRB (1982) Clinical trials of the efficacy and duration of antibacterial cover for elective resection in inflammatory bowel disease. *British Journal of Surgery* **69**: 215–217.

Harper PR, Truelove SC, Lee ECG, Kettlewell MGW & Jewell DP (1983) Split ileostomy and ileocolostomy for Crohn's disease of the colon and ulcerative colitis: a 20 year study. *Gut* **24**: 106–113.

Hawley PR (1988) Emergency surgery for ulcerative colitis. *World Journal of Surgery* **12**: 169–173.

Heimann TM, Greenstein AJ, Mechanic LK & Aufses AH (1985) Early complications following surgical treatment for Crohn's disease. *Annals of Surgery* **201**: 494–498.

Jewell DP & Truelove SC (1974) Azathioprine in ulcerative colitis: final report on a controlled therapeutic trial. *British Medical Journal* **2**: 627–628.

Jones HJ & Chapman M (1969) Definition of megacolon in colitis. *Gut* **10**: 562–564.

Lennard-Jones JE, Ritchie JK, Hilder W & Spicer CC (1975) Assessment of severity in colitis: a preliminary study. *Gut* **16**: 579–581.

Orda R, Goldwaser B & Wizintger T (1982) Free perforation of the colon in Crohn's disease: a report of a case and review of the literature. *Disease of the Colon and Rectum* **25**: 145–147.

Rao SSC, Holdsworth CD & Forrest ARW (1987) Small intestinal absorption and tolerance of enteral nutrition in acute colitis. *British Medical Journal* **295**: 698.

Sampson PA & Walker FC (1961) Dilatation of the colon in ulcerative colitis. *British Medical Journal* **2**: 1119–1123.

Saverymuttu SM, Carmilleu M, Rees H, Lavender JP, Hodgson HJF & Chadwick VS (1986) Indium-III granulocyte scanning in the assessment of disease extent and disease activity in inflammatory bowel disease. A comparison of colonoscopy, histology and fecal indium-III granulocyte excretion. *Gastroenterology* **90**: 1121–1128.

Sayfan J, Wilson DAL, Allan A, Andrews H & Alexander-Williams J (1989) Recurrence after strictureplasty or resection for Crohn's disease. *British Journal of Surgery* **76**: 335–338.

Tartter P, Driefuss RM, Malon AM, Heimann TM & Aufses AH (1988) Relationship of postoperative septic complications and blood transfusions in patients with Crohn's disease. *American Journal of Surgery* **155**: 43–47.

Truelove SC (1988) Medical management of ulcerative colitis and indications for colectomy. *World Journal of Surgery* **12**: 142–147.

Truelove SC & Marks CG (1981) Toxic megacolon. *Clinics in Gastroenterology* **i**: 107–110.

Truelove SC, Lee ECG, Willoughby CP & Kettlewell MGW (1978) Further experiences with the treatment of severe attacks of ulcerative colitis. *Lancet* **ii**: 1086–1088.

Turnbull RB, Hawk WA & Schofield P (1970) Choice of operation for the toxic megacolon phase of non-specific ulcerative colitis. *Surgical Clinics of North America* **50**: 1151–1153.

Turnbull RB, Hawkes WA & Wheakley FL (1971) Surgical treatment of toxic megacolon: ileostomy and colostomy to prepare patient for colectomy. *American Journal of Surgery* **122**: 325–331.

van Coevorden F (1989) *Surgical aspects of Crohn's disease*. Thesis, University of Amsterdam.

Zelas P & Jagelman DG (1980) Loop ileostomy in the management of Crohn's colitis in the debilitated patient. *Annals of Surgery* **191**: 164–168.

11

PROBLEMS OF INTESTINAL OBSTRUCTION

R. A. Cobb and R. C. N. Williamson

INTRODUCTION

The incidence of acute intestinal obstruction in adults in the United Kingdom decreased by approximately 50% between 1960 and 1980 (Bevan, 1982). Common causes of intestinal obstruction are listed in Table 1. The pattern of pathology seen in clinical practice has also changed: neglected hernias and obstructed colonic tumours have become less frequent, while adhesion obstruction of the small bowel has become more frequent not only in relation to the total number of emergency admissions but also in absolute numbers. Despite the reduction in numbers of admissions, intestinal obstruction remains a common general surgical emergency, accounting for 3% of emergency admissions (Bevan, 1982).

In this chapter the management of adult intestinal obstruction will be discussed both for the small intestine and the large intestine. Specific problems that arise in diagnosis and treatment will be explored.

TABLE 1
The causes of intestinal obstruction in adults

	Within lumen	In intestinal wall	Outside intestinal wall
Small intestine	Foreign body	Primary neoplasm	External hernia
	Gallstone	Secondary neoplasm	Internal hernia
	Food bolus	Crohn's disease	Adhesions
		Radiation enteropathy	Secondary neoplasm
		Intussusception	Volvulus
		Endometriosis	
Large intestine	Foreign body	Primary neoplasm	External hernia
		Secondary neoplasm	Volvulus
		Diverticulitis	
		Crohn's disease	
		Radiation colitis	
		Intussusception	
		Endometriosis	

SMALL BOWEL OBSTRUCTION

Clinical features

The classical symptoms of small bowel obstruction are abdominal pain, vomiting, abdominal distension and reduced bowel actions. The pain is usually peri-umbilical and colicky. The episodes of colic tend to be of higher frequency and shorter duration than those resulting from large bowel obstruction. Vomiting occurs early, especially if the level of the obstruction is in the upper small bowel (when pain and distension may not be prominent symptoms).

On examination the patient is often dehydrated. Tachycardia, pyrexia and abdominal tenderness are worrying signs that suggest strangulation. Abdominal examination must include a careful assessment of previous scars and hernial orifices for the presence of an irreducible hernia. Prolonged auscultation is often necessary to hear the classical high-pitched obstructive bowel sounds.

Investigations

The following investigations should be performed in all patients admitted with a clinical diagnosis of small bowel obstruction: haemoglobin; white cell count; serum urea and electrolytes; serum amylase; supine abdominal X-ray; erect chest X-ray.

The radiological features of obstructed small bowel, as opposed to large bowel, are a central distribution of dilated loops and valvulae conniventes (of jejunum) or featureless mucosa (of ileum). In addition the absence of a dilated caecum will differentiate between the two.

Traditionally, erect and supine abdominal films have been requested as the standard radiological investigations for many acute abdominal problems. A retrospective audit of requests for abdominal radiographs in an accident and emergency department revealed that 25% of patients had inappropriate X-rays for conditions such as acute appendicitis and gastrointestinal bleeding (Lacey et al, 1980). In a prospective study of 102 patients admitted with acute abdominal pain, the value of the erect abdominal film was assessed. It was found that all the abnormalities seen on the erect film were also evident on the supine film (Field et al, 1985). In support, in a series of 252 patients, the supine abdominal film combined with an erect chest X-ray achieved a correct diagnosis in 98% (Mirvis et al, 1986). The authors calculated that elimination of the erect film would save $128 000 000 per annum in the United States, besides reducing the gonadal irradiation by 207 mR in men and 437 mR in women.

Thus an erect abdominal X-ray is *not* essential in order to diagnose small bowel obstruction. Small bowel obstruction will always be evident on a good quality supine abdominal film. The observation of air/fluid levels on the erect or decubitus film merely confirms the diagnosis, though such confirmation may be useful in equivocal cases.

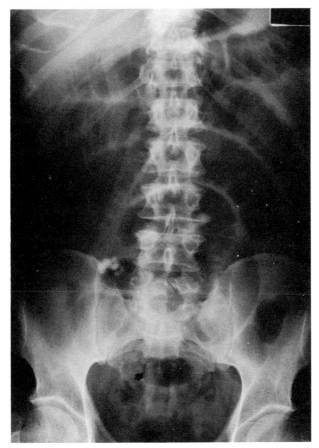

FIGURE 1 Small intestinal obstruction: distended loops are seen centrally located with valvulae conniventes. The opacity to the right of the lumbosacral joint is a calcified mesenteric lymph node.

Pathology

The increase in elective operations for hernia has markedly reduced the incidence of obstruction due to irreducible or strangulated hernias. In developing countries the pattern is different, with a high incidence of obstruction due to external hernias (Ellis, 1982). In the U.K. and the U.S.A. adhesions are now the commonest cause of small bowel obstruction, accounting for 60% of all admissions (Ellis, 1982) and nearly 50% of surgically managed cases (Mucha, 1987). In the latter series from the Mayo clinic, the causes of small bowel obstruction in 314 surgically managed cases were 49% adhesions, 16% neoplasms, 15% hernias and 20% miscellaneous. These figures are typical of western surgical practice.

The pathophysiology of postoperative adhesions

The traditional teaching was that postoperative adhesions are formed by organization of the fibrinous exudate that develops between loops of small bowel and other peritoneal surfaces where breaches of the parietal or visceral peritoneum have occurred. This theory led to the surgical practice of closing peritoneal defects at all costs. However, subsequent experiments demonstrated that raw peritoneal surfaces heal rapidly and that closing peritoneal defects does not reduce (but rather *increases*) the incidence of adhesions. Ellis then showed that tissue ischaemia was the critical event in the formation of most adhesions and that the role of these adhesions was to act as vascular grafts to preserve the viability of damaged tissues (Ellis, 1971). It is impossible to validate these data in man, but the adoption of a policy of leaving peritoneal defects open has not led to an increase in the incidence of postoperative adhesions in clinical surgical practice.

Apart from tissue ischaemia, adhesions may form in reaction to substances contaminating the peritoneal cavity. Talc was used in the manufacture of surgical gloves for many years until it was shown that talc particles could be identified within the dense adhesions that were found in many patients who had undergone laparotomy. Starch was introduced as an alternative lubricant for surgical gloves, but this agent can also be associated with adhesion formation, especially after sterilization by irradiation rather than by autoclaving. Fragments of surgical swabs and suture material and spilled gut contents have also been found in some adhesions.

Prevention of adhesion formation

Most patients form adhesions after abdominal operations, but only a few (less than 5%) develop problems as a consequence. Indeed, Ellis argues that the surgeon should 'regard adhesions as friends who occasionally misbehave, rather than his enemies' (Ellis, 1982). Certainly adhesions can preserve a precarious anastomosis that is ischaemic. Nevertheless the preventable causes of adhesions should be reduced to a minimum by the following means:

(1) Non-starch-coated gloves (such as Biogel®) should be employed if available. If only starch-lubricated gloves are available, then the method of Fraser (1982) should be used to wash off all the starch powder. After putting on surgical gloves, 10 ml of Betadine® is applied and the cleansing process is continued for 1 min. The gloves are then rinsed off over 30 s with 500 ml of sterile water, with effective removal of the starch being evident by an audible and palpable click on separation of the opposed thumb and forefinger. Fraser demonstrated that there were no residual starch granules seen by light microscopy in 16 out of 20 gloves treated by this method.

(2) Care should be taken not to leave suture and swab fragments inside the peritoneal cavity.

(3) Any spillage of intestinal contents should be meticulously cleansed. If there is generalized peritoneal contamination, copious lavage should be used.

(4) The bulk of the tissue beyond a ligature should be as small as is safe to prevent the ligature slipping off, so as to minimize the extent of ischaemic tissue available for the formation of adhesions.

Pathophysiology of radiation enteritis

Both the small and the large intestine are very radiosensitive. The acute gastrointestinal side effects reflect damage to the rapidly dividing epithelial cells. The symptoms of chronic radiation enteritis occur in 2–5% of patients who have had previous abdominopelvic radiotherapy (Allen-Mersh et al, 1986). Chronic radiation enteropathy results from damage to vascular connective tissue with a progressive obliterative vasculitis. This process leads to mural thickening and mucosal ulceration. Ulceration may extend through the bowel wall, leading to perforation, fistula and abscess. Resolution of the process results in stricture formation and also dense fibrotic intraperitoneal adhesions. Both the strictures and adhesions can cause intestinal obstruction.

Initial management of small bowel obstruction

Early surgical intervention is mandatory when an irreducible external hernia is the cause, when there are features of toxicity (fever, tachycardia, leucocytosis), or when there is abdominal tenderness. In children with adhesion obstruction early operation is indicated in any case, because there is a higher incidence of strangulation than in adults (Festen, 1982).

In the absence of all these features, conservative treatment may be indicated, i.e. nasogastric aspiration, intravenous fluids and regular clinical review. Nasogastric aspiration is as effective as long-tube gastrointestinal decompression (Bizer et al, 1981), although long tubes remain popular in the United States (Wolfson et al, 1985). Intravenous fluid and electrolyte replacement should take account of the considerable gastrointestinal losses that may occur in obstructed gut.

Up to two-thirds of patients with adhesion obstruction will settle with this conservative regimen, but if there is any deterioration to suggest strangulation or if there is no improvement within 72 h, operation is indicated without further delay.

Operations for small bowel obstruction

External hernias

The operative principles are straightforward. The contents of the hernia are exposed and assessed for viability. If viable, the contents are reduced and the hernia repaired. If the contents are not viable, resection is performed before repair of the hernia. Of a series of 190 strangulated external hernias 43% were inguinal, 38% were femoral, 14% were umbilical and 5% were incisional (Andrews, 1981). In this series, the effects of viability of the hernia contents on outcome were analysed for 163 of the cases (Table 2). From these figures it is obvious that non-viable hernia contents were associated with much higher morbidity and mortality rates than viable hernia contents. Operations for irreducible external hernias must be performed as early as possible after the onset of symptoms. Therefore the

TABLE 2
The effect of viability of hernia contents on outcome

	Bowel condition		
	Absent from sac	Incarcerated, viable	Resected, non-viable
Hospital stay (days)	7.7	12.3	19.3
Wound infection (%)	9.7	16.0	41.0
Mortality rate (%)	6.6	7.3	37.0

numbers of such emergency operations should be minimized by prompt elective operation for hernias.

For an inguinal hernia causing obstruction, the same approach should be used as for an elective operation. If the contents are not viable, resection of the ischaemic small bowel can usually be performed through the sac. Occasionally the access is inadequate, in which case resection should be performed through a separate incision.

The low approach to a femoral hernia is suitable for most elective operations, and in cases of obstruction when strangulation is unlikely. When strangulation of the intestine is predicted, any of the higher approaches (e.g. those of Henry, McEvedy on the approach via the inguinal canal) are preferable because ready access to the abdominal cavity can be achieved (Kirk and Williamson, 1987).

Adhesion obstruction

If an old vertical incision is present, the best policy is to reopen it; if possible the peritoneal cavity should be entered by extension beyond the old scar. Once entry has been gained to the abdomen, the viscera should be freed from the scar and any other areas of adhesions to the parietes. The patterns of adhesions encountered are a single band, diffuse adhesions and incisional on omental bowstring (Bevan, 1984). Apart from diffuse adhesions, these patterns often lead to a closed loop internal hernia, which may be visible as a localized distended loop on the plain abdominal X-ray. These localized types of adhesions present few technical difficulties at operation.

The difficult cases are those in which dense multiple adhesions are encountered. The goal of the surgeon is to free each loop of bowel from the ligament of Treitz to the ileocaecal valve. The dissection has to be undertaken with great care to avoid damage to the bowel wall. It is wise to advance on a broad front rather than to dissect in one area only, and to attempt to stay within avascular planes. If the mucosa is breached, the defect should be closed immediately. Areas of ischaemic or densely fibrotic bowel will need to be resected.

A few patients develop recurrent obstruction due to diffuse adhesions. Simply freeing the adhesions again is associated with a very high probability of future adhesion obstruction. In these cases, two techniques have been described to maintain the intestine in an orderly configuration whilst adhesions form.

Mesenteric plication Noble (1937) described a method of mesenteric and enteric plication by means of a running suture starting at the root of the mesentery to secure the free edges of two adjacent folds of mesentery, continuing along the mesenteric borders of adjacent loops of small bowel, then back to the root of the mesentery. This is repeated for adjacent loops along the length of the small bowel so that at the end of the procedure the intestine is fixed in the fashion of a closed fan. However, the method carries an appreciable risk of intraperitoneal sepsis and fistulation between adjacent loops of intestine. The enteric component of the plication was the cause of these complications, and several simplified methods of mesenteric plication have been reported (Childs and Phillips, 1960; MacCarthy and Sharf, 1965).

Intraluminal stenting This method was described by White (1956) and later by Baker (1959). A long catheter with a balloon at the lower end is introduced into the intestinal lumen (usually via a proximal jejunostomy) and passed along the small intestine and through the ileocaecal valve. The balloon is inflated in the caecum. The proximal end of the catheter is brought through the abdominal wall. The jejunostomy must be carefully affixed around the catheter and on to the abdominal wall. Most authors recommend that this catheter is left *in situ* for 2–3 weeks whilst adhesions form. Many minor variations to this method have been described.

The major hazards of the method arise from leaks around the jejunostomy, causing intra-abdominal sepsis. Occasionally the tube may be difficult to remove.

The results of these methods in the treatment of recurrent adhesion obstruction have recently been collated by Lavelle-Jones and Cuschieri (1990) (Table 3). It is apparent that mesenteric plication gave the best long-term results, albeit with a higher operative mortality rate than intraluminal intubation. Much of the morbidity and many of the operative deaths following mesenteric plication occurred when it was performed in the presence of intraperitoneal sepsis.

Crohn's disease

It is clearly established that cure cannot be achieved by either medical or surgical therapy. One-third of patients with Crohn's disease will require reoperation within 10 years for recurrent symptomatic disease (Hulten, 1988). The devastating effects of short bowel syndrome following extensive small bowel resections have led surgeons to restrict excision to the segment causing problems. The fears of increased morbidity when anastomoses use bowel involved with the disease have not been realized, and the fashion for frozen section examination to confirm normal intestine at resection margins has passed. The observation that anastomosis in the presence of disease was safe led to the adoption of 'strictureplasty' for

TABLE 3
Results of operations for recurrent adhesion obstruction

	Operative mortality	Reoperation rate
Division of adhesions alone	3.0%	10.2%
Mesenteric plication	8.4%	3.3%
Intraluminal intubation	4.2%	5.5%

relatively short fibrotic Crohn's strictures (Lee and Papaionnou, 1982; Alexander-Williams, 1986). This technique has been demonstrated to be safe (Dehn et al, 1989). The recurrence rate following strictureplasty, as assessed by the need for reoperation, is the same as for excisional surgery (Sayfan et al, 1989). Those who perform this technique emphasize that it should be employed only for short fibrotic strictures (especially if multiple). Longer inflammatory stenoses are best managed by excision.

Radiation enteritis

Operative treatment is hazardous for many reasons. The nutritional state of the patient may be poor, multiple adhesions are commonly associated with chronic radiation enteritis and the area of affected bowel is rarely discrete. Bowel normal to the naked eye may have a blood supply compromised by small vessel damage. In contrast to Crohn's disease, extensive resections are often necessary for radiation enteritis.

Bypass procedures have been advocated (Smith and De Cosse, 1986), but the unresected diseased segment may continue to cause symptoms. Resection and primary anastomosis of irradiated bowel have a high rate of anastomotic leakage and are associated with a high operative mortality rate (Galland and Spencer, 1987). Ideally both bowel ends used for an anastomosis should be free of disease. Some authors advise use of frozen section histology to identify uninvolved gut prior to primary anastomosis (Yeoh and Horowitz, 1988), but others have not found this helpful (Galland and Spencer, 1987). It is best to use intestine from outside the radiation field for at least one end of the anastomosis. By this means Galland and Spencer had only one leak in a series of 14 patients, and this was not a clinical problem.

Following pelvic irradiation, a few patients develop a frozen pelvis without recurrent disease. In this situation either a side-to-side bypass of small bowel involved in the radiation damage or a defunctioning colostomy for distal colonic strictures may be all that is feasible. Any stoma should be fashioned using gut from outside the original radiation field.

LARGE BOWEL OBSTRUCTION

Clinical features

Large bowel obstruction typically presents with change in bowel habit, abdominal distension and colicky suprapubic pain. When constipation becomes absolute, pain and abdominal distension increase. Vomiting occurs late in comparison with small bowel obstruction. On admission to hospital many patients are dehydrated. Clinical examination confirms the abdominal distension. Tenderness in the right lower quadrant is a worrying sign, suggesting imminent caecal perforation in the presence of a competent ileocaecal valve. Operation should be performed urgently if caecal tenderness is present.

Investigations

Most cases of large bowel obstruction do not require urgent laparotomy. Adequate resuscitation with replacement of fluid and correction of electrolyte abnormalities is a mandatory prerequisite. This interval between admission and operation must also be used to identify the level and cause of the obstruction by contrast studies and, in some instances, by endoscopy. A retrospective study of 91 patients who had undergone contrast examination included 79 patients with suspected mechanical obstruction of the large bowel and 12 patients with suspected pseudo-obstruction. Of the 79 thought to have a mechanical cause, no less than 29 (37%) had no lesion demonstrated. Of the 12 with suspected pseudo-obstruction, two had a carcinoma (Koruth et al, 1985a).

These findings were confirmed in a prospective study of 117 patients admitted with suspected large bowel obstruction (Stewart et al, 1984). Ninety-nine had a clinical diagnosis of mechanical obstruction and the remaining 18 of pseudo-obstruction. Urgent contrast studies confirmed mechanical obstruction in 63 cases, but 35 patients had free flow of contrast to the caecum; 11 of these were eventually diagnosed as pseudo-obstruction. Of the 18 patients with clinical pseudo-obstruction two had a mechanical cause. Contrast studies failed on two occasions in elderly patients who were unable to retain the contrast.

The message is clear; clinical diagnosis is fallible and radiological confirmation is necessary.

Operative options for colorectal carcinoma

Mortality and survival statistics for patients with obstructing carcinomas are worse than those with non-obstructing carcinomas. Irvin and Greaney (1977) recorded an operative mortality of 38% for obstructed cases, compared with 12% for elective resections. In a multicentre study in which data were accrued prospectively (Phillips et al, 1985), there was an operative mortality rate of 23% for obstructing cancers and 11% for non-obstructing cancers. The overall 5-year survival rates were 16–23% following resection of obstructing cancers compared with 37–42% for non-obstructing cases (Ohman, 1982; Irvin and Greaney, 1977; Phillips et al, 1985). Ohman explained this difference by the observation that 72% of obstructed cases were either Dukes stage C or had disseminated disease, whereas only 51% of elective cases were in these categories. Phillips et al (1985) argued that this discrepancy was not the sole factor responsible for the poor survival data because the survival curves were parallel after 18 months; they postulated that there may be a residual effect of prolonged illness in the first year following operation.

There is no debate about the procedure of choice for large bowel obstruction caused by right-sided colonic tumours: primary resection should be followed by ileocolic anastomosis. By contrast, there is considerable debate about the best approach to an obstructing left-sided colonic tumour, and our discussion will focus on this problem.

The traditional technique for left-sided colonic obstruction was a three-stage procedure comprising: (1) a defunctioning stoma; (2) resection and anastomosis;

(3) closure of stoma. The disadvantage of this approach is that it is unduly cumbersome, with a prolonged hospital stay (Irvin and Greaney, 1977) and cumulative morbidity and mortality rates that are at least the equivalent of two-stage procedures (Umpleby and Williamson, 1984; Phillips et al, 1985).

Immediate resection of the tumour with creation of a terminal colostomy and either closure of the rectal stump (Hartmann's operation) or formation of a mucous fistula reduces the number of operations from three to two. Its main drawback is that the second-stage anastomosis entails a major operation that may be difficult even with stapling devices. According to Koruth et al (1985b), 40% of patients are left with their stomas after Hartmann's operation.

The hazards of reversing either a Hartmann's operation or an end stoma with mucous fistula may be avoided by performing a primary anastomosis covered by a proximal defunctioning stoma. However, this primary anastomosis may be technically demanding because of the discrepancy in diameter of the proximal and distal large bowel. The column of faeces between the stoma and the anastomosis provides a serious hazard if there is an anastomotic leak.

Comparison of the three-stage approach against primary resection reveals conflicting results in retrospective studies. Earlier authors reported better results with a three-stage policy (Floyd and Cohn, 1967; Welch and Donaldson, 1974; Dutton et al, 1976), but several more recent series have shown the reverse (Fielding and Wells, 1974; Clark et al, 1975; Carson et al, 1977; Irvin and Greaney, 1977; Umpleby and Williamson, 1984; Buetcher et al, 1988). Phillips et al (1985) found that the operative mortality and survival rates were the same for primary and staged resection. However, there was a significantly lower wound complication rate and a shorter hospital stay after primary resection.

On-table colonic lavage, as described by Dudley et al (1980), may enable a primary anastomosis to be performed more safely after resection of obstructing tumours. This method is easy to learn, but with gross impaction of solid faeces above an obstruction it can take an hour to wash the colon clean. This extra operating time may not be justified in very frail patients. Moreover, poor technique risks serious contamination.

Another recent innovation is an intracolonic bypass tube developed by Ger and Ravo (1984) to protect anastomoses following colonic resections. This method has been used following resection of six obstructing left-sided colonic tumours (Keane et al, 1988). There were no postoperative anastomotic leaks nor deaths in this small series. More data are required to assess the role of this technique.

An alternative procedure for patients with obstructing carcinomas of the left colon is to perform an extended right hemicolectomy or subtotal colectomy with a primary ileosigmoid or ileorectal anastomosis (Klatt et al, 1981). This method avoids the colocolic anastomosis of a conventional resection for an obstructing left-sided cancer that has a leak rate of 18% and operative mortality rate of 22% (Phillips et al, 1985). The results of extended right hemicolectomy are summarized in Table 4. Among 53 cases the solitary leak and 9.5% operative mortality rate compare favourably with more limited resections for obstructing cancers.

Marston (1989) has recently advocated a policy of total colectomy and ileorectal anastomosis for *all* large bowel cancers, arguing that: (1) the operation is straightforward; (2) there is a low anastomotic leak rate; (3) the problem of synchronous or metachronous tumours is eliminated.

The first statement may be true for non-obstructed tumours, but a total

TABLE 4

Results of extended right hemicolectomy for obstructing left-sided colonic cancers

Author	Number of cases	Postoperative deaths	Clinical leaks	Other postoperative complications
Klatt et al (1981)	5	0	0	1 small bowel obstruction 1 wound infection
Deutsch et al (1983)	14	1	?1	2 wound infections 1 pneumonia 1 intraperitoneal abscess
Morgan et al (1985)	16	2	0	1 cerebrovascular accident
Wilson and Gollack (1989)	18	2	0	3 wound infections 5 chest infections
Total	53	5	?1	15

colectomy in the presence of gross large bowel obstruction can be a difficult operation. Since metachronous tumours occur in only 3.5–5% (Heald and Lockhart-Mummery, 1972; Cunliffe et al, 1984), 95% of patients will have an unnecessarily radical operation. The other disadvantages are that the resultant loose and frequent bowel actions may not be well tolerated by elderly patients, and that the functions of the large intestine (other than the absorption of water) are poorly understood (Moran et al, 1989).

We would reserve an extended right hemicolectomy for young patients with obstructing cancers no lower than the descending colon so that the anastomosis lies within reach of the 60 cm flexible sigmoidoscope for follow-up screening. We prefer to avoid more extensive colonic resections, especially in an elderly patient.

INTESTINAL OBSTRUCTION AS AN EARLY COMPLICATION OF LAPAROTOMY

After abdominal operations gastrointestinal activity returns to normal within 1 week in all but a few patients. In this worrying group the differential diagnosis is:

(1) Ileus owing to continued intra-abdominal sepsis or a leaking anastomosis
(2) Mechanical obstruction caused by early adhesion formation
(3) Prolonged paralytic ileus.

Distinguishing between these three is important in that the first two require operation whereas the third does not. Alas, the distinction is rarely straight-forward.

Continued sepsis or a closed loop obstruction may be evident with features of toxicity (high pulse, raised temperature, leucocytosis) and local or generalized abdominal tenderness. If sepsis is suspected without any obvious cause, pelvic and subphrenic abscesses should be sought clinically and radiologically and dealt with as appropriate (often by percutaneous aspiration under ultrasound guidance). If a gastrointestinal anastomosis was performed at the original operation, contrast studies may demonstrate a leak. If either continued generalized intra-abdominal sepsis or closed loop intestinal obstruction are suspected, early reexploration of the abdomen is mandatory.

Plain X-rays of the abdomen may be helpful in differentiating mechanical obstruction from paralytic ileus. Dilatation of small intestine with absence of colonic gas suggests mechanical intestinal obstruction, whereas gaseous distension of the entire intestine including the rectum supports the diagnosis of paralytic ileus.

When the cause of delayed return of gastrointestinal function after an abdominal operation is not apparent, we recommend a limited period of conservative management. This policy necessitates vigilant clinical review, maintenance of fluid balance and electrolyte status, and nasogastric aspiration. Parenteral nutrition should not be delayed for longer than 1 week after the original operation. If there are no signs of resolution of the ileus within 48 h, re-exploration is indicated.

VOLVULUS

Volvulus is defined as a torsion of part of the alimentary tract on its mesenteric axis. This may result in occlusion of the lumen and impairment of the blood supply. The commonest site for a volvulus to occur is in the sigmoid colon. It occurs rarely in the right colon and very occasionally in the transverse colon.

Sigmoid volvulus

Sigmoid volvulus accounted for about 4% of all intestinal obstructions in a series from Edinburgh (Anderson and Lee, 1981), an incidence that is typical for most western countries. In eastern Europe, Scandinavia, Africa and India the incidence is much higher. For example about 30% of admissions for intestinal obstruction in a series from India (Sinha, 1969) were due to sigmoid volvulus.

In a large series comprising 134 cases of sigmoid volvulus, 86% of patients were aged 50 years or older and 45% were over 70 years. Two-thirds of the patients had associated psychiatric or medical conditions (Anderson and Lee, 1981). These findings are typical of the experience in the west. The clinical features of sigmoid volvulus are essentially those of large bowel obstruction, as previously described, though generally of more rapid onset. Abdominal distension may be so marked as to impair respiratory or cardiac function. If the sigmoid loop has either strangulated or perforated, there will be signs of peritonitis.

Plain abdominal X-rays will confirm the diagnosis in 70% of cases (Anderson and Lee, 1981). The diagnostic features (Figure 2) are: (1) enormous dilatation of the sigmoid loop, which may extend right up to the diaphragm; (2) on an erect film two air/fluid levels may be seen (one in each limb of the obstructed loop); (3) occasionally the typical 'bird's beak' deformity (seen if contrast studies are performed) may be apparent on plain films.

General resuscitative measures should commence immediately on admission to hospital.

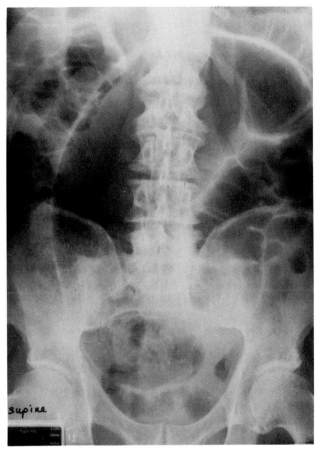

supine

FIGURE 2 Sigmoid volvulus: the massively distended sigmoid loop is clearly seen occupying most of the abdomen. Typical haustrations are seen at the apex of the loop.

Sigmoidoscopic tube decompression

Bruusgaard (1947) achieved satisfactory decompression in 90% of episodes of sigmoid volvulus. This Scandinavian method was subsequently adopted in the west, the previous practice being primary operative treatment which carried a high mortality rate; success was reported in 76–88% of cases (Shepherd, 1968; Anderson and Lee, 1981).

In Bruusgaard's description of the method, the patient is placed in the knee–elbow position and the sigmoidoscope is passed until the site of narrowing is encountered, usually within 25 cm of the anus. Sometimes passage of the sigmoidoscope will achieve decompression, but usually the passage of a well-lubricated rubber tube via the sigmoidoscope is required to release large quantities of flatus and fluid stool. If decompression occurs, the tube should be affixed to the perianal skin with adhesive tape and left *in situ* for 2–3 days.

If mucosa of dubious viability is seen through the sigmoidoscope or if decompression fails, early operative treatment is indicated. The recurrence rate for sigmoid volvulus after successful decompression is high (50% within 2–3 years according to Shepherd (1968)), so that elective resection should be considered for

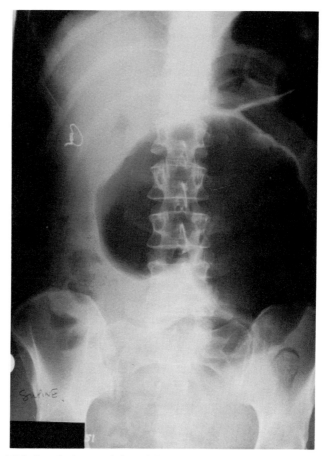

FIGURE 3 Caecal volvulus: the 'comma'-shaped distended caecal volvulus extends laterally to the left
flank and superiorly to the upper abdomen.

all cases. The decision to advise operation is not easy, since many of these patients
are elderly and often reside in long-term care institutions. It may therefore
be prudent to manage recurrent attacks in such patients by repeated tube
decompression.

Operative options

The simplest operation is merely to untwist the volvulus. The twist in the
sigmoid colon is usually anticlockwise, so that clockwise derotation should be
attempted first. Following untwisting, a rectal tube should be manoeuvred from
below by an assistant into the sigmoid loop to achieve decompression. Since the
recurrence rate of simple detorsion is 40% (with or without attempts to fix the
sigmoid colon), resection should be performed in all but the very unfit patient, and
it is essential if necrosis is present.

After resection, the options are: (1) a Paul–Mikulicz double-barrelled colostomy;
(2) a Hartmann's-type procedure with closure of the upper rectum and left iliac
fossa colostomy; (3) a primary anastomosis with or without a covering proximal
loop stoma.

Although the first option may be considered to be the most appropriate, bringing the distal limb of the stoma to the surface of the abdomen is never easy, and this limb tends to retract postoperatively. As discussed elsewhere in this chapter, the major disadvantage of Hartmann's operation is the difficulty of the subsequent restoration of colonic continuity. Thus in most patients the best option is a primary anastomosis covered by a proximal colostomy if necessary. The technique of on-table colonic lavage (and possibly the intraluminal bypass tube) mentioned on page 212 may reduce the number of patients who require a covering colostomy.

Caecal volvulus

Caecal volvulus is an uncommon condition in which all or part of an abnormally mobile caecum and ascending colon may rotate axially. The cause of the abnormal mobility may be either partial or complete failure of midgut rotation (which occurs at 6–9 weeks' gestation) or failure of the caecum to attach to the posterior abdominal wall. Failure of midgut rotation has been reported in 1–2% of the population (Keyes, 1939), and in 11 of 125 consecutive post-mortems the ascending colon was found to be 'insufficiently fixed allowing torsion' (Wolfer et al, 1942). The incidence of caecal volvulus is 2.8–7.1 per 10^6 per annum. Thus the anatomical prerequisite for caecal volvulus has been calculated as being 400 times as common as the clinical incidence of this event (Tejler and Jiborn, 1988). Additional factors thought to trigger the volvulus are previous operations, distal obstruction and pregnancy.

Caecal volvulus may present either as an acute emergency (strangulation of the twisted segment or small bowel obstruction) or as a rare cause of episodic obstruction. The radiological features (Figure 3) are absence of the caecum in the right iliac fossa, with the dilated viscus present in the midline or on the left side of the abdomen, together with small bowel obstruction.

Operative options

When strangulation is found, the surgical treatment is resection of the right colon. When strangulation has not developed, various other operations have been performed (simple detorsion, caecopexy or caecostomy). However the postoperative complication rate after these procedures is unacceptably high. Serious infections are common after both caecopexy and caecostomy, and recurrence of torsion has been recorded in 13% of patients treated by either simple detorsion or detorsion and caecopexy (Tejler and Jiborn, 1988). Thus a right hemicolectomy is the operation of choice for both viable and non-viable right colon involved in a volvulus.

GALLSTONE ILEUS

The pathological event is mechanical intestinal obstruction by one or more gallstones rather than an adynamic ileus. The gallstones reach the small intestine via a biliary-enteric fistula, usually between gallbladder and duodenum but sometimes between gallbladder and stomach. The gallstone usually impacts in the terminal ileum, where the lumen of the bowel is narrowest. Intestinal diseases that diminish the size of the lumen, such as Crohn's disease (Highman and Jagelman, 1981), may cause stones to lodge at the site of the narrowing. Impaction in the colon has also been described (Milsom and MacKeigan, 1985; Phillips and Doran, 1986).

The condition is uncommon, being responsible for only 1–5% of all intestinal obstructions. It occurs predominantly in the elderly, with the average age reported as 65 years or greater; 20% of cases of small bowel obstruction in patients over 65 years old are due to gallstone ileus (Hudspeth et al, 1970). Gallstone ileus is commoner in females than males (van Hillo et al, 1987; Day and Marks, 1975). The clinical features are of small bowel obstruction. Symptoms suggestive of biliary disease can be elicited from 30–70% of patients (the higher reported figures include findings elicited in retrospect) (Hudspeth et al, 1970). The diagnosis may be made on radiological grounds from a plain film of the abdomen (Figure 4) if two of the following three criteria are met: (1) intestinal obstruction; (2) air in the biliary tree; (3) an aberrantly located radiopaque gallstone. Day and Marks (1975) reviewed the

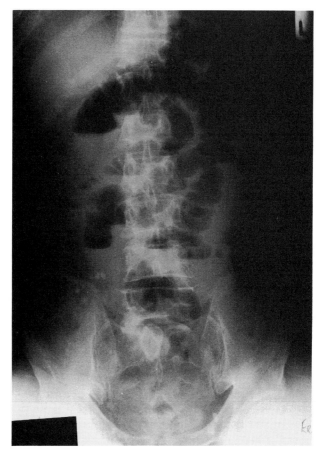

FIGURE 4 Gallstone ileus: there are distended loops of small intestine, with an aberrantly located gallstone seen overlying the lumbosacral region.

X-rays of the 34 patients in their series and identified intestinal obstruction in 18 (53%), air in the biliary tree in 12 (35%) and an aberrantly located gallstone in 14 (41%). In 13 (38%) of the cases two of the three criteria were present, but in only one case was the diagnosis of gallstone ileus made preoperatively.

Operations for gallstone ileus

The objective is to relieve the intestinal obstruction. This goal is achieved either by milking the stone into the caecum (and if feasible crushing the stone) or removal of the stone via an enterotomy, which is carried out either over the stone or just above it. The small bowel should be thoroughly checked for other stones in the lumen, which are found in 3–15% of cases (von Hillo et al, 1987). The entire bowel must also be checked for strictures.

In most patients this procedure is sufficient. The biliary-enteric fistula should be left alone because only a few patients will have further related problems. Recurrent gallstone impaction has been reported in approximately 5% of cases, and ascending cholangitis can also occur (Day and Marks, 1975). Cholecystectomy with closure of the fistula may then be undertaken as a second procedure. If the fistula is closed at the time of presentation with obstruction by an impacted gallstone, the operation is technically difficult and has a much higher morbidity and mortality rate than simple relief of obstruction, owing to the age and poor condition of the patient. There have been some reports of successful cholecystectomy in the presence of gallstone obstruction, but only in fit patients with well-defined fistulas and accessible gall bladders (Berliner & Burson, 1965; Hudspeth et al, 1970; Day and Marks, 1975).

RARER CAUSES OF INTESTINAL OBSTRUCTION

Bolus obstruction

By food

This is liable to occur after a partial gastrectomy if food is not masticated well. Oranges, dried fruits and similar fibrous fruits and vegetables are the common foodstuffs that cause the obstruction.

By worms

An aggregation of *Ascaris lumbricoides* is a rare cause of intestinal obstruction seen in the tropics, most commonly after administration of an anti-helminthic. At operation, the bolus of food or worms can usually be squeezed into the caecum. If this manoeuvre is unsuccessful, an enterotomy must be performed to remove the bolus.

Tumours of the small intestine

Benign neoplasms

Adenomas, lipomas, leiomyomas and the hamartomatous polyps of Peutz–Jegher syndrome have all been reported as causing small bowel obstruction, usually by intussusception (Harding Rains and Mann, 1988).

Malignant neoplasms

In a series of 171 small bowel tumours, 65% of patients with primary small intestinal carcinomas and 59% of patients with lymphomas of the small intestine presented with clinical features of intestinal obstruction (Williamson et al, 1983).

Intussusception

This condition is most commonly seen in infants. In adults, colo-colic intussusception is a rare presentation of primary colonic cancer. Any of the small intestinal neoplasms listed above may cause intussusception (Williamson et al, 1983), likewise invagination of a Meckel's diverticulum (Williamson et al, 1984). Idiopathic intussusception has been reported in Egypt following the Mohammedan fasting season (Harding Rains and Mann, 1988).

Non-specific small bowel ulceration

The clinical features of this rare condition are of acute or chronic gastrointestinal haemorrhage (five out of six cases in our experience) and mild obstructive symptoms (four out of six cases). The most productive investigations for establishing the diagnosis in this group of patients were selective visceral angiography and small bowel enemas (Thomas and Williamson, 1985). As with all rare causes of small intestinal obstruction, the diagnosis is usually made at operation (Strodel et al, 1981).

Endometriosis

Intestinal obstruction has been reported as a rare complication of endometriosis. In a review of 1573 cases of endometriosis (Prytowsky et al, 1988) 85 patients had gastrointestinal involvement. In this series there were two cases of ileal involvement causing small bowel obstruction, and also three cases of involvement of the sigmoid colon causing strictures.

Internal hernias

These can occur at any of the following sites, and can present with small intestinal obstruction (Harding Rains and Mann, 1988): the foramen of Winslow; a hole in the small bowel mesentery, transverse mesocolon or omentum; a defect in the broad ligament; congenital or acquired diaphragmatic hernias; fossae around the duodenum, caecum and appendix; the intersigmoid and supravesical fossae.

External hernias

Obturator hernias

Ninety per cent occur in elderly females. The diagnosis can be established preoperatively if there is a history of pain radiating from groin to knee, a lump in Scarpa's triangle or a mass palpable in the region of the obturator foramen on vaginal examination.

Sciatic, gluteal, interstitial and lumbar hernias

These are all extremely rare causes of intestinal obstruction.

PSEUDO-OBSTRUCTION

The term pseudo-obstruction was introduced by Dudley in 1958 to describe a group of patients who presented with appearances resembling acute mechanical obstruction but in whom no mechanical cause was found. The condition is due to abnormal gut motility and affects predominantly the large bowel.

The pathophysiological basis of pseudo-obstruction is either excessive sympathetic inhibition or a decreased stimulatory effect of the parasympathetic system. The causes can be classified as: (1) idiopathic; (2) systemic disease; (3) local disease. Using this classification a full list of causes is given in Table 5 (Paterson-Brown and Dudley, 1990; Isaacs and Keshavarzian, 1985).

The incidence of pseudo-obstruction is unknown. On the basis of contrast enema studies in large bowel obstruction (Stewart et al, 1984; Koruth et al, 1985a), 25–31% of patients admitted with a clinical diagnosis of large bowel obstruction have no mechanical lesion. The mean age in all series is in the sixth decade. There is no predisposition for either sex.

The clinical features are those of intestinal obstruction. Abdominal distension occurs in association with diminished passage of flatus and faeces. There may be abdominal pain, although this is often not a marked symptom unless caecal perforation has occurred. Bowel sounds may become high pitched, as with mechanical obstruction.

The plain abdominal film resembles mechanical obstruction, with distended large bowel and absence of rectal gas. Presence of gas beyond the splenic flexure in association with distension of small and/or large bowel is suggestive but not diagnostic of pseudo-obstruction. Contrast enema examination is therefore mandatory. If the contrast study is equivocal, colonoscopy should be performed.

It is essential to establish the diagnosis of pseudo-obstruction because the

TABLE 5

Causes of pseudo-obstruction

Idiopathic
Systemic causes
Electrolyte abnormalities
Cardiac disease
Renal disease
Hypovolaemia
Hypoxia
Alcoholic liver disease
Burns
Lead and other heavy metal poisoning
Puerperium
Myxoedema
Drugs
Local causes
Gut nerve dysfunction
   Toxic—drugs, heavy metals, insecticides
   Metabolic—diabetes mellitus, paraneoplastic, amyloidosis, porphyria
   Inflammatory—Chagas' disease, varicella, Kawasaki disease
   Genetic—congenital and familial visceral neuropathy
Gut muscle dysfunction
   Familial visceral myopathy
   Dystrophia myotonica
   Polymyositis
Disorders affecting gut muscle and nerve function
   Phaeochromocytoma
   Congenital hypoparathyroidism
   Pregnancy
   Enteroglucagonoma
   Blunt abdominal trauma
   Jejuno-ileal bypass
Disorders of gut collagen and interstitium
   Scleroderma
   Radiation
   Strongyloidiasis
   Ehlers–Danlos syndrome
   Mesenteric panniculitis

treatment is non-operative, in contrast to obstruction from a mechanical cause. Rehydration, correction of electrolyte abnormalities and adequate oxygenation often leads to a resolution of symptoms. Parenteral nutrition is advised in malnourished patients or if pseudo-obstruction persists for more than 5 days. Therapeutic endoscopy has been used for many years in the management of sigmoid volvulus. The advent of the flexible fibre-optic colonoscope has enabled better decompression for sigmoid volvulus and also of the dilated colon in pseudo-obstruction. Prolonged decompression has been successful, using the colonoscope to pass a long tube either alongside (Groff, 1983) or over the instrument (Burke and Shellito, 1987).

A regimen of guanethidine and physostigmine originally reported for use in patients with prolonged postoperative ileus (Catchpole, 1969) may be of benefit in some cases of pseudo-obstruction.

As with mechanical obstruction, the caecum may distend massively and eventually rupture. Caecal perforation is associated with a mortality rate of 45% (Gierson et al, 1975), so that progressive distension of the right colon beyond 9 cm diameter (as assessed by serial plain X-rays) requires operative relief. The best procedure for either impending or established caecal rupture is to formally exteriorize the caecum (Bachulis and Smith, 1978); tube caecostomy is unsatisfactory.

Contrast studies occasionally give false positive results, so that at operation the surgeon may encounter distended colon without mechanical obstruction. In this circumstance the colon can be decompressed by on-table colonoscopy, insertion into the colon of a 19-gauge needle attached to suction apparatus, or formation of a formal caecostomy. Tube caecostomy and transverse colostomy should be avoided

CONCLUSIONS AND THE WAY FORWARD

Future trends in small bowel obstruction

Prevention

Elective repair of all external hernias would reduce the world-wide incidence of small bowel obstruction. In reality, this is an impossible aim. In the west, the increased proportion of the population undergoing laparotomy has led to a remarkable rise in the incidence of adhesion obstruction. Use of new processes in the manufacture of surgical gloves will reduce the contamination of the peritoneal cavity at operation. Whether this leads to a decrease in the incidence of adhesion obstruction remains to be seen.

Abdominopelvic radiotherapy is being administered to an increasing number of patients. Awareness of the problems of chronic radiation enteritis may lead to better technical methods to avoid inclusion of the intestine within the radiation field.

Surgery

The management of recurrent diffuse adhesions remains controversial. A direct comparison between plication and intraluminal intubation would resolve the issue, but it is unlikely that such a trial would ever be satisfactory. Most other surgical aspects of small bowel obstruction are straightforward.

Future trends in large bowel obstruction

Prevention—screening for colorectal cancers

The aim of screening for colorectal cancers is early detection with eradication of neoplasms at the adenoma stage. If this objective were achieved there should be a significant reduction in the incidence of malignant large bowel obstruction. Long-term results from studies of faecal occult blood screening of large populations (Nivatongs et al, 1982; Hardcastle et al, 1983) may provide such evidence. However, faecal occult blood testing may prove to be limited by insensitivity and lack of specificity in predicting colonic neoplasia.

Rigid proctosigmoidoscopy will detect early distal colonic or rectal cancers (Gilbertsen, 1974), but later studies from the same institution (Nivatongs et al, 1982) demonstrated that examination of the large bowel to the sigmoid colon would only detect 56% of large bowel cancers.

The alternative approach is to screen large populations by colonoscopy as advocated by Reasbeck (1987), but the costs and logistics of this would seem to be prohibitive.

Established large bowel obstruction

The major problem in management is that the operative results for obstructed tumours are worse than for non-obstructed tumours. Phillips et al (1985) showed that the results achieved by consultants were better than those achieved by surgeons in training in this context. Better training and supervision should lead to an improvement in the operative results for colorectal cancer, especially when obstruction is present.

Decompression of colonic obstruction by new therapeutic techniques performed via the colonoscope has been reported in the management of advanced colorectal cancer (Mathus-Vliegen and Tytgat, 1986). Use of these techniques to relieve obstruction before surgical resection could result in an improved outcome similar to that seen after sigmoidoscopic decompression was introduced for sigmoid volvulus.

Laser therapy Colonoscopy combined with the use of neodymium yttrium–aluminium–garnet (Nd YAG) lasers has been used to debulk obstructing advanced colorectal tumours by photoablation. In a review of 181 patients treated for advanced colorectal cancers in seven centres by laser therapy (Mathus-Vliegen and Tytgat, 1986), 55% of patients had symptoms of obstruction. Good palliation of obstruction was achieved in 87%, with a procedure-related mortality rate of only 3.4%. This method has also been used as a preoperative measure in 27 selected patients, with only one death (Kiefhaber et al, 1986).

Low power Nd YAG laser energy delivered by fibres inserted directly into colonic tumours in rats have also been used to destroy the tumour by local hyperthermia (Mathewson et al, 1988).

Photodynamic therapy The basis of this method is the selective uptake of haematoporphyrin derivatives in malignant tissues. Application of red light (from a laser source) to the tumour after pretreatment with these agents results in cell death, probably by the production of free oxygen radicals. This method is in the early stages of development, and data are scanty (Bown, 1988).

Randomized controlled studies are needed to establish whether application of these new endoscopic techniques to relieve obstruction before definitive operation has a significant effect on morbidity, mortality and survival rates.

Conclusion

Intestinal obstruction remains a common surgical problem. The pattern of pathological causes has changed in developed countries, in that neglected external hernias have become less common and adhesions more common. World-wide, hernias and colonic volvulus remain the commonest cause of small and large bowel obstruction.

We advocate the adoption of rational management protocols for intestinal obstruction as illustrated in Figures 5 and 6. When conservative management of small bowel is appropriate we emphasize the importance of careful and regular clinical review. Of the causes of small bowel obstruction, adhesions are the most difficult to manage.

We strongly recommend that all patients suspected of having large bowel obstruction on the basis of the clinical and plain abdominal X-ray findings should have contrast studies performed to exclude pseudo-obstruction. If contrast examination is equivocal, colonoscopy is advised.

The high morbidity and mortality rates after operations for large bowel obstruction compared with operations on the non-obstructed colon may be improved by better technique. In the future decompression of large bowel obstruction before operation by new methods such as laser therapy may also improve the operative results.

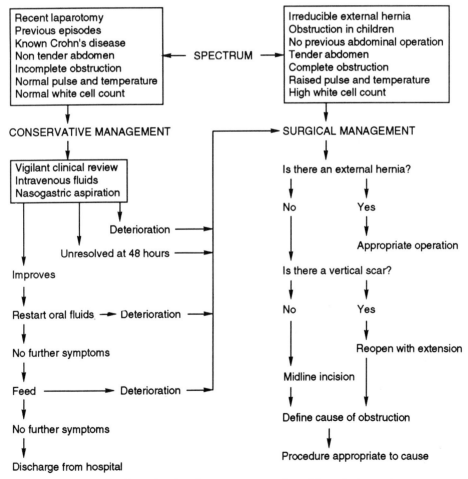

FIGURE 5 Algorithm for the management of small bowel obstruction.

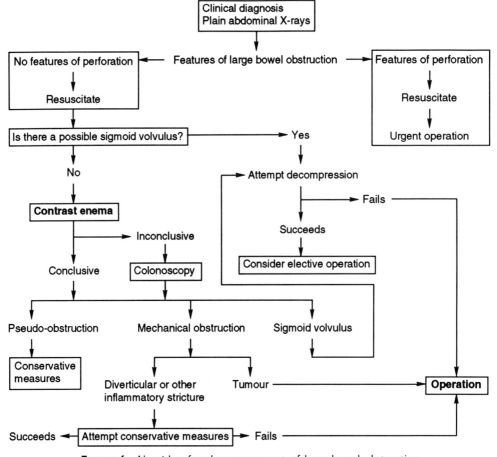

FIGURE 6 Algorithm for the management of large bowel obstruction.

REFERENCES

Alexander-Williams J (1986) The technique of intestinal strictureplasty. *International Journal of Colorectal Disease* **1**: 54–57.

Allen-Mersh TG, Wilson EJ, Hope-Stone HF & Mann CV (1986). Has the incidence of radiation-induced bowel damage following treatment of uterine carcinoma changed in the last 20 years? *Journal of the Royal Society of Medicine* **79**: 387–390.

Anderson JR & Lee D (1981) The management of acute sigmoid volvulus. *British Journal of Surgery* **68**: 117–120.

Andrews NJ (1981) Presentation and outcome of strangulated external hernia in a district general hospital. *British Journal of Surgery* **68**: 329–332.

Bachulis BL & Smith PE (1978) Pseudo-obstruction of the colon. *American Journal of Surgery* **136**: 66–72.

Baker JW (1959) A long jejunostomy tube for decompressing intestinal obstruction. *Surgery Gynecology and Obstetrics* **109**: 519–520.

Berliner SD & Burson LC (1965) One stage repair for cholecyst-duodenal fistula and gallstone ileus. *Archives of Surgery* **90**: 313–316.

Bevan PG (1982) Acute intestinal obstruction in the adult. *British Journal of Hospital Medicine* **28**: 258–265.

Bevan PG (1984) Adhesive obstruction. *Annals of the Royal College of Surgeons of England* **66**: 164–169.

Bizer LS, Liebling RW, Delany HM & Gliedman ML (1981) Small bowel obstruction: the role of non operative treatment in simple intestinal obstruction and the predictive criteria for strangulation obstruction. *Surgery* **89**: 407–413.

Bown SG (1988) The future of lasers in cancer therapy. *British Journal of Hospital Medicine* **40**: 161.

Bruusgaard C (1947) Volvulus of the sigmoid colon and its treatment. *Surgery* **22**: 466–478.

Buetcher KJ, Boustany C, Caillouette R & Cohn I (1988) Surgical management of the acutely obstructed colon: a review of 127 cases. *American Journal of Surgery* **156**: 163–168.

Burke G & Shellito PC (1987) Treatment of recurrent colonic pseudo-obstruction by endoscopic placement of a fenestrated overtube. *Diseases of the Colon and Rectum* **30**: 615–619.

Carson SN, Poticha SM & Shileds TW (1977) Carcinoma obstructing the left side of the colon. *Archives of Surgery* **112**: 523–526.

Catchpole BN (1969) Ileus: use of sympathetic blocking agents in its treatment. *Surgery* **66**: 811–820.

Childs WA & Phillips RB (1960) Experience with intestinal plication and a proposed modification. *Annals of Surgery* **152**: 258–265.

Clarke J, Hall AW & Moossa AR (1975) Treatment of obstructing cancer of the colon and rectum. *Surgery Gynecology and Obstetrics* **141**: 541–544.

Cunliffe WJ, Hasleton PS, Tweedle DEF & Schofield PF (1984) Incidence of synchronous and metachronous colorectal carcinoma. *British Journal of Surgery* **71**: 941–943.

Day EA & Marks C (1975) Gallstone ileus. *American Journal of Surgery* **129**: 552–558.

Dehn TCB, Kettlewell MGW, Mortensen NJMcC, Lee ECG & Jewell DP (1989) Ten year experience of strictureplasty for obstructive Crohn's disease. *British Journal of Surgery* **76**: 339–341.

Deutsch AA, Zlikovski A, Sternberg A & Reiss R (1983) One-stage subtotal colectomy with anastomosis for obstructing carcinoma of the left colon. *Diseases of the Colon and Rectum* **26**: 227–230.

Dudley HAF, Sinclair ISR, McLaren IF, McNair TJ & Newsam JE (1958) Intestinal pseudo-obstruction. *Journal of the Royal College of Surgeons of Edinburgh* **3**: 206–217.

Dudley HAF, Radcliffe AG & McGeehan D (1980) Intraoperative irrigation of the colon to permit primary anastomosis. *British Journal of Surgery* **67**: 80–81.

Dutton JW, Hreno A & Hampson LG (1976) Mortality and prognosis of obstructing carcinoma of the large bowel. *American Journal of Surgery* **131**: 36–41.

Ellis H (1971) The cause and prevention of postoperative intraperitoneal adhesions. *Surgery Gynecology and Obstetrics* **133**: 497–511.

Ellis H (1982) The causes and prevention of intestinal adhesions. *British Journal of Surgery* **69**: 241–243.

Festen C (1982) Postoperative small bowel obstruction in infants and children. *Annals of Surgery* **196**: 580–583.

Field S, Guy PJ, Upsdell SM & Scourfield AE (1985) The erect abdominal radiograph in the acute abdomen: should its routine use be abandoned? *British Medical Journal* **290**: 1934–1936.

Fielding LP & Wells BW (1974) Survival after primary and staged resection for large bowel obstruction caused by cancer. *British Journal of Surgery* **64**: 741–744.

Floyd CE & Cohn I (1967) Obstruction in cancer of the colon. *Annals of Surgery* **165**: 721–731.

Fraser I (1982) Simple and effective method of removing starch powder from surgical gloves. *British Medical Journal* **284**: 1835.

Galland RB & Spencer J (1987) Natural history and surgical management of radiation enteritis. *British Journal of Surgery* **74**: 742–747.

Ger R & Ravo B (1984) Prevention and treatment of intestinal dehiscence by an intraluminal bypass graft. *British Journal of Surgery* **71**: 726–729.

Gierson ED, Storm FK, Shaw W & Coyne SK (1975) Caecal rupture due to colonic ileus. *British Journal of Surgery* **62**: 383–386.

Gilbertsen VA (1974) Proctosigmoidoscopy and polypectomy in reducing the incidence of rectal cancer. *Cancer* **34**: 936–939.

Groff W (1983) Colonoscopic decompression and intubation of the cecum for Ogilvie's syndrome. *Diseases of the Colon and Rectum* **26**: 503–506.

Hardcastle JD, Farrands PA, Balfour TW, Chamberlain J, Amar SS & Sheldon MG (1983) Controlled trial of faecal occult blood testing in the detection of colorectal cancer. *Lancet* **ii**: 1–4.

Harding Rains AJ & Mann CV (1988) *Bailey and Love's Short Practice of Surgery*, 20th edn. London: Lewis.

Heald RJ & Lockhart-Mummery HE (1972) The lesion of the second cancer of the large bowel. *British Journal of Surgery* **59**: 16–19.

Highman L & Jagelman DG (1981) Gallstone ileus complicating terminal ileal Crohn's disease. *British Journal of Surgery* **68**: 201–202.

Hudspeth AS, McGuirt WF & Winston-Salem NC (1970) Gall stone ileus, a continuing surgical problem. *Archives of Surgery* **100**: 668–672.

Hulten L (1988) Surgical treatment of Crohn's disease of the small bowel or ileocaecum. *World Journal of Surgery* **12**: 180–185.

Irvin TT & Greaney MG (1977) The treatment of colonic cancer presenting with intestinal obstruction. *British Journal of Surgery* **64**: 741–744.

Isaacs P & Keshavarzian A (1985) Intestinal pseudo-obstruction. *Postgraduate Medical Journal* **61**: 1033–1038.

Keane PF, Ohri SR, Wood CB & Sackier JM (1988) Management of the obstructed left colon by the one-stage intracolonic bypass procedure. *Diseases of the Colon and Rectum* **31**: 948–951.

Keyes EI (1939) Anomalous fixation of the mesentery: report of two cases. *Archives of Surgery* **38**: 99–106.

Kiefhaber P, Kiefhaber K & Huber F (1986) Preoperative Neodymium-YAG laser treatment of obstructive colon cancer. *Endoscopy* **18**: 44–46.

Kirk RM & Williamson RCN (1987) *General Surgical Operations*, 2nd edn. London: Churchill Livingstone.

Klatt GR, Martin WH & Gilespie JT (1981) Subtotal colectomy with primary anastomosis without diversion in the treatment of obstructing carcinoma of the left colon. *American Journal of Surgery* **141**: 577–578.

Koruth NM, Koruth A & Matheson NA (1985a) The place of contrast enema in the management of large bowel obstruction. *Journal of the Royal College of Surgeons of Edinburgh* **30**: 258–260.

Koruth NM, Hunter DC, Krukowski ZH & Matheson NA (1985b) Immediate resection in emergency large bowel surgery: a 7 year audit. *British Journal of Surgery* **72**: 703–707.

Lacey GJ, Bignall BK, Bradbrooke S, Reidy J, Hussain S & Cramer B (1980) Rationalising abdominal radiography in the accident and emergency department. *Clinical Radiology* **31**: 453–455.

Lavelle-Jones M & Cuschieri A (1990) Adhesion obstruction of the small bowel. In Williamson RCN & Cooper MJ (eds) *Emergency Abdominal Surgery*. Edinburgh: Churchill Livingstone.

Lee ECG & Papaionnou N (1982) Minimal surgery for chronic obstruction in Crohn's disease. *Annals of the Royal College of Surgeons of England* **64**: 229–233.

McCarthy JD & Sharf TJ (1965) A simple intestinal plication. *Surgery, Gynecology and Obstetrics* **121**: 1340–1342.

Marson A (1989) Treatment of cancer of the colon: a non-specialist's point of view. *British Journal of Surgery* **76**: 71.

Mathewson K, Barton T, Lein MR, O'Sullivan JP, Northfield TC & Bown SG (1988) Low power interstitial laser photocoagulation in normal and neoplastic rat colon. *Gut* **29**: 27–34.

Mathus-Vliegen EMH & Tytgat GNJ (1986) Nd:YAG laser photocoagulation in gastroenterology—its role in palliation of colorectal cancer. *Lasers in Medical Science* **1**: 75–80.

Milsom JW & MacKeigan JM (1985) Gallstone obstruction of the colon. *Diseases of the Colon and Rectum* **28**: 367–370.

Mirvis SE, Young JWR, Keramati B, McCrea ES & Tarr R (1986) Plain film evaluation of patients with abdominal pain: are three radiographs necessary? *American Journal of Radiology* **147**: 501–503.

Moran BJ, Jackson AA & Karran SJ (1989) Subtotal colectomy or colonic preservation in the treatment of colonic cancer? *British Journal of Surgery* **76**: 421 (letter).

Morgan WP, Jenkins N, Lewis P & Aubrey A (1985) Management of obstructing carcinoma of the left colon by extended right hemicolectomy. *American Journal of Surgery* **149**: 327–329.

Mucha P (1987) Small intestinal obstruction. *Surgical Clinics of North America* **67**: 597–620.

Nivatongs S, Gilbertsen VA, Goldberg SM & Williams SE (1982) Distribution of large bowel cancers detected by occult blood test in asymptomatic patients. *Diseases of the Colon and Rectum* **25**: 420–421.

Noble TB (1937) Plication of the small intestine as prophylaxis against adhesions. *American Journal of Surgery* **35**: 41–44.

Ohman U (1982) Prognosis in patients with obstructing colorectal carcinoma. *American Journal of Surgery* **143**: 742–747.

Paterson-Brown S & Dudley HAF (1990) Colonic pseudo-obstruction. In Williamson RCN & Cooper MJ (eds) *Emergency Abdominal Surgery*.

Phillips DE & Doran J (1986) Obstruction of the colon by a giant gallstone. *British Journal of Hospital Medicine* **36**: 444.

Phillips RKS, Hittinger R, Fry JS & Fielding LP (1985) Malignant large bowel obstruction. *British Journal of Surgery* **72**: 296–302.

Prytowsky JB, Stryker SJ, Ujiki GT & Poticha SM (1988) Gastrointestinal endometriosis: incidence and indications for resection. *Archives of Surgery* **123**: 855–858.

Reasbeck PG (1987) Colrectal cancer: the case for endoscopic screening. *British Journal of Surgery* **74**: 12–17.

Sayfan J, Wilson DAL, Allan A, Andrews H & Alexander-Williams J (1989) Recurrence after strictureplasty or resection for Crohn's disease. *British Journal of Surgery* **76**: 335–338.

Shepherd JJ (1968) Treatment of volvulus of the sigmoid colon: a review of 425 cases. *British Medical Journal* **1**: 280–283.

Sinha RS (1969) A clinical appraisal of volvulus of the pelvic colon with special reference to aetiology and treatment. *British Journal of Surgery* **56**: 838–840.

Smith DH & De Cosse JJ (1986) Radiation damage to the small intestine. *World Journal of Surgery* **10**: 189–194.

Stewart J, Fiana PJ, Courtney DF & Brennan TG (1984) Does a water soluble contrast enema assist in the management of acute large bowel obstruction: a prospective study of 117 cases. *British Journal of Surgery* **71**: 799–801.

Strodel WE, Eckhauser FE & Simmons JL (1981) Primary ulceration of the ileum. *Diseases of the Colon and Rectum* **24**: 183.

Tejler G & Jiborn H (1988) Volvulus of the caecum: report of 26 cases and review of the literature. *Diseases of the Colon and Rectum* **31**: 445–449.

Thomas WEG & Williamson RCN (1985) Nonspecific small bowel ulceration. *Postgraduate Medical Journal* **61**: 587–591.

Umpleby HC & Williamson RCN (1984) Survival in acute obstructing colorectal carcinoma. *Diseases of the Colon and Rectum* **27**: 299–304.

van Hillo M, van der Vliet JA, Wiggers T, Obertop H, Terpstra OT & Greep JM (1987) Gallstone obstruction of the intestine: an analysis of ten patients and a review of the literature. *Surgery* **101**: 273–276.

Welch JP & Donaldson GA (1974) Management of severe obstruction of the large bowel due to malignant disease. *American Journal of Surgery* **127**: 492–499.

White RR (1956) Prevention of recurrent small bowel obstruction due to adhesions. *Annals of Surgery* **143**: 714–719.

Williamson RCN, Welch CE & Malt RA (1983) Adenocarcinoma and lymphoma of the small intestine: distribution and etiologic associations. *Annals of Surgery* **197**: 172–178.

Williamson, RCN, Cooper MJ & Thomas WEG (1984) Intussusception of invaginated Meckel's diverticulum. *Journal of the Royal Society of Medicine* **77**: 652–655.

Wilson RG & Gollock JM (1989) Obstructing carcinoma of the left colon managed by subtotal colectomy. *Journal of the Royal College of Surgeons of Edinburgh* **34**: 25–26.

Wolfer JA, Beaton LE & Anson BJ (1942) Volvulus of the cecum. Anatomical factors in its etiology: report of a case. *Surgery, Gynaecology and Obstetrics* **74**: 882–894.

Wolfson PJ, Bauer JJ & Gelernj IM (1985) Use of the long tube in the management of patients with small intestinal obstruction due to adhesions. *Archives of Surgery* **120**: 1001–1006.

Yeoh E & Horowitz M (1988) Radiation enteritis. *British Journal of Hospital Medicine* **39**: 498–504.

12

ACUTE INFLAMMATORY CONDITIONS OF THE ALIMENTARY TRACT

John L. Duncan and Christopher J. Stoddard

ACUTE CHOLECYSTITIS

Acute cholecystitis is the second commonest cause, after acute appendicitis, of acute inflammatory intra-abdominal conditions that precipitate emergency admission to hospitals in western countries. Almost 100 000 cholecystectomies are performed annually in the United Kingdom and many of these patients present initially with acute cholecystitis.

Gallstones may be asymptomatic. Their prevalence increases with age, being commoner in females at all ages (Figure 1). Of patients discovered to have asymptomatic gallstones, 10% will become symptomatic within 5 years and 18% within 20 years (Gracie and Ransohoff, 1982). Of 781 patients with symptomatic stones followed for between 1 and 11 years, Wenckert and Robertson (1966) found 49% had few or no symptoms after the initial cholecystogram, 33% developed chronic cholecystitis and 18% had complications related to their gallstones.

Major advances have been made in the diagnosis and treatment of gallstones and gallstone-related diseases in the last 10 years. Rapid confirmation of diagnosis by ultrasonography or scintigraphy may be followed by early cholecystectomy; alternative treatments by stone dissolution or extracorporeal shock wave lithotripsy, and relief of cholangitis and jaundice by endoscopic papillotomy, have become common. In the last few years minimally invasive surgery has appeared with percutaneous stone extraction and laparoscopic cholecystectomy. Treatment of all aspects of gallstones is changing, including the indications for surgery.

Pathophysiology

Acute cholecystitis usually follows an attack of biliary pain lasting several hours and in over 90% of cases is caused by obstruction of the cystic duct by a gallstone. However, impaction of a gallstone in the cystic duct may lead to the development of a mucocoele rather than cause acute cholecystitis. Experimentally, cystic duct

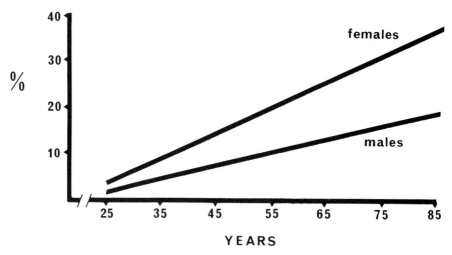

FIGURE I   The prevalence of gallstones according to age.

ligation or implantation of gallstones into the gallbladder alone do not cause acute cholecystitis but it can be induced by a combination of cystic duct ligation with intraluminal administration of a number of different irritant solutions (Roslyn et al, 1980). Acute cholecystitis is due to the interaction of both luminal and mucosal factors. Between 5% and 10% of patients have no gallstones. Acalculous cholecystitis may follow major surgery such as oesophagectomy or gastrectomy or can occur in patients with major burns or those receiving assisted ventilation or intravenous nutrition (Williamson, 1988).

Bacteria can be cultured from the bile of 40–60% of patients with acute cholecystitis (Patti and Pellegrini, 1989). It is probable that bacterial infection is a secondary, rather than a primary, event. Patients with sterile bile have identical symptoms, signs and pathological changes in the gallbladder to those with infected bile. Bile that is supersaturated or has a high proportion of deoxycholate can induce acute cholecystitis in the obstructed gallbladder (Morris et al, 1952). Duct obstruction with active gallbladder contraction leads to increased intraluminal pressure and this in turn to active secretion of fluid into the lumen by the mucosa. This secretion is mediated by intramural non-adrenergic, non-cholinergic nerves and by increased protaglandin production by the mucosa of the inflamed gallbladder. Opiate agonists and prostaglandin synthesis inhibitors will reduce intraluminal fluid secretion and pressure and thus reduce pain due to biliary distension (Jivegard et al, 1987).

Clinical presentation

Acute cholecystitis is characterized by upper abdominal pain, often radiating to the right scapular region, fever between 37.5°C and 38.5°C, tenderness over the gallbladder and a neutrophil leucocytosis. There may be a history of preceding episodes of biliary colic. The pain may be exacerbated by movement but is less severe than ureteric colic or peritonitis due to perforation of a peptic ulcer.

On examination the temperature is raised. A fever above 38.5°C is more likely to be due to a suppurative cholangitis with or without septicaemia. When symptoms have been present for over 24 h, Murphy's sign may be present or a tender mass may be palpable in the right subcostal area. Shoulder tip pain or tenderness extending down the right paracolic gutter may occur in acute cholecystitis but in an elderly patient, or when symptoms have been present for a few days, gangrenous perforation of the gallbladder with biliary peritonitis should be considered. There may be mild jaundice or a trace of bilirubin in the urine from oedema in the porta hepatis with extrinsic compression of the common hepatic duct or, more likely, a stone within the bile duct.

The diagnosis of acute cholecystitis is usually not difficult but other intra-abdominal conditions may cause similar symptoms and signs. The commonest are a perforated duodenal or gastric ulcer, acute pancreatitis, acute appendicitis in a patient with a long retrocaecal appendix or undescended caecum, or less frequently, diverticular disease or a perforated carcinoma in the region of the hepatic flexure. A past history of ulcer symptoms or treatment with ulcerogenic drugs such as non-steroidal anti-inflammatory agents should be sought. Acute pancreatitis is often due either to gallstones or alcohol abuse.

Initial diagnosis and treatment

Initial investigation

Initial investigation is aimed at excluding other causes of acute right upper quadrant pain followed later by confirmation of acute cholecystitis. On admission, all patients should have blood taken for haemoglobin and white cell count, looking particularly for a neutrophil leucocytosis, a serum amylase, to exclude acute pancreatitis, and urea and electrolytes in elderly patients, those taking diuretics or when vomiting has been a prominent symptom. The serum amylase may be marginally raised in acute cholecystitis, but a concentration three times greater than the upper limit of normal is very suggestive of acute pancreatitis. An erect chest X-ray should be performed, looking for subphrenic air from a perforated peptic ulcer, and a supine abdominal film. Ten per cent of gallstones are radio-opaque.

Initial treatment

Having reasonably excluded other acute intra-abdominal conditions, and before confirmation of the diagnosis of acute cholecystitis, the initial treatment should be to relieve pain, rest the gallbladder and reduce the risk of infective complications. An intravenous infusion of a crystalloid solution such as dextrose/saline should be commenced. Patients should be kept fasted. This will reduce cholecystokinin release from the upper small bowel, hence gallbladder contraction, and mucosal fluid production and gallbladder distension. Opiate analgesics should be given to relieve pain. By inhibition of intramural nerves they may also reduce gallbladder mucosal secretion. Pethidine, although reported to cause less spasm of the sphincter of Oddi than other opiates, has too short a duration of action to recommend its use. Papaveretum (omnopon) or morphine is more effective. Prostaglandin synthesis inhibitors will relieve biliary pain and reduce intraluminal gallbladder pressure but are not used routinely.

The role of antibiotics in acute cholecystitis remains controversial. The likelihood of patients with biliary tract disease having bacteria in the bile is dependent on a number of risk factors (Table 1). Cultures of normal bile in the absence of gallstones are usually sterile. Bacteria are present in the bile of 10–20 per cent of patients undergoing elective cholecystectomy for chronic cholecystitis, 40 to 60 per cent of patients with acute cholecystitis and over 70 per cent with obstructive jaundice. Biliary bacteria are commonest in patients over the age of 70 years and in those with a non-functioning gallbladder. The commonest organisms isolated from bile are *Escherichia coli*, *Klebsiella pneumoniae* and *Streptococcus faecalis*. Anaerobic bacteria such as *Bacteroides fragilis* or *Clostridium perfringens* are generally found only in patients with positive aerobic cultures.

It is common practice to prescribe antibiotics in acute cholecystitis. They will not sterilize the bile but may reduce the inflammation in the gallbladder wall, the risk of cholangitis and, if surgery is performed, the wound infection rate (Keighley, 1977). Parenteral cephalosporins such as cefazolin 1 g or cefuroxime 750 mg 8-hourly are the most commonly used antibiotics for biliary infections (Willis et al, 1984). Ciprofloxacin, other cephalosporins or a combination of ampicillin with gentamicin have been used with equally good results.

Confirmation of the diagnosis and operative treatment

The time-honoured treatment for acute cholecystitis has been intravenous fluids, analgesics and antibiotics followed by elective cholecystectomy 6–8 weeks later. This policy was advocated by many, including Du Plessis and Jerskey (1973), because of the uncertainty of the clinical diagnosis in the early stages, the risks of surgery in patients with an acutely inflamed gallbladder, particularly in the elderly and diabetics, and the fact that the mortality rate of acute cholecystitis is low. Patients would be subjected to laparotomy only if there were signs of spreading peritonitis suggesting gallbladder perforation, inability to control pain or the development of an empyema.

There has been a trend towards more aggressive surgery in recent years and many have advocated early operation within 48 h of admission (McArthur et al, 1975; Norrby et al, 1983; Addison and Finan, 1988). The advantages of early

TABLE I
Factors associated with an increased risk of biliary infection

Age over 70 years
Acute cholecystitis
Obstructive jaundice
Acute cholangitis
Choledocholithiasis
Previous biliary surgery

operation are: (1) early relief of pain; (2) decreased total duration of illness and disability; (3) avoidance of the serious complications of delayed treatment such as perforation and empyema; (4) some patients will not return for the planned cholecystectomy. Economically, early intervention is more advantageous to both patient and hospital (Fowkes and Gunn, 1980).

Rapid and accurate diagnosis is critical in cases of suspected acute cholecystitis if patients are to be offered early cholecystectomy and unnecessary laparotomy avoided (Schofield et al, 1986). Of patients admitted to hospital with a clinical diagnosis of acute cholecystitis, between 6% and 33% prove not to have gallbladder disease on further investigation (Herlin et al, 1984).

Techniques for diagnosis of acute cholecystitis

A number of different imaging techniques can be used for rapid diagnostic assessment of acute cholecystitis (Marton and Doubilet, 1988). Choice of investigation will depend on availability of a specific technique, the ease with which it can be performed, its sensitivity and specificity. Many of these methods depend on failure of the gallbladder to function and hence produce only indirect evidence of disease.

Ultrasonography Ultrasonography is the most commonly used test. It is readily available in most hospitals, non-invasive, easy to perform, safe and accurate (Figure 2). In addition it provides information about the liver, kidneys and pancreas, and other sources of non-biliary right upper quadrant pain. Obesity, intestinal gas and severe right upper quadrant tenderness may make examination

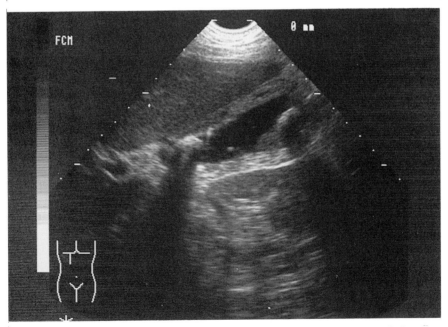

FIGURE 2 Ultrasound scan of a patient with acute cholecystitis showing thick walled oedematous gallbladder and gallstones.

difficult. Small gallstones less than 5 mm diameter may be missed and the sensitivity of the test is partly dependent on the equipment and operator skill and experience.

Cholecystography Oral cholecystography is of little value in acute cholecystitis when a rapid diagnosis is required. The patient may not tolerate oral fluids or absorb the contrast material and if opacification of the gallbladder fails to occur with the first study a repeat examination is required before the gallbladder can be considered pathological. Infusion cholangiography overcomes many of these problems and provides a result within a few hours (Dykes et al, 1984). In the presence of visualized ducts, failure of the gallbladder to opacify after 4 h indicates cystic duct obstruction. Technical failure occurs in up to 20% of studies.

Radio-isotope scanning Radionuclide scanning with iminodiacetic acid derivatives (HIDA) can be used for assessment of cystic duct patency. The isotope is given intravenously and the biliary region scanned with a gamma camera. Failure of the gallbladder to opacify confirms gallbladder disease but does not differentiate between acute cholecystitis and a non-functioning gallbladder in chronic disease. Gamma camera facilities and an out-of-hours service are not always available.

Contrast tomography Thickening of the gallbladder wall, indicative of acute cholecystitis, can be demonstrated by tomography following infusion of an appropriate contrast material. The thickening is a function of the hypervascularity of the inflammed gallbladder and this provides direct evidence of acute cholecystitis (Herlin et al, 1984). Contrast tomography does not depend on hepatic excretion and can be used even in the presence of jaundice.

Because of its availability and safety, ultrasonography is the procedure of choice for initial investigation of patients with suspected acute cholecystitis. Radionuclide scanning or contrast tomography should be used when ultrasonography gives equivocal results. Cholescintigraphy is safer and less observer dependent than contrast tomography. Acalculous cholecystitis may be difficult to confirm with ultrasonography or radionuclide scanning.

Surgical treatment

Having confirmed the suspected diagnosis of acute cholecystitis, patients may be treated by early cholecystectomy within a maximum of 7 days from onset of symptoms or by delayed operation 6–8 weeks later. Provided that the operation is performed by an experienced surgeon there is no increased morbidity or mortality with early cholecystectomy (McArthur et al, 1975; Norrby et al, 1983). Infective complications can be reduced by prophylactic antibiotics. Intra-operative blood loss may be greater. Economically there are sound reasons for advocating early cholecystectomy (Fowkes and Gunn, 1980). Patients over the age of 70 years frequently present with more serious complications of acute gallbladder disease and have an operative mortality rate of approximately 10% (Addison and Finan, 1988). There is no place for operation performed by inexperienced surgical staff in the middle of the night.

Of patients offered delayed cholecystectomy, 10–15% will not return for surgery and up to 27% will be readmitted with a recurrence of acute gallbladder disease before the planned date for elective surgery. Emergency cholecystectomy should be reserved for patients with suspected gallbladder perforation and biliary peritonitis. In patients with severe concurrent medical problems and acute cholecystitis, cholecystostomy is an alternative to cholecystectomy, if necessary under local anaesthesia.

Treatment of gallstones other than by cholecystectomy

Avoidance of early cholecystectomy in the initial treatment of acute cholecystitis leaves the option open for subsequent treatment of the gallstone disease by other methods such as laparoscopic cholecystectomy, percutaneous gallstone removal (Kellett et al, 1988), attempted gallstone dissolution or extracorporeal shock wave lithotripsy (ESWL) (Heberer et al, 1988; Keane and Tanner, 1988).

ACUTE CHOLANGITIS

In over 80% per cent of patients acute cholangitis is due to biliary infection in the presence of stones in the bile duct. Less frequently the biliary obstruction is due to a benign bile duct stricture or carcinoma of the extrahepatic biliary tree. Acute cholangitis may follow instrumentation of the biliary tree either after endoscopic retrograde cholangiopancreatography (ERCP) or as a complication of percutaneous transhepatic biliary drainage. In one large series, 7% of patients developed acute cholangitis following ERCP, most of whom had a malignant biliary obstruction and were febrile prior to ERCP (Lai et al, 1989). Cholangitis following percutaneous transhepatic biliary drainage is often due to infection with *Staphylococcus aureus* from the skin at the puncture site rather than the usual biliary organisms, and may present as late as 1 month after the procedure. The principal risk factors are malignant strictures, multiple biliary obstructions, neoplastic invasion of the bile duct and duodenal compression (Audisio et al, 1988).

Clinical presentation

Patients with acute cholangitis present with right upper quadrant pain, a high fever usually above 38.5°C and jaundice. They are frequently elderly, choledocholithiasis being commoner in this age group. Obstruction of the extrahepatic bile ducts by calculi produces stasis, biliary infection and later reflux of bacteria into the bloodstream. There is a direct correlation between increased pressure in the common bile duct (CBD) and cholangiovenous reflux. The normal CBD pressure is 10–12 cmH$_2$O but is higher in patients with acute suppurative cholangitis secondary to cholelithiasis than either in patients with no CBD stones or those with CBD stones but no pus (Csendes et al, 1988). Hepatocyte secretion of bile ceases when the CBD pressure exceeds 30 cmH$_2$O.

Differential diagnosis

Distinction should be made between acute cholecystitis and acute cholangitis. The former requires confirmation of diagnosis followed, in most cases, by laparotomy and cholecystectomy, whereas operation may not be required in the latter (*vide infra*). A fever over 38.5°C and the presence of jaundice favour acute cholangitis. Fever, jaundice and abdominal pain may occur in cirrhotic patients with infected ascites. The duration of jaundice, past history of liver disease and alcohol intake should be sought. With infected ascitic fluid the patient may be deeply jaundiced and abdominal tenderness is generalized rather than confined to the right upper quadrant. Acute pancreatitis may progress to formation of a pancreatic abscess and mild jaundice due to compression of the common bile duct.

Investigation and treatment

Acute cholangitis may be lethal. The bacteraemia which follows biliary obstruction may lead to Gram-negative septicaemia, hypotension, acute renal failure, multisystem failure and death. The time-honoured treatment with antibiotics followed by urgent surgical decompression of the biliary tree has been superseded by ERCP and endoscopic sphincterotomy.

On admission, blood should be taken for a full blood count, urea and electrolytes, serum amylase, liver function tests and bacteriological culture. As in patients with acute cholecystitis, an erect chest X-ray and supine abdominal X-ray should be performed. An intravenous infusion of a crystalloid solution is commenced and pulse, blood pressure and urine output monitored hourly after insertion of a urinary catheter. Hypotension should be corrected with adequate intravenous fluid infusion and peripheral tissue perfusion maintained. If more than 4 l of fluid are required in 24 h, half should be given as colloid. When large volumes of fluid are required, central venous pressure monitoring may be necessary, especially in elderly patients with cardiac problems where it may be critical to prevent fluid overload and iatrogenic cardiac failure.

Intravenous antibiotics should be given immediately without waiting until the infecting organism has been identified from the blood culture. A cephalosporin such as cefuroxime or cefotaxime is the usual choice. Whenever possible the combination of ampicillin and gentamicin should be avoided in patients with cholangitis because of the risks of acute renal failure and aminoglycoside nephrotoxicity. When an aminoglycoside is used the serum creatinine and pre- and post-aminoglycoside levels should be checked daily and the antibiotic dose adjusted accordingly.

If acute cholangitis is suspected, ultrasonography of the liver and biliary system should be performed within 24 h of admission to confirm the diagnosis of gallstones, to assess the bile duct, to look for choledocholithiasis and exclude, as far as possible, hepatic and pancreatic abscesses.

Most patients with acute cholangitis will respond to this treatment but 10–30% continue with high fever, hypotension and often poor urine output and need urgent decompression of the biliary tree (Patti and Pellegrini, 1989). Female sex, those over 50 years, acute renal failure, liver abscess, biliary stricture, cirrhosis and cholangitis after percutaneous transhepatic cholangiography are risk factors for failure of response to medical treatment (Gigot et al, 1989).

In patients failing to respond to medical treatment, early decompression of the common bile duct and extraction of stones is required. Endoscopic sphincterotomy is the treatment of choice. Surgical decompression is associated with a higher mortality (21%) than early endoscopic sphincterotomy (roughly 5%), even in older patients and those with more medical risk factors (Leese et al, 1986).

The need for subsequent cholecystectomy after endoscopic sphincterotomy for cholangitis is controversial. In some series (Leese et al, 1986; Olaison et al, 1987) only 6–8% of patients have further biliary pain requiring cholecystectomy, whereas other authors recommend cholecystectomy after endoscopic sphincterotomy in patients with concomitant cholelithiasis (Tanaka et al, 1987).

ACUTE ILEITIS

The symptoms and signs of acute ileitis can mimic acute appendicitis. Frequently patients with acute ileitis are subjected to laparotomy on the basis of a preoperative diagnosis of acute appendicitis. The commonest cause of acute ileitis is not Crohn's disease but an infection with bacteria of the *Yersinia* group. The majority of patients with acute ileitis do not subsequently develop Crohn's disease (Gump et al, 1967). Tuberculous ileitis is seen more frequently in Third World countries. It is important to distinguish between bacterial ileitis and Crohn's disease from the point of view of treatment and prognosis.

Yersinial ileitis

Bacteria of the *Yersinia* group are responsible for a number of gastrointestinal conditions whose severity range from mild to life threatening. As with many conditions, the very young, very old and the immunocompromised are at greatest risk.

Bacteriological characteristics

The *Yersinia* bacteria are members of the Enterobacteriaceae family. *Y. entero-colitica* and *Y. pseudotuberculosis* are the principal pathogens.

Transmission of infection is by ingestion of contaminated food, principally meat and vegetable products. The ability of *Yersinia* to grow at low temperature, even as low as the normal refrigeration temperatures of 4°C, explains the persistence of organisms in affected foodstuffs and may partly explain the seasonal variation in clinical infections which are most frequent in autumn and winter. The growth characteristics may also be related to the geographical variations in yersinial infections. They are commoner in the cooler climates of Scandinavia and other northern European countries than in warmer countries. Most infections are sporadic but epidemics from infected drinking water and milk have been reported (Mair, 1977).

Clinical presentation

Yersinial terminal ileitis is usually due to *Y. enterocolitica*, serotype 0:9. Patients present with symptoms and signs similar to acute appendicitis. There may have been a preceding gastrointestinal upset with diarrhoea and associated malaise. On examination there is usually a low grade fever and signs of peritoneal irritation in the right iliac fossa. Acute ileitis, Crohn's disease and an appendix mass/abscess should be considered if a localized tender mass is palpable beneath McBurney's point. Long-standing gastrointestinal symptoms, weight loss and past history of anorectal sepsis are more in favour of Crohn's disease. Differentiation of yersinial ileitis and Crohn's disease at laparotomy can be extremely difficult. With both conditions the bowel wall is thickened and hyperaemic and the serosal surface may be covered with a serosanguinous exudate which causes adherence between adjacent loops of small intestine. The presence of skip lesions in the small bowel, encroachment of fat from mesentery on to the bowel wall and extension of disease into the right colon favour Crohn's disease. Pathological differentiation of the two conditions can also be difficult. A chronic non-specific inflammatory infiltrate with monouclear cells, lymphocytes and few polymorphs occurs in both and sarcoid-like granulomas and microabscesses can be found in lymphoid tissue in the gut wall and infected lympth nodes in *Yersinia* ileitis.

Despite the pathological similarities there is no definite association between *Yersinia* infection and either Crohn's disease or ulcerative colitis (Jess, 1981). However, there are undoubted cases of chronic, non-specific inflammatory bowel disease which are the result of an infection with *Y. enterocolitica* (Vantrappen et al, 1977). Infection with *Y. enterocolitica* and *Y. pseudotuberculosis* has been associated with acute appendicitis. Bacteria have been cultured and a rise, followed by a fall, in specific serum antibody levels to *Y. enterocolitica* have been observed in patients with acute appendicitis. Attwood et al (1989) were able to demonstrate infection with *Y. pseudotuberculosis* in 27% of patients with acute appendicitis. It is possible that many patients with acute abdominal pain have a *Yersinia* infection in the lymphoid tissue which may either resolve or progress to mesenteric adenitis, acute appendicitis or chronic right iliac fossa pain (Attwood et al, 1987).

Mesenteric adenitis is often due to *Y. pseudotuberculosis* (usually serotype I) or *Y. enterocolitica* (Saebo, 1983). *Y. enterocolitica* may also be responsible for non-specific abdominal pain, especially in children, many of whom have an associated pharyngitis from which the organism can be cultured. *Yersinia* species can also have a number of rare non-gastrointestinal manifestations. They can cause suppurative infections such as lung abscesses, osteomyelitis, pneumonia, cerebral abscesses, pyomyositis and lymphadenitis. *Yersinia* has also been implicated in a number of non-suppurative inflammatory conditions thought to be immunologically mediated. The commonest of these is an acute arthritis but ankylosing spondylitis, Reiter's syndrome, thyroiditis and glomerulonephritis have been described.

Diagnosis and treatment

Unequivocal proof of *Yersinia* infection depends on organism culture and demonstration of an appropriate rise and later fall in specific serum antibody titres (Bottone and Sheehan, 1983). In practice this is difficult to achieve. The infected site may be relatively inaccessible (mesenteric adenitis), strict culture conditions must be observed and it is important to check for changes in antibody titre for each pathogenic *Yersinia* serotype. However, for laboratories with an interest in *Yersinia* infections the specificity of techniques for antibody detection is very high. An enzyme-linked immunosorbent assay is the most accurate but detection of specific

IgA and IgM antibodies and tube agglutination are alternative methods (Cafferkey and Buckley, 1987). A fourfold rise in antibody titre or high level with subsequent fall are diagnostic of infection. The rise in antibody titre occurs within 1 week of infection and remains elevated for 1–3 months.

If a laparotomy is performed through a grid-iron/Lanz incision on the basis of a preoperative diagnosis of acute appendicitis and the patient is found to have terminal ileitis or Crohn's disease, an appendicectomy should be performed. The risk of a postoperative intestinal fistula in a patient with Crohn's disease is no greater after appendicectomy than if the appendix is not removed. If terminal ileitis due to *Yersinia* is suspected, an attempt should be made to culture the organism from the luminal contents of the appendix and a blood sample sent for serology.

Yersinia species are sensitive to tetracyclines, cotrimoxazole, aminoglycosides and choloramphenicol. In patients with *Yersinia*-related appendicitis no treatment other than appendicectomy is necessary. In those patients with terminal ileitis or persistent postoperative right iliac fossa pain in whom the diagnosis of *Yersinia* infection has been confirmed serologically the antibiotics of choice are tetracycline (except in children) or cotrimoxazole (Attwood et al, 1989).

Tuberculous ileitis

Abdominal tuberculosis is an uncommon condition in Britain. Any part of the gastrointestinal tract may be involved but most frequently it is the terminal ileum, right colon or peritoneum that is affected. Patients with abdominal tuberculosis usually present with symptoms of malaise, anorexia, abdominal pain, weight loss and diarrhoea extending back over a few months, but in the United Kingdom up to one-third present with acute symptoms requiring emergency laparotomy (Lambrianides et al, 1980).

Although tuberculosis is now uncommon in the indigenous population, largely as a result of the eradication of bovine tuberculosis and a decline in pulmonary tuberculosis, the disease has not disappeared. In 1980, 2289 cases of non-respiratory tuberculosis were notified in England, this representing approximately 25% of the total number of cases (Health and Personal Social Service Statistics for England, 1982). Tuberculosis is still a problem in underdeveloped countries and the majority of cases in the UK occur in immigrants of Asian or African descent.

Destruction of muscle and mucosa with fibrosis leads to mucosal ulceration, thickening of the bowel wall and eventually stricture formation. Spread of the organisms through the gut wall leads to the formation of tuberculous nodules (tubercles) on the visceral and parietal peritoneum, often with ascites.

Clinical presentation

The symptoms and signs of patients with abdominal tuberculosis who present acutely are similar to other intra-abdominal conditions such as acute appendicitis, perforated peptic ulcer or intestinal obstruction. Usually the diagnosis is not suspected preoperatively and is made at laparotomy. Abdominal tuberculosis should be considered in areas with a high immigrant population or where there is a poor standard of living. Ideally the diagnosis should be made without laparotomy and the patient treated medically with antituberculous drugs.

Diagnosis and treatment

The preoperative diagnosis of abdominal tuberculosis can be difficult. Laparotomy which provides tissue for culture and histological examination is often necessary to differentiate tuberculosis from Crohn's disease, small bowel lymphoma or colonic carcinoma. Mantoux testing is positive in only 30% of cases; a strongly positive test is very suggestive of tuberculosis. A leucocytosis is uncommon and less than 50% of patients have active pulmonary tuberculosis.

The diagnosis of abdominal tuberculosis is usually immediately obvious if a patient with acute symptoms is subjected to emergency laparotomy. The commonest finding is multiple tubercles over the serosal surface of the terminal ileum and caecum. It may be difficult to differentiate tubercles from metastatic deposits of adenocarcinoma. Tubercles tend to be larger, fewer in number and concentrated around the terminal ileum compared with deposits of carcinoma which are small, hard and often disseminated throughout the peritoneal cavity. If there is doubt, intraoperative frozen section examination of an excised nodule will be helpful. Mesenteric lymphadenopathy, an ileocaecal mass and tuberculous ascites are other frequent findings. A 'plastic peritonitis' is uncommon.

If tuberculosis is suspected at laparotomy, and there are no intestinal complications, surgery should be restricted to excision of a tubercle and removal of a sample of ascitic fluid, both for histological and bacteriological examination. Stenotic narrowing of the gut sufficient to produce intestinal obstruction or perforation requires resection of the affected bowel with end-to-end anastomosis.

Postoperatively antituberculous drugs should be commenced as soon as the diagnosis is confirmed. A number of different drug regimes have been used. Rifampicin and isoniazid plus ethambutol or streptomycin for 2 months followed by rifampicin and isoniazid alone for a further 7 months is usual treatment. Rifampicin 600 mg and isoniazid 300 mg daily for 1 month followed by rifampicin 600 mg and isoniazid 900 mg three times weekly for a further 8 months has also been reported to be successful and avoids the potential side effects of streptomycin (Dutt et al, 1986).

Postoperatively patients should be given other supportive treatment as appropriate (blood transfusion, correction of electrolyte disturbances, and enteral or parenteral nutrition). Family and other contacts should be screened for tuberculosis by the community health department.

Typhoid fever

Perforation of the terminal ileum may occur as a complication of typhoid fever and patients with this condition may present with fever and initially a localized peritonitis in the right iliac fossa. The differential diagnosis at this stage includes perforated appendicitis or peptic ulcer.

Bacteriology and pathology

Typhoid fever is caused by a Gram-negative bacillus *Salmonella typhi* and is contracted by ingestion of contaminated water or food. The ingested bacteria enter the blood stream via the Peyer's patches, multiply in the reticuloendothelial system during the next 10–14 days and then spread haematogenously, this phase corresponding with the onset of clinical symptoms. Bacteria reach the gut wall via the bloodstream or bile and concentrate in the Peyer's patches of the terminal ileum which swell. There is an associated mesenteric adenitis. Ulceration of the Peyer's patches in the craniocaudal axis of the bowel occurs and may be complicated by haemorrhage or perforation, which, most frequently, is on the anti-mesenteric border of the terminal ileum. Perforation usually occurs 8–11 days after the onset of clinical symptoms (Eggleston et al, 1979).

Clinical presentation

Typhoid is a disease of underdeveloped countries with poor sanitation but cases do occur in the United Kingdom in patients who have recently entered the country from an infected area. The characteristic signs are a very high fever (38.5–40°C), splenomegaly and rose spots on the upper abdomen. Patients may complain of diarrhoea or constipation, headaches, respiratory symptoms and develop a bradycardia and confusion. Increasing abdominal pain beginning in the right iliac fossa and exacerbated by movement is suggestive of small bowel perforation. The typical signs of a gastrointestinal perforation may not be present in a very toxic patient and regular abdominal examination is necessary in this group.

Diagnosis and treatment

The diagnosis of typhoid infection is made by culture of the organism from the blood during the first or second weeks or from urine or faeces from day 8 onwards. A Widal test becomes positive by the end of the second week. In cases of ileal perforation subdiaphragmatic air is present in approximately 70% of patients. The diagnosis of typhoid should be made on the basis of the preceding history of fever, the clinical signs of typhoid described and the presence of peritonitis in the right iliac fossa.

The mortality rate of typhoid perforations is high, figures from 40% to 60% being reported (Gibney, 1989). The treatment is operation after aggressive preoperative resuscitation with correction of fluid and electrolyte abnormalities based on clinical signs and laboratory results. Pulse, blood pressure and urine output should be carefully monitored and when fluid balance is critical central venous pressure monitoring should be performed.

Intravenous antibiotics should be given to all patients with a suspected diagnosis of typhoid fever. Chloramphenicol 500 mg 4-hourly (or 50 mg/kg/day) is the most effective and should be combined with ampicillin and metronidazole in the case of an ileal perforation.

Laparotomy is performed, preferably through a vertical lower abdominal incision, once the patient has been adequately resuscitated. Operative treatment depends on the number of intestinal perforations. A thorough laparotomy should be performed to assess the number of perforations and drain any localized collections of pus. With one or two perforations, closure of the perforation in two layers after excision of the ulcer is the treatment of choice. Bowel resection with end-to-end anastomosis is recommended if there are three or more perforations. All areas of doubtful viability should be oversewn to minimize the risk of postoperative reperforations that may occur with the paralytic ileus that frequently follows. Postoperatively antibiotics should be continued for a minimum of 14 days, at which stage blood, faeces and urine should be recultured to ensure eradication of the infection. Persistence of infection with continued excretion of bacteria is not an uncommon problem.

Crohn's ileitis

The diagnosis and management of patients with Crohn's ileitis is considered in Chapters 10 and 11.

ACUTE APPENDICITIS

Acute appendicitis presents the surgeon with a disease whose timely diagnosis and treatment can result in a short straightforward recovery, but one in which delay in diagnosis is the primary cause of much morbidity and some mortality. Approximately 150 patients die of appendicitis each year in England and Wales and although the majority of them are in the older age groups, deaths still occur in small numbers throughout the whole age spectrum. The classical presentation is familiar to all, the diagnosis being made predominantly clinically with investigations playing only a peripheral role. The numerous unusual presentations can, however, cause difficulties to even the most experienced clinician.

Acute appendicitis, a term coined by Fitz at Harvard in 1886, was only recognized as a primary inflammation of the appendix in the last 20 years of the nineteenth century. The incidence of the disease appears to have peaked in the first half of this century and is slowly declining (presently 10 per 10 000 per year). It is an uncommon problem in children under 3 years and rises to a peak incidence in the second decade, decreasing again thereafter (Andersen et al, 1980; Macfee 1982; Pieper and Kager, 1982). When it does occur at either extremity of the age range, the diagnosis may not be considered by the patient, their family or their doctor until the condition is advanced.

Aetiology

The aetiology of the disease is poorly understood. It is a disease of westernized society, but which features of this lifestyle are important is speculative.

Pathology

The primary cause of the inflammation seen in acute appendicitis is thought to be due to obstruction of the lumen with consequent increase in pressure (Pieper et al, 1982b) enabling bacteria from the lumen to invade the wall and initiate the inflammatory process. The obstruction is due to a faecolith in about 40% of cases (Shaw, 1965) and in the remainder is most probably caused by swelling of lymphoid tissue in the wall, producing a functional obstruction of the lumen. Gangrene with perforation is commoner in those with a faecolith (75%) than in those without (40%) (Shaw, 1965). Inflammation progresses to gangrene and then perforation with consequent peritonitis. Perforation is responsible for the major complications of the disease so that expeditious diagnosis and treatment, resulting in appendicectomy prior to perforation, should prevent most of the morbidity and mortality associated with the disease.

Infants have a particularly wide appendicular lumen which may be the cause of the low incidence in the early years of life. With ageing, the vascularity of the appendix decreases and, as the distal appendix is supplied by functional end arteries, it is not difficult to explain the higher incidence of perforation in the elderly (Lindgren and Aho, 1969).

Clinical presentation

History

The classical presentation is of colicky central abdominal pain caused by appendicular distension. As the inflammation progresses, discomfort, increasing to pain, develops in the right iliac fossa as the peritoneum is involved. Twenty-five per cent of patients, however, will start with the right iliac fossa pain, often made worse by movement and never have the central abdominal component (Winsey and Jones, 1967; Pieper et al, 1982a). Vomiting is seen in over 50% of adult patients and most patients lose their appetite. Bowel actions are often normal, or there may be constipation. Diarrhoea is an important symptom as 15–20% of patients with appendicitis will complain of it (often those with pelvic appendicitis) and it is also a symptom of a number of important diseases in the differential diagnosis, particularly *Yersinia* infection (Winsey and Jones, 1967; Jones, 1969; Pieper et al, 1982a).

Examination

The importance of careful examination of all systems cannot be overemphasized as diseases of almost every system enter the differential diagnosis. Low grade pyrexia and tachycardia are often present but some patients will have neither (Winsey and Jones, 1967). Furring of the tongue and a foetid breath will be present in many, but up to 40% will have neither.

The single consistent sign in acute appendicitis is local tenderness (Jones, 1976). In many cases this tenderness will be around McBurney's point ($1\frac{1}{2}$–2 inches from the anterior, superior iliac spine on a line to the umbilicus) but in retrocaecal appendicitis it will be quite far lateral and superior. In a pelvic appendicitis there may be little to find in the abdomen at all, with tenderness only elicited on rectal examination (Winsey and Jones, 1967; Jones, 1976; Pieper et al, 1982a). Involuntary guarding is a very useful sign and is much more specific for peritoneal inflammation than is tenderness alone, though guarding will be absent in up to 10% of patients. In retro-ileal inflammation there is also tenderness quite far medially without guarding and it is in this situation that release tenderness (rebound tenderness) may help in differentiation.

Rectal examination is vital in those patients (even children) where a confident positive diagnosis cannot be made on abdominal examination alone. This is particularly true in the case of patients with abdominal pain and diarrhoea (Winsey and Jones, 1967).

The concept of 'active observation' developed by Jones (1976) is extremely useful when there is any doubt about the diagnosis (Thomson and Jones, 1986). This approach does not discourage an immediate decision to operate, but rather is designed for those patients where the clinical condition is not clear cut. Repeated assessment is made by the same individual, initially after a short period but then over progressively longer intervals until either a decision to operate is made or the diagnosis has been excluded and an alternative treatment plan initiated.

Investigations

Leucocytosis is present in only 60% of patients with appendicitis (Winsey and Jones, 1967; Pieper et al, 1982a), so that its presence may reinforce a clinical diagnosis but its absence has little relevance. Microscopy of the urine is important, but again some patients with appendicitis have pyuria (Andersen et al, 1980). There are no pathognomonic X-ray signs of appendicitis and plain films are used (if at all) to exclude other conditions.

Differential diagnosis

The number of conditions in the differential diagnosis of patients with acute right iliac fossa pain is enormous. The main areas of potential difficulty are in the elderly and amongst young women, where as many will have a gynaecological condition as will have appendicitis (Walmsley et al, 1977).

The main gynaecological conditions that must be considered are rupture of a Graafian follicle, pelvic inflammatory disease (Bongard et al, 1985) and ectopic pregnancy (Macfee, 1982). The occurrence of lower abdominal pain at or just after the midcycle, combined with the acute onset of the pain should suggest the diagnosis of ruptured follicle. A short period of observation usually shows a marked improvement in symptoms. Pelvic inflammatory disease is suggested by fevers, vaginal discharge, predominantly suprapubic tenderness and tenderness on cervical excitation during rectal examination. Vaginal examination can then be combined with the taking of a high vaginal or endocervical swab, blood for *Clamydia* serology and definitive treatment.

Ectopic pregnancy should always be considered in women of reproductive years and the date of the last menstrual period must be sought. The history of investigation for infertility or the presence of an intra-uterine contraceptive device may also be pointers. Ninety per cent of women with an ectopic pregnancy will have had vaginal bleeding but this may have been quite mild in nature (Hughes, 1979). Tests for pregnancy should be performed.

In the elderly the diagnoses most frequently confused with appendicitis are diverticulitis (q.v.), where the sigmoid can lie over towards the right and perforation of a caecal carcinoma or other viscus. Rupture of an aortic aneurysm must also be considered as it is exactly the type of condition which will be missed if not considered.

Treatment

Timely appendicectomy is clearly the best treatment for the disease, but especially so in the very young and in the elderly. In almost all patients, but especially at the extremes of the age range, several hours preparing the patient for anaesthesia and operation may make all the difference between a smooth and stormy convalescence. As many patients have been taking little fluid for some hours and most have been vomiting, considerable quantities of intravenous fluids may be necessary to restore the fluid balance. Antibiotics should be given either as therapy or prophylactically depending on the severity of the case. (If the latter, metronidazole by suppository has the advantage of economy.)

Technique

Incision In the vast majority of cases a right iliac fossa muscle splitting incision will be best, as it gives excellent exposure, is easily extended and the majority of the conditions likely to be encountered can be dealt with through it (Gilmore et al, 1975). In the elderly, where the diagnosis can sometimes be only tentative, it is still best to use the quadrant incision but be prepared to extend it or to close it and make a midline incision, whichever is more appropriate.

Procedure In many cases the appendix is untethered and can simply be delivered and excised. The mesoappendix may be thickened and friable and is usually best dealt with by ligation and subsequent division without clamps. The stump is then inverted using a pursestring suture or Z stitch. It is much safer to leave the stump unburied than to attempt to bury a bulky stump into an oedematous friable caecum (Sinha, 1977). The operation is concluded with a check on haemostasis and vigorous peritoneal lavage with isotonic saline using tetracycline in the final litre.

There is often doubt about the best course of action when terminal ileitis is found. Many of these cases have *Yersinia* infection (Attwood et al, 1989) but some do have Crohn's disease. There is no substitute for the assessment of the bowel by an experienced surgeon in determining the appropriate operative strategy. Most often if the caecum is relatively normal the appendix only should be removed and a culture swab taken from its lumen looking for *Yersinia* infection. Postoperatively stool culture and *Yersinia* serology should enable a positive diagnosis to be made. Kewenter et al (1974) found that 85% of these patients had no signs of Crohn's disease 5 years later. A small number of patients do have Crohn's disease presenting acutely and in these a localized resection may be the most straightforward approach in the long term. Identification of these depends on experience in assessing the diseased bowel.

Occasionally an appendiceal tumour may be found. Adenocarcinoma of the appendix occurs rarely. It usually presents as an emergency and is perforated in over half of the cases reported. Right hemicolectomy is the treatment of choice but the prognosis is often poor (Gilhome et al, 1984; Cerame, 1988). Carcinoids are rarely recognized as such at operation, but their size determines prognosis (Anderson and Wilson, 1985). If the tumour is larger than 2 cm in diameter it should probably be treated by a right hemicolectomy.

The normal appendix

Even in the best hands a small proportion of patients will be found to have a normal appendix—around 20% in adults (Gilmore et al, 1975) but as low as 10% in children after active observation (Jones, 1976) (The following figures in brackets refer to the frequency of each finding from Gilmore et al (1975), Andersen et al (1980) and Pieper et al (1982a). If there is no peritoneal contamination the terminal ileum should be inspected looking for terminal ileitis (2–7%), a Meckel's diverticulum (1–2% in adults, but up to 14% in children (Jones, 1976)) or mesenteric adenitis (25–50%). The caecum should be inspected looking for caecal diverticulitis or a carcinoma. In the female the right fallopian tube and ovary should be carefully inspected. If disease is found (10–20%) a conservative approach is usually best. The removal of an ovary for a non-malignant condition in a woman of reproductive years may be a disaster for her. If there is doubt a gynaecological opinion should be sought. In those women with salpingitis, an intraperitoneal and an endocervical swab taken at the end of the procedure will allow treatment to progress postoperatively.

When there is peritoneal contamination or a retroperitoneal haematoma, a more thorough laparotomy is necessary and a vertical incision is mandatory. The primary problem can then be dealt with on its merits.

Appendicitis in the elderly

With larger numbers of patients in the older age groups so appendicitis is seen more often in the elderly. The history is usually less dramatic with generalized abdominal pain and constipation, often no shift of pain and commonly abdominal distension (Pieper et al, 1982a). Because of their age and the non-specific nature of many of the symptoms, presentation is often late and the diagnosis less sure (Burns et al, 1985; Sherlock, 1985). Sherlock (1985) felt that the higher perforation rate in those patients over 60 was due to delay in diagnosis after admission. Despite these concerns abut early operation to prevent perforation, it is vital that these elderly people are thoroughly assessed and prepared for operation in view of the prevalence of general medical conditions. It is notable, however, that one of the two deaths in Pieper's study was an elderly patient who, at operation, had a normal appendix (Pieper et al, 1982a).

Appendicitis in pregnancy

There are numerous potential problems when these two common clinical entities coincide. It has been calculated that this occurs in about one in every 1500–2000 deliveries so that individual surgeons are going to meet this problem rarely. Two of the physiological changes of pregnancy make the diagnosis more difficult. The lower pole of the caecum is displaced upwards and laterally by the enlarging uterus. The abdominal muscle relaxation necessary to accommodate the gravid uterus means that guarding is absent or reduced. The two cardinal signs of appendicitis, local tenderness and guarding, are difficult to evaluate. The major differential diagnosis is between appendicitis and a right-sided pyelitis. Microscopy of the urine is therefore vital.

The operative approach will depend on the gestation but a muscle-splitting incision centred on the area of maximal tenderness will give best access and ought to give the least problems later in pregnancy. Appendicectomy early in the course of pregnancy is a relatively safe procedure for the mother. Similarly, the removal of a normal appendix did not result in any fetal loss in the study by Finch and Lee (1974). Morbidity and fetal loss occur in the later stages of the disease and Finch and Lee also found a higher percentage of perforated or gangrenous appendices in pregnant women compared to non-pregnant women, perhaps indicating later diagnosis. Overall a fetal loss rate of 5–7% seems to be expected but this would be less with earlier diagnosis (Finch and Lee, 1974 ; Masters et al, 1984).

Complications

With early operation, prophylactic and therapeutic antibiotics and peritoneal lavage, complications are rare following appendicectomy. Wound infection should be uncommon (less than 10%; Krukowski et al, 1986) but a small number of pelvic and intraperitoneal abscesses still arise, as does adhesive intestinal obstruction (1–2%) (Pieper et al, 1982a).

Complications particular to appendicectomy are rupture of a stump abscess or stump rupture with a faecal leak. In the former an abscess forms under the pursestring stitch but does not communicate with the bowel (0.2%) (Sinha, 1977); if it does the result will be a faecal leak. Both of these are very rare and will require reoperation. Peritoneal toilet and drainage will be sufficient for rupture of an abscess but a faecal leak will require either a caecostomy or a resection. Whether anastomosis is performed after resection will depend on the state of the peritoneal cavity and the patient's general condition.

THE APPENDIX MASS

Occasionally patients, presenting with a history that would fit with appendicitis, have a tender mass in the right iliac fossa. If there is a fever and constitutional symptoms it is likely that pus is present and this should be drained. An ultrasound may confirm the diagnosis. Sometimes there is no fever and apart from a slightly tender mass the patient is well. Depending on the age group it may be important to consider other diagnoses such as Crohn's disease or a carcinoma of the caecum. A period of observation will demonstrate either resolution or progression to fever and increased tenderness. In the latter, the abscess can be drained and the underlying pathology treated on its merits. In the former case a barium enema will exclude a carcinoma. Whether or not an interval appendicectomy is performed is a matter of debate.

SOLITARY CAECAL DIVERTICULITIS

Inflammation of a solitary caecal diverticulum is a distinct entity separate from diverticulitis of the ascending colon. The diverticulum is a true one, usually close to the ileocaecal valve on the medial wall and probably congenital in origin. In many series this condition is confused with, and incorporated along with, cases of diverticulosis coli affecting the ascending colon.

The majority of patients are young adults. The presentation is indistinguishable from appendicitis and the differentiation at operation from carcinoma can be difficult. The choice of operation, because of the position close to the ileocaecal valve, and the difficulty differentiating the mass from carcinoma, is usually resection. The condition is often not recognized for what it is and a right hemicolectomy performed (Riseman and Wichterman, 1989). Less radical surgery is said to be safer if the condition is recognized and local excision, or no excision, is performed (Anscombe et al, 1967). This reluctance to perform formal resection seems to relate to previous rates of morbidity and mortality that would now be unacceptable, and resection ought to be a safe option (Riseman and Wichterman, 1989).

MECKEL'S DIVERTICULUM

Although the vast majority of Meckel's diverticula cause no complications, those complications which do occur can be life threatening and, especially in the adult, difficult to diagnose. The commonest congenital abnormality in the gastrointestinal tract, it arises because of a failure of obliteration of the vitellointestinal duct which, at 8 weeks of intra-uteric life, joins the yolksac to the small bowel. In three out of four cases Meckel's diverticulum will not be attached to another structure, the remainder being attached to the mesentery or the umbilicus with various portions remaining potentially patent.

Although the majority will lie within 100 cm of the ileocaecal valve, they can occur more cranially. Most are small (5 cm or less) but much longer structures are occasionally seen. By Meckel's original definition they have their own blood supply (omphalomesenteric artery) crossing the ileum from the mesentery to the wall of the diverticulum.

One to two per cent of the population have this anomaly but very few will experience complications. Perhaps as few as 4% of Meckel's ever become symptomatic and three-quarters of these will be within the first 15 years of life (Leijonmarck et al, 1986). The complications which do occur are intestinal obstruction, peptic ulceration and diverticulitis. The majority of the patients with obstructions have a band obstruction or volvulus round an attached band. The diverticulum can also become the apex of an ileo-ileal intussusception with diverticular knots and stenosis occurring very rarely.

Ectopic gastric mucosa occurs in 20–40% of diverticula and may give rise to ulceration, usually around the base of the diverticulum. In children there are a limited number of causes of painless melaena so that the condition will be thought of early and a technetium pertechnetate scan will show the ectopic mucosa as a hot spot in the mid-abdomen (Berquist et al, 1976). In adults, where there are a larger number of potential causes of this symptom complex, other commoner diagnoses should be excluded first, but a technetium scan should certainly precede arteriography. It is very rare for the peptic ulcer to perforate.

Diverticulitis may unusually occur in a Meckel's diverticulum. The history will be so similar to that of acute appendicitis that a correct preoperative diagnosis is unlikely. The appendix is normal or shows only superficial serosal inflammation as part of a generalized peritonitis. When sufficient ileum is delivered into the wound, the offending lesion will be found and can be excised. The presence of a diverticulum in a strangulated hernia was described by Alexis Littré but is rare (Meyerowitz, 1958).

The diverticulum found incidentally in a patient below the age of 20 years carries a 4–5% lifetime chance of complications, falling to 2% at 30 years and 1% by 60 years (Leijonmarck et al, 1986). In adults, unless it is attached to another structure, is particularly long or has a narrow base, it is probably best left alone (Soltero and Bill, 1976).

Operative treatment

Preoperative preparation will depend on the indication for operation. When found, the diverticulum should be excised by dividing or, better, underrunning the omphalomesenteric artery on the side of the ileum and excising the diverticulum along with a small portion of the ileal wall around the base. This latter precaution ensures that the 5% of ulcers which occur in the ileum adjacent to the neck of the diverticulum are also excised (Cobb, 1936). If the defect in the wall is closed obliquely or transversely there should be no luminal narrowing.

If it is thought necessary to excise a diverticulum found incidentally, it can probably be safely performed by clamping the base, with excision and oversewing, so that the bowel need never be opened.

DIVERTICULAR DISEASE OF THE COLON

Introduction

The presence of acquired colonic diverticula is common in developed countries, especially in people of the older age groups. Fortunately the majority of those with diverticular disease (diverticulosis) never present with either symptoms or complications of the condition (Parks, 1969a). The small minority of patients who do develop one of the complications of the disease are at risk of considerable morbidity and significant mortality. The prevalence of colonic diverticula rises with age and in western countries has risen during this century from about 5% in 1910 to over 50% now (Almy and Howell, 1980). Fifty to 75% of individuals over the age of 80 have diverticula (Cranston et al, 1988).

Pathology

The incidence is inversely related to dietary fibre (Manousos et al, 1985) and the postulated pathogenesis of smooth muscle spasm and thickening, generating short segments of high pressure which in turn cause pulsion diverticula, is well known (Painter, 1985). An ultrastructural study has recently shown that the primary abnormality may in fact be an increase in elastin in the taeniae, with consequent shortening (Whiteway and Morson, 1985). This may predispose to high pressures generated over a short length of colon during segmentation contractions. These in turn cause pulsion diverticula at the weak points in the colonic wall where the arteries traverse the muscularis propria.

The overwhelming majority of diverticula never give rise to any complication. A tiny minority become infected, probably by a faecolith obstructing one with a narrow neck. The bacteria in the enclosed mucus and faeces proliferate and, after mucosal damage has occurred, gain entry to the colonic wall or mesentery. Depending on the virulence of the organisms, and perhaps on the vascularity of the bowel, an abscess forms.

It is probable that many small abscesses discharge back into the colon enabling the inflammatory episode to settle either spontaneously or under conservative treatment. If the abscess develops slowly, adhesions may have formed to surrounding organs or omentum keeping the abscess confined. This pericolic collection will then present as a tender mass, usually with fever and leucocytosis. Alternatively, the abscess may perforate into an adjacent viscus, producing a fistula (e.g. bladder, vagina or bowel). Fistulas are present in about 20% of patients coming to surgery for diverticular disease (Woods et al, 1988) with about 65% of these being colovesical, 25% colovaginal and the remainder are coloenteric or colouterine. The uterus and broad ligament protect the bladder to some extent, explaining the strong male predominance for colovesical fistulas in most series; in women over 50% are seen in those who have previously undergone a hysterectomy (Woods et al, 1988). If the abscess develops quickly adhesions will not have formed so that perforation will be more likely to occur into the peritoneal cavity, giving rise to either a localized or generalized peritonitis. Whether this peritonitis is faecal or merely purulent will depend on whether the abscess cavity, however small, also communicates with the colon. This is sometimes termed a 'communicating perforation'. In some cases there appears little evidence of a preceding abscess when a faecal peritonitis has developed, there being only a small hole in the colonic wall in an area of diverticular disease. In these cases presumably the inflammation produces thrombosis of a vessel resulting in ischaemic necrosis and perforation. Corder (1987) has drawn attention to the association between septic complications of diverticular disease and the use of corticosteroids and non-steroidal anti-inflammatory drugs.

Various classifications of the septic complications of diverticular disease have been suggested. The most useful would appear to be that suggested by Krukowski and Matheson (1988) (Table 2). It is more useful than that proposed by Hinchey et al (1978) in the USA in that it differentiates generalized from localized peritonitis both purulent and faecal. Clearly this differentiation is vital in terms of prognosis, treatment and also in the comparison of results.

The pathology of bleeding from diverticular disease seems to relate to the

TABLE 2
Classification of septic complication of diverticular disease (Krukowski and Matheson, 1988)

(1) Acute diverticulitis with no visible pus
(2) Pus present
(a) Localized
(i) Abscess
(ii) Localized purulent peritonitis
(b) Generalized purulent peritonitis
(3) Faecal peritonitis
(a) Localized
(b) Generalized

anatomy of the vasa recti and their relationship to the wall of the diverticulum (Meyers et al, 1976). When pericolic inflammation has resolved, it is not surprising that fibrosis, in combination with the shortening and narrowing of the lumen seen in uncomplicated diverticular disease, can result in obstruction. It is often difficult to differentiate this type of obstruction from carcinoma. Occasionally Crohn's disease and diverticular disease coexist and the transmural inflammation of the Crohn's disease predisposes to peridiverticulitis and complications (Meyers et al, 1978).

Clinical presentation

As in appendicitis, the importance of the clinical assessment of these patients cannot be overemphasized. The presentation covers a wide range of severity and the initial assessment, the monitoring of response to treatment and decision to operate all require experience and familiarity with the condition. Krukowski and Matheson (1984) have emphasized the relative infrequency with which these patients are seen and it is clear that decisions should be taken by a senior surgeon and not delegated to a more junior one.

The typical presentation is of a middle-aged or elderly patient with lower abdominal pain, usually in the left iliac fossa. The onset is acute with no previous bowel symptoms (Parks, 1969b; Parks and Connell, 1970) but there may be non-specific malaise and anorexia, and some constipation is common. In the less severe case there is tenderness in the left iliac fossa but the remainder of the abdomen is soft. There may be a pyrexia and dehydration. Rectal examination is usually normal but occasionally an inflammatory mass can be felt in the pelvis. Sigmoidoscopy is usually unhelpful and the examination is often limited by faeces or discomfort at the level of the rectosigmoid junction. A leucocytosis may be present and plain abdominal films are usually unremarkable.

This presentation fits well with an acute diverticulitis with no large collection of pus. The vast majority of these patients settle with conservative treatment if it is timely and intensive (Krukowski and Matheson, 1988). Some present later with fever and a larger, more tender mass and in these patients pericolic abscess should be considered.

In the minority of patients who present with perforation (10–15%) (Parks and

Connell, 1970; Kyle and Davidson, 1975) the onset will be more dramatic and there is usually little doubt that the patient has generalized peritonitis. One patient will have generalized faecal peritonitis for every four with generalized purulent peritonitis (Shephard and Keighley, 1986) and less than half of these patients will have subdiaphragmatic gas (Nagorney et al, 1985). One of the most important features of this group of patients is that there is a high incidence of other diseases known to increase surgical risk (Alanis et al, 1989) notably cardiorespiratory disease, in addition to a significant proportion taking corticosteroid therapy (Nagorney et al, 1985).

Investigation

Investigations in the acute illness have usually been limited to blood tests and plain X-rays, contrast studies being avoided for fear of stimulating or further complicating the inflammation. If the patient settles, a barium enema can then be performed as an out-patient to confirm the diagnosis and exclude carcinoma. This course of action is satisfactory in the majority of patients, but where there is doubt about the diagnosis or concern about abscess formation, further radiological investigations are often necessary. Ultrasonic scanning may well detect a paracolic collection, as may computed tomography. Recently the use of water-soluble contrast studies has been examined and it would appear that the reluctance to use a contrast enema is unfounded. Kourtesis et al (1988) used contrast studies in 48 patients during the first week of hospitalization without complication. Krukowski and Matheson (1988) have also found this a useful and safe investigation to confirm or refute the diagnosis, identify complications such as perforation, and help to exclude coexisting carcinomata. Johnson et al, (1987) found contrast enema more accurate than CT scanning which seldom leads to a change in management.

Treatment

Almost all patients presenting with uncomplicated acute diverticulitis can be managed with 'medical treatment'. A careful assessment of the patient's general condition is important because of the frequency of concurrent illness, especially cardiorespiratory disease (Nagorney et al, 1985). Dehydration must be corrected and urine output measured. More invasive monitoring may be necessary if there is any element of cardiac failure of dysrhythmia. Anaemia should also be corrected.

Antibiotics will be the mainstay of supportive treatment. The agents used will depend on local policy but a combination of a cephalosporin or gentamicin with ampicillin and metronidazole will cover all likely organisms. Intravenous fluids should be continued after rehydration with only small amounts of oral fluid until clear improvement is occurring. Whether a water-soluble barium enema is performed at this stage or deferred, it is vital that carcinoma is excluded as 20–25% of patients having resections for diverticular disease in fact have carcinoma (Krukowski et al, 1986). The use of colonoscopy or flexible sigmoidoscopy to assess a stricture seen on barium enema will help reduce the number of patients in whom there is uncertainty, but if doubt remains, resection must be advised if the patient's condition permits.

An expectant policy with acute diverticulitis is likely to result in a low operative rate in these patients. Krukowski and Matheson (1988) operated on only 15% of their patients presenting with acute diverticulitis during that admission and none within 48 h of admission. If this type of policy is to be pursued a high level of experience and consistency of assessment are necessary.

Presentation as appendicitis

From time to time, at laparotomy for appendicitis, even after careful assessment, uncomplicated sigmoid diverticulitis will be found. The right thing to do in this situation is to remove the appendix, assess the remainder of the peritoneum and close the abdomen after peritoneal lavage (Ryan, 1983; Krukowski and Matheson, 1988). Postoperative antibiotics should be given.

Operative treatment

The main indications for operation are the development of a pericolic abscess that cannot be drained percutaneously and spreading peritonitis despite intensive supportive treatment. If it is possible to drain an abscess extraperitoneally, this can be done through a small incision over the mass followed by the insertion of a tube drain. However, this is exactly the type of abscess easiest to deal with percutaneously under radiological control so that this indication for operation is becoming less frequent. If drained percutaneously, investigation must then proceed to exclude carcinoma. Once excluded, the decision abut elective resection can be taken by reference to the patient's symptoms, age and general condition. Although some would suggest that percutaneous drainage of more complicated sepsis would allow more patients to have a single stage resection (Mueller et al, 1987), this has not been clearly proved. Those patients with spreading peritonitis, those with more complex sepsis or a free perforation will require a laparotomy.

In those patients who present with generalized peritonitis a few hours spent preparing them for surgery is seldom wasted. The mortality of this complication, even in reported series, lies between 10% and 25% (Krukowski and Matheson, 1984) and many of the patients are elderly, often with general medical problems. A long midline incision will enable adequate peritoneal toilet and lavage to be performed. Once the majority of the contamination has been removed it is wise rapidly to assess the remainder of the abdomen and exclude concurrent pathology before focusing attention on the affected colon, almost always the sigmoid.

Immediate versus staged resection

Formerly there was little doubt that the procedure of choice in dealing with the complications of sigmoid diverticular disease was a defunctioning colostomy and drainage followed by staged resection. Immediate resection is now the treatment of choice for the complications of diverticular disease. Resection carries the advantages that the source of contamination has been removed and with it the lingering doubt about the presence of carcinoma. A 'defunctioning' colostomy alone still leaves faeces between the colostomy and the diseased bowel which may potentiate sepsis. It leaves the patient facing one or more further procedures depending on the timing of closure of the colostomy. Twenty to 40% of the patients who have a defunctioning colostomy never have the stoma closed or have a resection (Shephard and Keighley, 1986; Finlay and Carter, 1987) and there is an increased chance of fistula formation in the defunctioned segment (Finlay and Carter, 1987). Few patients who really needed the procedure originally can simply have the colostomy closed without resection and a proportion of these require further operation at a later date.

The level of division of the vascular pedicle when resecting the sigmoid in these circumstances is debatable. The mesentery is usually thickened, shortened and difficult to transilluminate. Ideally, as there will often be a possibility of an occult carcinoma, high ligation of the inferior mesenteric artery would be preferable. The evidence that a 'high tie' of the inferior mesenteric artery is beneficial is weak (Surtees et al, 1990) and if the colon has perforated then the resection is, in any case, technically palliative.

The most crucial technical points are the upper and lower level of division of bowel as these must be through normal, pliable colon. At the lower end this almost always means division at the rectosigmoid junction or in the upper rectum above the peritoneal reflection; a Paul Mickulicz-type resection therefore is impossible. As in any resection of this type the left ureter and gonadal vessels are identified and preserved.

Peritoneal lavage

The value of peritoneal toilet has been studied. Hudspeth (1975) reported no intraperitoneal sepsis following radical debridement of the peritoneum but Polk and Fry (1980) showed no benefit from radical removal (including sharp dissection) of all fibrinous exudate when thorough lavage had also been performed. It seems reasonable, therefore, to perform thorough lavage, remove all particulate matter but not damage the serosa by trying to remove densely adherent fibrin plaques. Many of these will separate with a gentle wipe with a moist swab, but more vigorous cleaning may be counterproductive.

We use saline in large quantities for peritoneal toilet and add tetracycline (1 g/l, i.e. 0.1% solution) to the final litre. There is good scientific evidence to support both the dilutional effect of lavage and the effectiveness of topical tetracycline (Krukowski et al, 1986). Although bacteriostatic in normal serum concentrations, tetracycline becomes bacteriocidal at concentrations in the peritoneal cavity. Evidence that adhesion formation is increased by the use of tetracycline has never been produced. It can be shown by electron microscopy that damage to the peritoneum can occur after its use but whether this is greater than that caused by a generalized peritonitis is dubious.

Delayed versus primary anastomosis

The question of staged versus primary excision having been settled, debate has now shifted to the place of primary anastomosis. Hartmann's procedure consists of a sigmoid resection with end colostomy and closure of the rectal stump. The rectal stump can be closed with staples, or more economically with one or two layers of sutures. It is often helpful to use silk or polyamide which is easily identified when reanastomosis is subsequently performed. The descending colon is mobilized sufficiently to be brought out transperitoneally in the left iliac fossa without tension. The procedure is then completed by further peritoneal lavage.

The decision regarding the safety of primary anastomosis is contentious and often difficult in the individual case. The patient may be in suboptimal condition, the bowel will usually be unprepared and there will often be peritoneal contamination. If anastomosis is to be performed most would regard on-table washout as being beneficial (Dudley et al, 1980; Koruth et al, 1985; Krukowski and Matheson, 1988; Saadia and Schein, 1989), indeed mandatory. The technique of anastomosis is similar to anterior resection in general. The splenic flexure is mobilized, all diseased bowel excised, good vascularity ensured and a tension-free anastomosis performed. Whether this anastomosis is in one layer or two is more related to individual familiarity than dogma. In general terms, the results of primary anastomosis are better than Hartmann's procedure (Krukowski and Matheson, 1984; Alanis et al, 1989). Primary anastomosis is safe in patients whose general condition is good, who do not have generalized peritonitis and in whom, after on-table lavage, an experienced colonic surgeon is to perform the anastomosis. Few would perform an anastomosis in the presence of generalized peritonitis.

Prognosis

Prognosis will depend on the patient's age, general condition and the extent of disease. Kyle (1968) has shown that only two-thirds of all patients will be alive 5 years later and that 60% of these deaths are due to cardiovascular or cerebrovascular disease. Two-thirds of the survivors will be symptom free. The patients who require operation (Finlay and Carter, 1987) have a much higher mortality than those who can be treated medically. If these patients survive the procedure their prospect of good quality life is as good, or better than those patients treated medically (Parks and Connell, 1970).

Right-sided diverticulitis

Amongst people of oriental origin, diverticular disease of the ascending colon seems to be a distinct clinical entity (Gouge et al, 1983; Tan et al, 1984; Graham and Ballantyne, 1987). This condition may be confused with solitary caecal diverticulum which is a separate, distinct disease. The presentation is very similar to appendicitis and patients often have a laparotomy on that basis. If the disease is considered, a barium enema shows characteristic appearances (Gouge et al, 1983) and most patients will settle with antibiotics. If found at operation, right hemicolectomy seems safe and should be performed (Graham and Ballantyne, 1987).

CONCLUSIONS AND THE WAY FORWARD

All these acute inflammatory conditions of the abdominal cavity require the same careful clinical evaluation, judicious use of modern investigations, and, where appropriate, thoughtful and planned operative management. In several areas, particularly the biliary tract, laparoscopic, peroral endoscopic and percutaneous techniques are likely to play an increasing role in the future.

REFERENCES

Addison NW & Finan RJ (1988) Urgent and early cholecystectomy for acute gall bladder disease. *British Journal of Surgery* **75**: 141–143.

Alanis A, Papanicolaou GK, Tadros RR & Fielding P (1989) Primary resection and anastomosis for treatment of acute diverticulitis. *Diseases of Colon and Rectum* **32**: 933–939.

Almy TP & Howell DA (1980) Diverticular disease of the colon. *New England Journal of Medicine* **302**: 324–331.

Andersen M, Lilja T, Lundell L & Thulin A (1980) Clinical and laboratory findings in patients subjected to laparotomy for suspected acute appendicitis. *Acta Chirurgica Scandinavica* **146**: 55–63.

Anderson JR & Wilson BG (1985) Carcinoid tumours of the appendix. *British Journal of Surgery* **72**: 545–546.

Anscombe AR, Keddie NC & Schofield PF (1967) Solitary ulcers and diverticulitis of the caecum. *British Journal of Surgery* 553–557.

Attwood SEA, Mealy K, Cafferkey MT et al (1987) Yersinia infection and acute abdominal pain. *Lancet* **i**: 529–533.

Attwood SEA, Cafferkey MT & Keane FBV (1989) Yersinia infections in surgical practice. *British Journal of Surgery* **76**: 499–504.

Audisio RA, Bozzetti F, Severini A, Bellesotti L, Bellomi M, Cozzi G, Pisani P, Callegaria L, Doci R, Gennari L (1988) The occurrence of cholangitis after percutaneous biliary drainage: evaluation of some risk factors. *Surgery* **103**: 507–512.

Berquist TH, Nolan NG, Stephens DH & Carlson HC (1976) Specificity of ^{99}Tc-pertechnetate in scintigraphic diagnosis of Meckel's diverticulum: Review of 100 cases. *Journal of Nuclear Medicine* **17**: 465–469.

Bongard F, Landers DV & Lewis F (1985) Differential diagnosis of appendicitis and pelvic inflammatory disease: a prospective study. *American Journal of Surgery* **150**: 90–95.

Bottone GJ & Sheehan DJ (1983) *Yersinia enterocolitica*: guidelines for serological diagnosis of human infections *Review of Infectious Diseases* **5**: 898–906.

Burns RP, Cochran JL, Russell WL & Bard RM (1985) Appendicitis in mature patients. *Annals of Surgery* **201**: 695–702.

Cafferkey MT & Buckley TF (1987) Comparison of saline agglutination anti human globulin and immunofluorescence tests in the routine serological diagnosis of yersiniosis. *Journal of Infectious Diseases* **156**: 845–848.

Cerame MA (1988) A 25 year review of adenocarcinoma of the appendix. *Diseases of Colon and Rectum* **31**: 145–150.

Cobb DB (1936) Meckel's diverticulum with peptic ulcer. *Annals of Surgery* **103**: 747–751.

Corder A (1987) Steroids, non-steroidal anti-inflammatory drugs, and serious septic complications of diverticular disease. *British Medical Journal* **295**: 1238

Cranston D, McWhinnie D & Collin J (1988) Dietary fibre and gastrointestinal disease. *British Journal of Surgery* **75**: 508–572.

Csendes A, Sepulvera A, Burdiles P, Braghetto J, Bastias J, Schutte H, Diaz J-C, Harmuch J & Maluenda F (1988) Common bile duct pressure in patients with common bile duct stones with or without acute suppurative cholangitis. *Archives of Surgery* **123**: 697–699.

Dudley HAF, Radcliffe AG & McGeehan D (1980) Intraoperative irrigation of the colon to permit primary anastomosis. *British Journal of Surgery* **67**: 80–81.

Du Plessis DJ & Jersky J (1973) The management of acute cholecystitis. *Surgical Clinics of North America* **53**: 1071–1077.

Dutt AK, Moers D & Stead WW (1986) Short course chemotherapy for extrapulmonary tuberculosis. *Annals of Internal Medicine* **104**: 7–12.

Dykes EH, Stewart I, Gray H, Simpson C, Davidson S & McArdle CS (1984) Infusion cholecystography in the early diagnosis of acute gall bladder disease. *British Journal of Surgery* **71**: 854–855.

Eggleston FC, Santoshi B & Singh CM (1979) Typhoid perforation of the bowel: experience in 78 cases. *Annals of Surgery* **190**: 31–35.

Finch DRA & Lee E (1974) Acute appendicitis complicating pregnancy in the Oxford Region. *British Journal of Surgery* **61**: 129–132.

Finlay IG & Carter DC (1987) A comparison of emergency resection and staged management in perforated diverticular disease. *Diseases of Colon and Rectum* **30**: 929–933.

Fowkes FGR & Gunn AA (1980) The management of acute cholecystitis and its hospital cost. *British Journal of Surgery* **67**: 613–617.

Gibney EJ (1989) Typhoid perforation. *British Journal of Surgery* **76**: 887–889.

Gigot JF, Leese T, Dereme T, Coutinhyo J, Castaing D & Bismuth H (1989) Acute cholangitis: Multivariate analysis of risk factors. *Annals of Surgery* **209**: 435–438.

Gilhome RW, Johnston DH, Clark J & Kyle J (1984) Primary adenocarcinoma of the vermiform appendix: report of a series of ten cases and review of the literature. *British Journal of Surgery* **71**: 553–555.

Gilmore OJA, Brodribb AJM, Browett JP et al (1975) Appendicitis and mimicking conditions. *Lancet* **2**: 421–424.

Gouge TH, Coppa GF, Eng K, Ranson JHC & Localio SA (1983) Management of diverticulitis of the ascending colon. *American Journal of Surgery* **145**: 387–391.

Gracie WA & Ransohoff DF (1982) The natural history of silent gallstones; the innocent gall stone is not a myth. *New England Journal of Medicine* **307**: 798–800.

Graham SM & Ballantyne GH (1987) Cecal diverticulitis: a review of the American experience. *Disease of Colon and Rectum* **30**: 821–826.

Gump FE, Lepore M & Richter HS (1967) A revised concept of acute regional enteritis. *Annals of Surgery* **166**: 942.

Health and Personal Social Services Statistics for England (1982) Department of Health and Social Security HMSO 127.

Heberer G, Paumgartner G, Sauerbruch T, Sackmann M, Kramling H-J, Delius M & Brendel W (1988) A retrospective analysis of 3 years experience of an interdisciplinary approach to gallstone disease including shock-waves. *Annals of Surgery* **208**: 274–278.

Herlin P, Alinder G, Karp W & Holmin T (1984) Contrast tomography of the gall bladder wall and ultrasonography in the diagnosis of acute cholecystitis. *British Journal of Surgery* **71**: 850–853.

Hinchey J, Schaal PG & Richards GK (1978) Treatment of perforated diverticular disease of the colon. *Advances in Surgery* **12**: 85–109.

Hudspeth AS (1975) Radical surgical debridement in the treatment of advanced generalized bacterial peritonitis. *Archives of Surgery* **110**: 1233–1236.

Hughes GJ (1979) The early diagnosis of ectopic pregnancy. *British Journal of Surgery* **66**: 789–792.

Jess P (1981) Acute terminal ileitis. A review of recent literature on the relationship to Crohn's disease. *Scandinavian Journal of Surgery* **16**: 321–324.

Jivegard L, Thornell E & Svanvik J (1987) Pathophysiology of acute obstructive cholecystitis. *British Journal of Surgery* **74**: 1084–1086.

Johnson CD, Baker ME, Rice RP, Silverman P & Thompson WM (1987) Diagnosis of acute colonic diverticulitis: a comparison of barium enema and CT. *American Journal of Radiology* **148**: 541–546.

Jones PF (1969) Acute abdominal pain in childhood with special reference to cases not due to acute appendicitis. *British Medical Journal* 1: 284–286.

Jones PF (1976) Active observation in management of acute abdominal pain in childhood. *British Medical Journal* 2: 551–553.

Keane FBV & Tanner WA (1988) Extracorporeal lithotripsy for gall stones. *British Journal of Surgery* 75: 506–507.

Keighley MRB (1977) Micro organisms in the bile. A preventable cause of sepsis after biliary surgery. *Annals Royal College of Surgeons of England* 59: 328–334.

Kellett MJ, Wickham JEA & Russell RCG (1988) Percutaneous cholecystolithotomy. *British Medical Journal* 296: 453–455.

Kewenter J, Hultén L & Kock NG (1974) Relationship and epidemiology of acute terminal ileitis and Crohn's disease. *Gut* 15: 801–804.

Koruth NM, Krukowski ZH, Youngson G et al (1985) Intra-operative colonic irrigation in the management of left-sided large bowel emergencies. *British Journal of Surgery* 72: 708–711.

Kourtesis GJ, Williams RA & Wilson SF (1988) Acute diverticulitis: safety and value of contrast studies in predicting need for operation. *Australian and New Zealand Journal of Surgery* 50, 801–804.

Krukowski ZH & Matheson NA (1984) Emergency surgery for diverticular disease complicated by generalized and faecal peritonitis: a review. *British Journal of Surgery* 71: 921–927.

Krukowski ZH & Matheson NA (1988) Acute diverticulitis. In Russell RCG (ed.) *Recent Advances in Surgery*, No 13, pp 125–141. Edinburgh: Churchill Livingstone.

Krukowski ZH, Koruth NM & Matheson NA (1986) Antibiotic lavage in emergency surgery for peritoneal sepsis. *Journal of the Royal College of Surgeons of Edinburgh* 31, 1–6.

Kyle J (1968) Prognosis in diverticulitis. *Journal of the Royal College of Surgeons of Edinburgh* 13: 136–141.

Kyle J & Davidson AI (1975) The changing pattern of hospital admissions for diverticular disease of the colon. *British Journal of Surgery* 62: 537–541.

Lai ECS, Lo C-M, Choi FK, Cheng W-K, Fan S-T & Wong J (1989) Urgent biliary decompression after endoscopic retrograde cholangiopancreatography. *American Journal of Surgery* 157: 121–125.

Lambrianides AL, Ackroyd N & Shorey BA (1980) Abdominal tuberculosis. *British Journal of Surgery* 67: 887–889.

Leese T, Neoptolemos JP, Baker AR & Carr-Locke DL (1986) Management of acute cholangitis and the impact of endoscopic sphincterotomy. *British Journal of Surgery* 72: 988–992.

Leijonmarck CE, Bonman-Sandelin K, Frisell J & Räf L (1986) Meckel's diverticulum in the adult. *British Journal of Surgery* 73: 146–149.

Lindgren I & Aho AJ (1969) Microangiographic investigations on acute appendicitis. *Acta Chirurgica Scandinavia* 135: 77–82.

McArthur P, Cuschieri A, Sells RA & Shields R (1975) Controlled clinical trial comparing early with interval cholecystectomy for acute cholecystitis. *British Journal of Surgery* 62: 850–852.

Macfee CAJ (1982) Ectopic pregnancy. *British Journal of Hospital Medicine* 28: 246–247.

Mair NS (1977) Yersinia infections. In Truelove SC & Lee E (eds) *Topics in Gastroenterology*, vol 5, pp 325–328. Oxford: Blackwell.

Manousos O, Day NE, Tzonou A, Papadimitriou C & Kapetanakis A (1985) Diet and other factors in the aetiology of diverticulosis: an epidemiological study in Greece. *Gut* 26: 544–549.

Marton KI & Doubilet P (1988) How to image the gall bladder in suspected cholecystitis. *Annals of Internal Medicine* 109: 722–729.

Masters K, Lerne BA, Gaskill HV & Sirinek KR (1984) Diagnosing appendicitis during pregnancy. *American Journal of Surgery* **148**: 768–771.

Meyerowitz BR (1958) Littré's hernia. *British Medical Journal* **1**: 1154.

Meyers MA, Alonso DR, Gray GF & Baer JW (1976) Pathogenesis of bleeding colonic diverticulosis. *Gastroenterology* **71**: 577–583.

Meyers MA, Alonson DR, Morson BC & Bartram C (1978) Pathogenesis of diverticulitis complicating granulomatous colitis. *Gastroenterology* **74**: 24–31.

Morris CR, Hohf RPO & Ivy AC (1952) An experimental study of the role of stasis in the etiology of cholecystitis. *Surgery* **32**: 673–685.

Mueller PR, Saini S & Wittenburg J (1987) Sigmoid diverticular abscesses: percutaneous drainage as an adjunct to surgical resection in 24 cases. *Radiology* **164**: 321–326.

Nagorney DM, Adson MA & Pemberton JH (1985) Sigmoid diverticulitis with perforation and generalized peritonitis. *Diseases of the Colon and Rectum* **28**: 71–75.

Norrby S, Herlin P, Holmin T, Sjodahl R & Tagesson C (1983) Early or delayed cholecystectomy in acute cholecystitis? A clinical trial. *British Journal of Surgery* **70**: 163–165.

Olaison G, Kald B, Karlqvist P-Å, Lindström E & Anderberg B (1987) Endoscopic removal of common bile duct stones without subsequent cholecystectomy. *Acta Chirurgica Scandinavica* **153**: 541–543.

Painter NS (1985) The cause of diverticular disease of the colon, its symptoms and its complications. *Journal of the Royal College of Surgeons of Edinburgh* **30**: 118–122.

Parks TG (1969a) Natural history of diverticular disease of the colon. A review of 521 cases. *British Medical Journal* **4**: 639–642.

Parks TG (1969b) Reappraisal of clinical features of diverticular disease of the colon. *British Medical Journal* **4**: 642–645.

Parks TG & Connell AM (1970) The outcome in 455 patients admitted for treatment of diverticular disease of the colon. *British Journal of Surgery* **57**: 775–778.

Patti MG & Pellegrini CA (1989) Biliary infections. *Current Opinions in Gastroenterology* **5**: 624–629.

Pieper R & Kager L (1982) The incidence of acute appendicitis and appendicectomy. *Acta Chirurgica Scandinavica* **148**: 45–49.

Pieper R, Kager L & Näsman P (1982a) Acute appendicitis: a clinical study of 1018 cases of emergency appendicectomy. *Acta Chirurgica Scandinavica* **148**: 51–62.

Pieper R, Kager L & Tidefeldt U (1982b) Obstruction of appendix vermiformis causing acute appendicitis. *Acta Chirurgica Scandinavica* **148**: 73.

Polk HC & Fry DE (1980) Radical peritoneal debridement for established peritonitis. *Annals of Surgery* **192**: 350–353.

Riseman JA & Wichterman K (1989) Evaluation of right hemicolectomy for unexpected cecal mass. *Archives of Surgery* **124**: 1043–1044.

Roslyn JJ, Den Besten L, Thompson JE & Silverman BF (1980) Roles of lithogenic bile and cystic duct occlusion in the pathogenesis of acute cholecystitis. *American Journal of Surgery* **140**: 126–130.

Ryan P (1983) Changing concepts in diverticular disease. *Diseases of the Colon and Rectum* **26**: 12–18.

Saadia R & Schein M (1989) The place of intraoperative antegrade colonic irrigation in emergency left-sided colonic surgery. *Diseases of the Colon and Rectum* **32**: 78–81.

Saebo A (1983) The *Yersinia enterolitica* infection in acute abdominal surgery. A clinical study with a 5 year follow-up. *Annals of Surgery* **6**: 760–764.

Schofield PF, Nulton NR & Baildam AD (1986) Is it acute cholecystitis? *Annals of the Royal College of Surgeons of England* **68**: 14–16.

Shaw RE (1965) Appendix calculi and acute appendicitis. *British Journal of Surgery* **52**: 451–459.

Shephard AA & Keighley MRB (1986) Audit on complicated diverticular disease. *Annals of the Royal College of Surgeons of England* **68**: 8–10.

Sherlock DJ (1985) Acute appendicitis in the over-sixty age group. *British Journal of Surgery* **72**: 245–246.

Sinha AP (1977) Appendicectomy: an assessment of the advisability of stump invagination. *British Journal of Surgery* **64**: 499–500.

Soltero MJ & Bill AH (1976) The natural history of Meckel's diverticulum and its relation to incidental removal. *American Journal of Surgery* **132**: 168–171.

Surtees P, Ritchie JK & Phillips RKS (1990) High versus low ligation of the inferior mesenteric artery in rectal cancer. *British Journal of Surgery* **77**: 618–621.

Tan EC, Tung KH, Tan K & Wee A (1984) Diverticulitis of caecum and ascending colon in Singapore. *Journal of the Royal College of Surgeons of Edinburgh* **29**: 373–375.

Tanaka M, Ikeda S, Yoshimoto H & Matsumoto (1987) The long term fate of the gall bladder after endoscopic sphincterotomy: complete follow-up study of 122 patients. *American Journal of Surgery* **154**: 505–509.

Thomson HJ & Jones PF (1986) Active observation in acute abdominal pain. *American Journal of Surgery* **152**: 522–525.

Walmsley GL, Wilson DH & Gunn AA (1977) Computer-aided diagnosis of lower abdominal pain in women. *British Journal of Surgery* **64**: 538–541.

Vantrappen G, Agg HO, Panette E et al (1977) Yersinia enteritis and enterocolitis: gastroenterological aspects. *Gastroenterology* **72**: 220–227.

Wenckert A & Robertson B (1966) The natural course of gallstone disease. Eleven year review of 781 non-operated cases. *Gastroenterology* **50**: 376–381.

Whiteway J & Morson BC (1985) Elastosis in diverticular disease of the sigmoid colon. *Gut* **26**: 258–266.

Williamson RCN (1988) Acalculous disease of the gall bladder. *Gut* **29**: 860–872.

Willis RG, Lawson WC, Hoare EM, Kingston RD & Sykes PA (1984) Are bile bacteria relevant to septic complications following biliary surgery? *British Journal of Surgery* **71**: 845–849.

Winsey HS & Jones PF (1967) Acute abdominal pain in childhood: analysis of a year's admissions. *British Medical Journal* **1**: 653–655.

Woods RJ, Lavery IC, Fazio VM et al (1988) Internal fistulas in diverticular disease. *Diseases of the Colon and Rectum* **31**: 591–596.

13

ACUTE SEPTIC CONDITIONS IN THE ABDOMINAL CAVITY

M. Lavelle-Jones and A. Cuschieri

INTRODUCTION

Most acute septic conditions in the peritoneal cavity are a consequence of bacterial contamination originating either from a diseased intraperitoneal viscus, from an infected retroperitoneal organ, or following a penetrating injury. Usually the infection is rapidly disseminated and leads to a generalized secondary bacterial peritonitis. Should the infection remain localized, an intra-abdominal abscess will develop, and in about one-third of patients abscess formation will be the sequel to an episode of generalized peritonitis.

The importance of prompt surgical intervention in these patients is emphasized by the high mortality rates (greater than 80%) in patients with neglected intra-abdominal sepsis who do not undergo surgical drainage. However, despite many advances in critical care medicine and in surgical technique mortality rates in patients with severe intra-abdominal sepsis remain between 10% and 30%. In the last decade, attempts to improve survival have centred on the development of a number of aggressive surgical procedures designed to achieve more effective surgical drainage of the septic abdomen together with the introduction of effective percutaneous drainage techniques enabling the interventional radiologist to provide a safe alternative to open drainage in patients with intra-abdominal abscess. This chapter will review the role of these recent developments in the treatment of patients with focal and diffuse intra-abdominal sepsis and will consider in detail the management of postoperative and retroperitoneal sepsis and their associated complications which are some of the most challenging intra-abdominal conditions the surgeon is likely to encounter.

ACUTE SECONDARY BACTERIAL PERITONITIS

Secondary bacterial peritonitis is the commonest cause of intraperitoneal infection and is the result of bacterial contamination usually from a septic focus within the abdomen—often a perforated viscus—or as a complication of elective surgery. Less commonly in the UK the source may originate from penetrating trauma (Table 1).

TABLE I
Common causes of peritonitis

Severity	Cause
Mild	Appendicitis
	Perforated peptic ulcers
	Acute salpingitis
Moderate	Small bowel perforation
	Gangrenous cholecystitis
	Intra-abdominal trauma
	Diverticulitis
Severe	Large bowel perforation
	Ischaemic bowel
	Infected necrotizing pancreatitis
	Postoperative complications

(After Boey and Dunphy, 1985.)

Diagnosis

Diffuse peritonitis is characterized by prostration, severe abdominal pain and the manifestations of systemic infection. In addition, there may be localizing symptoms and signs caused by the underlying injury. Septic shock (oliguria, hypotension and tachypnoea) is evident in about 10% of patients (Lygidakis, 1986). The most important physical finding is muscle guarding with or without rebound tenderness (Flint, 1982). The presence of bowel sounds does not exclude the diagnosis of generalized peritonitis. Diaphragmatic irritation, if present, can produce shoulder tip or subscapular pain. Any or all of these physical signs may be masked in the elderly patient with a lax abdominal wall, in patients with neglected peritonitis where a reactive intra-abdominal effusion has developed or in patients who are immunosuppressed.

Although most patients with generalized peritonitis will have a significant leucocytosis (greater than $15 \times 10^9/l$), spuriously low white cell counts or a normal count with a left shifted differential may be evident in the immunosuppressed, overwhelmingly septic or debilitated patient (Flint, 1982). Plain abdominal radiographs may be similarly non-specific and free air will be encountered only in a proportion of erect chest films and only then if the patient has been allowed to remain upright for 10 min prior to exposure (Flint, 1982).

Occasionally, despite these 'routine' investigations, particularly in those individuals with multiple medical problems or in whom a medical history is unreliable and abdominal findings difficult to interpret, the surgeon may be faced with the patient in whom the need for operation is uncertain. In these individuals, diagnostic peritoneal lavage may be of value (Richardson et al, 1983). A sample of peritoneal fluid is obtained after instilling 1 l of isotonic saline into the peritoneal cavity via a disposable peritoneal dialysis catheter inserted under local anaesthesia (Richardson et al, 1983). If one or more of the following criteria are present, the lavage is considered positive: (1) a leucocyte count greater than $500/mm^3$; (2) an erythrocyte count greater than $100\,000/mm^3$; (3) the presence of bile. Using these criteria, the false positive rate was 10% in a group of 138 patients evaluated by lavage and only one patient had a false negative result suggesting that the procedure is useful in the detection of peritonitis in critically ill patients in whom the standard diagnostic criteria are absent or equivocal. In addition, the lavage fluid amylase can be measured. An amylase content twice that of the serum amylase is considered significant and in keeping with the diagnosis of acute pancreatitis (Flint, 1982).

The laparoscope provides an alternative approach in those patients in whom coexistant medical disease makes a negative laparotomy unacceptable. Although there is little doubt that laparoscopy is of value in the diagnosis of patients with chronic abdominal pain its use has been less widely accepted in the evaluation of the acute abdomen (Cuschieri, 1980). However, a recent study has demonstrated its effectiveness as an adjunct to decision making in the acute abdomen (Paterson-Brown et al, 1986). In this study of 125 patients with abdominal pain, the need for laparotomy was uncertain in 31 individuals. Urgent laparoscopy in this subgroup obviated six inappropriate operative decisions. Had all patients undergone laparoscopy, a further 11 incorrect management decisions could have been avoided, underlining the value of laparoscopy in evaluating the 'acute' abdomen with equivocal abdominal findings. As yet the role of the laparoscope in the evaluation of sepsis in the postoperative abdomen has not been evaluated but it is likely that technical difficulties will limit its application under these conditions.

Scoring systems

The interpretation of many recent therapeutic trials has been hampered by a lack of patient stratification and the uncontrolled nature of many studies (Lavori et al, 1983). As a result, a number of scoring systems have been devised to aid comparison between groups of patients. Most are based on the APACHE system which consists of a two part assessment taking into account the physiological response to the underlying insult (AP) and a chronic health evaluation (CHE) reflecting the patients preadmission health status. This system designed by Knaus et al (1981) to describe the mortality risk in populations of intensive care patients has subsequently been simplified (APACHE II score) (Knaus et al, 1985) and validated prospectively in abdominal sepsis (Bohnen et al, 1988). More recently, it has been used to stratify patients in several sepsis studies (Garcia-Sabrido et al, 1988; Schein et al, 1988). Although these sepsis scores can usefully provide a comparison between groups of patients they are only of limited value in assisting the clinician in the assessment and management of individual patients (Dellinger, 1988).

Preoperative preparation

Resuscitation

Adequate preoperative preparation of the patient with diffuse peritonitis is vital. Inevitably, there will be massive and continuing losses of extracellular fluid into the peritoneal cavity and volume restoration is the first consideration in these critically ill patients. We prefer to begin infusion via large-bore peripheral lines sited on the upper limbs reserving subclavian or internal jugular vein catheterization until the initial phase of resuscitation is under way. In the critically ill shocked patient a 2 l intravenous infusion of isotonic saline or balanced salt solution is rapidly administered (15–20 min) and the response assessed. All patients should undergo urinary catheterization and the restoration of a urine output (30–50 ml/h) is the best indicator of an adequate initial resuscitation. Once this initial phase is underway, central venous access either by the jugular or subclavian route is established to allow monitoring of central venous pressure and volume replacement. It is our practice to restrict the use of colloid until the initial resuscitation has been completed using salt solutions. Thereafter colloid is introduced as necessary to maintain the central venous pressure and the urine output. In the elderly patient or those with significant cardiac disease placement of a pulmonary artery Swan–Ganz catheter will allow measurement of cardiac output, mixed venous oxygen levels and right and left atrial pressures (O'Quinn and Marini, 1983) which will help fine tune therapy in septic shock particularly if inotropic agents such as dopamine or dobutamine are employed.

Once the initial resuscitation has been carried out, any delay in definitive treatment will only lead to clinical deterioration. In the critically ill patient, prolonged preoperative preparation can be counterproductive and under these circumstances early operative intervention is mandatory.

Antibiotics

Successful treatment ultimately depends upon effective, early surgery together with appropriate intensive supportive care. Antibiotics have a secondary, although important, role in the management of patients with severe intra-abdominal sepsis. Most intraperitoneal infections are polymicrobial. In patients with colonic perforation or intestinal necrosis the infecting inoculum is usually large and contains anaerobes and aerobes whereas infection following an upper gastrointestinal perforation is usually caused by aerobes (Lygidakis, 1986). The commonest infecting organisms are E. coli and Baceroides fragilis which are present in about 60% and 45%, respectively, of all cases of intra-abdominal sepsis (Table 2) (Solomkin et al, 1988). Any antibiotic regimen chosen should be active against these organisms, and currently most clinicians will opt for a broad spectrum preoperative cover using metronidazole in combination with an aminoglycoside and a penicillin derivative. Using these regimens, a near 100% cure rate has been achieved when combined with adequate surgery (Solomkin, 1988). Recently, the use of 'triple therapy' as a gold standard has been challenged by the development of single broad spectrum agents such as the second and third generation cephalosporins (beta-lactams) as a means to avoid the nephrotoxic and ototoxic side effects associated with aminoglycosides. Despite many beta-lactams having a reduced spectrum of sensitivity against certain intra-abdominal organisms, for example Bacteroides sp, and Pseudomonas aeruginosa, they still appear to be clinically effective (Solomkin, 1988). In particular, recent studies using imipenem (Leaper et al, 1987) or cefotetan (Huizinga et al, 1988) have demonstrated the efficacy of single agent antimicrobial therapy without the development of enterococcus superinfection or coagulation disturbances noted with earlier beta-lactams

TABLE 2
Bacterial species identified in intra-abdominal sepsis

Species	% of cases
Aerobes	
Escherichia coli	62
Klebsiella spp.	15
Proteus spp.	15
Pseudomonas spp.	8
Enterobacter spp.	5
Other Gram negatives	16
Enterococci	22
Other *Staphylococcus*/*Streptococcus* spp.	19
Staphylococcus aureus	9
Anaerobes	
Bacteroides fragilis	46
Bacteroides spp.	38
Clostridium spp.	23
Peptococcus/*Peptostreptococcus*	22
Fusobacterium	5
Other anaerobes	16

(After Solomkin, 1988.)

(Solomkin, 1988). Collectively, these studies in which beta-lactam antibiotic therapy was used as an adjunct to appropriate surgical intervention have shown that antibiotic monotherapy is as effective but no better than existing combination chemotherapy. Ultimately, their major advantage may simply be one of convenience avoiding the need to administer multiple agents or monitor serum antibiotic levels on a busy surgical unit.

Operative management

Operation

A midline abdominal incision is the most useful approach in the patient with diffuse peritonitis of undiagnosed origin. A complete examination of the peritoneal cavity is carried out, a specimen of pus obtained for aerobic and anaerobic culture, and the primary lesion dealt with, the precise details depending upon the actual pathology. In general terms, operation for a diffuse spreading peritonitis should be designed to limit the spread of infection either by closure, resection or exteriorization of the ruptured viscus. Anastomosis in the presence of sepsis should be avoided at all costs. Once contamination is controlled, the peritoneal cavity is meticulously debrided of peritoneal exudate and debris and thereafter a variety of adjunctive operative measures may be considered in an attempt to pre-empt the development of recurrent intra-abdominal sepsis. These are summarized in Table 3.

TABLE 3
Surgical options in intra-abdominal sepsis

Intra-operative lavage
Postoperative lavage
Intra-abdominal drains
Radical peritoneal debridement
Elective relaparotomy
Open draining—mesh/zipper techniques

Intra-operative lavage

Intraoperative lavage using copious amounts of warm isotonic saline is now widely accepted as being beneficial. The procedure is effective because it removes a significant proportion of the bacterial inoculum along with toxins and contaminants such as faeces and haemoglobin which support the growth of bacteria and compromise the peritoneal defence mechanisms (Hau et al, 1978). The value of adding antibiotics to the lavage is less clear, but in a recent study the sepsis-related mortality rate was less than 4% in a series of 276 emergency 'dirty' operations in which preoperative antibiotic lavage using tetracycline 1 mg/ml was employed (Krukowski et al, 1986), thus supporting the contention that the addition of an antibiotic to preoperative lavage is beneficial. Once completed, the lavage fluid with or without antibiotics should be aspirated as completely as possible to prevent impairment of the naturally occurring defence mechanisms (e.g. by diluting opsonins).

Drains and intra-abdominal sepsis

Random drainage of the peritoneal cavity following laparotomy for generalized peritonitis in order to prevent postoperative intra-abdominal sepsis is undesirable and is usually ineffective. Drains placed for this purpose are rapidly walled off and may themselves act as a conduit for exogenous contamination. Furthermore, abscesses rarely recur at drain sites (Flint, 1982). In our view, a dubious anastomosis which requires prophylactic drainage in a septic abdomen should probably not have been constructed, and the septic site is probably better dealt with by exteriorization. Perhaps the only indication for draining a septic abdomen occurs if there is an abscess cavity which cannot be obliterated or if there is a residual focus of infection which cannot be resected. Under these circumstances, dependent drainage or low grade suction sump drainage systems should be used.

Post-operative lavage

Since intra-operative cleaning of the peritoneal cavity is beneficial, it seems logical that lavage continued into the postoperative period may help reduce septic intra-abdominal complications by preventing reaccumulation of fluid and necrotic debris (and hence bacterial proliferation) after laparotomy. Although several animal studies have supported this hypothesis (Douglas, 1972; Rosato et al, 1972) clinical reports have been unconvincing. In a recent critical review of 39 studies (Leiboff and Soroff, 1987) the results of 2746 patients receiving continuous postoperative lavage (CPPL) were compared to those of 648 patients who did not receive CPPL. Although there was a 9.4% difference in overall mortality rates favouring CPPL (13.7% vs 23.1%), mortality rates in each group were similar (CPPL, 22.6%, no CPPL, 23.1%) when the data were carefully stratified by eliminating patients with a significantly lower mortality risk, for example acute appendicitis. Indeed, the only groups of patients with peritonitis who appeared to benefit from CPPL were those with post-operative peritonitis or peritonitis secondary to gynaecological pathology (Leiboff and Soroff, 1987).

Numerous technical variations for postoperative CPPL have been described. Currently, most authors seem to use two inflow catheters directed to the subphrenic spaces and two outflow catheters placed in the pelvis. Patients are lavaged usually with isotonic saline to which a wide variety of antibiotics have been added. Thereafter, continuous or intermittent lavage is performed usually for 2–5 days. Various complications have been described including fluid overload and antibiotic toxicity, and in some studies up to 15% of patients have to discontinue treatment because of the technical complications or complaints of abdominal discomfort (Hallerback et al, 1986).

Radical surgery

Despite the measures outlined above, mortality rates in patients with severe intra-abdominal sepsis remain in the range of 30–40%. Mortality rates are higher in patients over 60 years of age, those with multiple septic foci, and those with preoperative organ failure (Butler et al, 1987). In most instances, failure to control intra-abdominal sepsis will lead to a multiple system organ failure and results in a mortality rate approaching 100% (Hinsdale and Jaffe, 1984). In an effort to improve this dismal outlook, a variety of aggressive surgical manoeuvres have been proposed, namely radical peritoneal debridement, planned reoperation and laparostomy/open drainage.

Radical peritoneal debridement Hudspeth (1975) first described this technique, which involves the methodical removal of all fibrin membranes, lysis of all intra-abdominal adhesions and excision of all abscess cavities, in the treatment of diffuse bacterial peritonitis in a series of 100 patients without mortality. However, these promising results were not confirmed when the technique was evaluated prospectively in a randomized trial (Polk and Fry, 1980). In this study the technique may itself have contributed to several of the deaths in patients over 60 years of age, possibly due to increased blood loss encountered during extensive debridement. As a result, the technique cannot be recommended.

More recently, interest has focused on the impact of electively staged multiple laparotomies and the technique of laparostomy or open drainage of the abdomen on the management of patients with severe intra-abdominal sepsis.

Planned reoperation Staged or planned laparotomies have been proposed to treat patients with severe intra-abdominal sepsis because of the poor results obtained when patients with ongoing or recurrent sepsis undergo repeated laparotomy based purely on clinical or radiological evidence of recurrent sepsis (Harbrecht et al, 1984). In addition, several reports have suggested a survival advantage in patients with perforated colonic diverticular disease treated by a programme of elective relaparotomies (Sakai et al, 1981). However, the superiority of this aggressive treatment policy has not been clearly established. In a prospective study, mortality rates were similar (38% and 45%, respectively) in a group of 77 patients undergoing either planned or 'as required' laparotomy for severe generalized intra-abdominal infection (Andrus et al, 1986). More recently, Schein and his colleagues (1988) reported a mortality rate of 32% in a series of 22 patients with severe diffuse peritonitis and were unable to show any clear benefit in a similar programme of repeated laparotomies.

Proponents of electively staged multiple relaparotomy recommend re-exploration at 24–72 h intervals, the decision to discontinue being made when the peritoneal cavity is free of purulent collections or necrotic debris. Although negative laparotomy rates approach 30% in most series, most authors feel that this does not contribute directly to the mortality rate (Schein et al, 1988). However, difficulties associated with repeatedly opening and closing an abdominal wound, repeated anaesthesia and 'in hospital' transfer of a critically ill patient may well contribute to the overall morbidity in this group of patients (Andrus et al, 1986). Although 'programmed relaparotomy' can effectively eradicate intra-abdominal sepsis, multiple system organ failure still occurs and was the cause of death in more than 75% of the treatment failures undergoing electively staged multiple laparotomy (Schein et al, 1988).

Laparostomy or open abdomen drainage The disappointing results achieved following elective relaparotomy, radical debridement or after postoperative lavage have been interpreted by some as a failure to eradicate or adequately drain septic foci within the abdomen which in turn has led to multiple organ failure and death (Garcia-Sabrido et al, 1988). It has been suggested that mortality rates in these patients could be reduced if recurrent intra-abdominal collections were prevented from forming by providing wide open drainage of the abdomen. The theoretical advantages to 'laparostomy' also include a reduction in intra-abdominal pressure leading to improved diaphragmatic excursion and better kidney perfusion (Richards et al, 1983) and the prevention of abdominal wall necrosis caused by forceful and repeated closure during programmed relaparotomy (Schein et al, 1988).

A variety of innovative techniques have been described to prevent the massive fluid losses, evisceration and small bowel fistulation which can complicate open abdominal drainage (Walsh et al, 1988). To date, the most effective temporary control of the abdominal wound has been achieved using a Marlex (polypropylene) mesh (Wouters, 1983) in conjunction with a zipper mechanism to permit daily reinspection of the peritoneal cavity (Walsh et al, 1988).

Numerous technical variations have been described (Walsh et al, 1988). Usually, the mesh is trimmed to fit the wound circumferentially and is secured either to the abdominal fascia or the skin. Wherever possible the omentum is interposed between the mesh and the bowel to prevent fistulation. Once secured the mesh is covered with saline-soaked gauze. Thereafter all re-explorations can be performed on the surgical intensive care unit using epidural anaesthesia or intravenous sedation. At the first re-exploration, the Marlex sheath is incised along the midline and the abdominal cavity thoroughly re-explored, debrided and lavaged. At the end of the first re-exploration, the abdomen is closed by suturing a commercially available gas sterilized nylon zipper to the cut edges of the mesh. Proponents of this technique recommend that re-exploration be performed up to three times each day until signs of local and systemic sepsis have abated (Walsh et al, 1988). In general, the development of healthy granulation tissue suggests the control of infection, and when a complete mat of granulation tissue overlies the viscera the mesh and zipper are removed (Walsh et al, 1988). Thereafter, the wound is usually left to heal by secondary intention. Incisional hernias are common and small bowel fistulas, when they develop, are difficult to treat (Garcia-Sabrido et al, 1989; Schein et al, 1988).

In a recent review (Schein et al, 1988) the mortality rate in over 500 patients treated by the open technique was 32% almost identical to the mortality rates (30–40%) reported in several recent series for intra-abdominal sepsis treated either by planned daily relaparotomy or reoperation based on clinical or radiological grounds.

Although these data collectively suggest that patients undergoing aggressive surgery for intra-abdominal sepsis do not benefit either from programmed relaparotomy or open drainage techniques, few studies have been large enough to stratify outcome with the underlying cause of the intra-abdominal infection. However, the evidence to date suggests that these techniques may have a role in the management of severe pancreatic sepsis (*vide infra*). The failure of these ultraradical techniques to improve survival in patients with other causes of severe intra-abdominal sepsis suggests that these patients are better managed by a single operation, meticulously performed by an experienced surgeon with re-exploration being restricted to those patients who develop clinical or radiological evidence of recurrent or ongoing infection.

One possible explanation for the failure of more radical measures to improve survival in patients with severe intra-abdominal sepsis may be related to the changes in intestinal function which occur during critical illness (Wilmore et al, 1988). In these patients, the integrity of the intestinal mucosal barrier assumes central importance and recent studies have shown that even a brief single exposure of normal gut to circulating endotoxin can lead to increased intestinal permeability which promotes, in turn, further bacterial translocation from the gut into the bloodstream (O'Dwyer et al, 1988). This increase in permeability may be mediated directly by the endotoxin or by locally released cytokines such as tumour necrosis factor (O'Dwyer et al, 1988) and may account for the observation that some critically ill patients in whom no focus of infection can be found even after laparotomy will continue to demonstrate the clinical signs of sepsis and will ultimately die from multisystem organ failure (Wilmore et al, 1988).

Special problems

Retroperitoneal sepsis

This is defined as sepsis restricted to the retroperitoneum, a potential space bounded by the diaphragms above, pelvis inferiorly and the quadratus lumborum muscles laterally. Retroperitoneal sepsis is uncommon but is important because, unlike intraperitoneal sepsis, it is often clinically silent and is associated with an insidious, occult, prolonged illness. In a recent review, 13 days were required, on average, to reach a diagnosis of retroperitoneal infection in a cohort of 50 patients

(Crepps et al, 1987). Almost one half of the episodes occurred in patients with renal disease (perinephric abscess) or were a postoperative complication. In this series, routine laboratory and radiological studies were of no value and may have contributed to the delay in establishing the diagnosis. In contrast, CT scanning, when employed, was the single most useful diagnostic test with 100% sensitivity. The results of this and other studies suggest that this condition is best dealt with by retroperitoneal drainage either by formal surgery (85% success rate) (Crepps et al, 1987) or by percutaneous techniques (Sheinfield et al, 1987). Transperitoneal drainage is less effective with recurrent abscess formation contributing to a 67% failure rate (Crepps et al, 1987).

Despite aggressive surgical treatment, up to 50% of patients with isolated retroperitoneal sepsis will suffer a major complication (organ failure, recurrent abscess) which contributes to the high mortality rate (22–46%) associated with the condition (Harris and Sparks, 1980).

Intraperitoneal and retroperitoneal sepsis

One of the most difficult septic complications a surgeon is likely to encounter is the combination of intra- and retroperitoneal sepsis which exists in patients with infected necrotizing pancreatitis. With non-operative management mortality rates in this group of patients (5–16% of all patients with acute pancreatitis) approaches 100%, the majority succumbing to septic complications and multisystem organ failure (Beger et al, 1988). High resolution contrast enhanced CT scanning is the most effective means of diagnosing pancreatic necrosis (Kivisaari et al, 1984). More recently, Gerzof et al (1987) have used this technique in combination with percutaneous needle aspiration followed by immediate Gram staining to reliably diagnose infected necrosis.

The poor results achieved with conventional surgical techniques in these patients, i.e. laparotomy, limited debridement and closed abdominal drainage, have led to a renewed interest in the surgical treatment of necrotizing pancreatitis, and recent studies in Europe and North America suggest that aggressive surgical debridement (necrosectomy) is the way ahead in dealing with patients with infected necrotizing pancreatitis. As described necrosectomy implies the removal, usually by blunt finger dissection, of necrotic peri- and intrapancreatic tissue together with the evacuation of any intra- and peripancreatic and retroperitoneal fluid collections (Beger et al, 1988). Proponents of this technique stress the importance of exploring the entire peritoneal cavity and retroperitoneum followed by meticulous debridement and drainage. It is essential not to overlook any dendritic extensions of the necrotic process, for example around the colonic flexures or in the pararenal spaces, as these areas frequently can be the site of recurrent lethal sepsis (Nicholson et al, 1988). It is this group of patients in whom promising results have been achieved with aggressive surgical techniques such as open abdominal drainage or postoperative lavage.

In a group of 95 patients with necrotizing pancreatitis treated by necrosectomy and local lavage Beger et al. (1988) reduced mortality rates to 8.4%. Equally impressive results were achieved when necrosectomy was combined with open drainage in a series of 28 patients with similar disease severity. In this series, there were only three deaths (11%), none of which were due to uncontrollable sepsis (Bradley, 1987).

Postoperative intra-abdominal sepsis

Postoperative intra-abdominal sepsis complicates between 1% and 4% of all laparotomies (Hinsdale and Jaffe, 1984) and accounts for 50% of the expected morbidity from elective gastric, biliary and colorectal operations (Flint, 1982). It is particularly common following certain types of operation, for example laparotomy for the septic complications of diverticular disease where mortality rates may approach 25% (Lambert et al, 1986). Most episodes of postoperative sepsis are either the result of anastomotic breakdown or are the sequel to inadequate primary treatment of established peritonitis and, as such, are potentially avoidable (Krukowski, 1988). In a recent series of 87 re-explorations for intra-abdominal sepsis in which the commonest peroperative findings were multiple abscesses (54%) and suture line leak (26%), the overall mortality rate was 43% (Hinsdale and Jaffe, 1984).

Diagnosis The onset of postoperative sepsis is often insidious and is most frequently marked by a fever, localized tenderness and absent bowel sounds (Hinsdale and Jaffe, 1984). These clinical signs are, however, not infrequent in the postoperative patient and can be present for reasons other than sepsis. In a recent series the predictive value of significant temperature elevations (greater than $38.5°C$ on two successive occasions) or a leucocytosis (greater than $12 \times 10^9/1$) was poor with infection being proved in only 27% and 45% of patients, respectively (Freischlag and Busuttil, 1983). The development of unexplained hypotension, changes in respiratory rate, pulmonary or systemic oedema, mental confusion, leucopenia, thrombocytopenia or the development of disseminated intravascular coagulation in the postoperative patient is more sinister (Ayres, 1985). In these individuals a diagnosis of intra-abdominal sepsis must be considered once an obvious septic focus in the chest or urinary tract has been excluded.

Although the interpretation of symptoms and physical signs can be difficult after abdominal surgery, their importance cannot be overemphasized. In a recent series, a thorough history and examination provided sufficient information to allow localization of the septic focus by a single diagnostic test in 74% of all patients with proven infection (Freischlag and Busuttil, 1983).

As yet, there is no specific biochemical screening test that will help predict the development of a postoperative septic complication although serial changes in circulating C-reactive proteins in patients with infective complications (positive predictive value of around 70%) appear promising (Mustard et al, 1987).

The importance of establishing an early diagnosis in patients with postoperative intra-abdominal sepsis is clear—any delay which results in progressive organ failure is usually fatal (Bohnen et al, 1983).

Imaging Ultrasound and CT scanning are generally held to be the most useful investigations (Rogers and Wright, 1987), particularly if an intra-abdominal abscess is suspected. They are far more sensitive than plain abdominal X-rays or a chest radiograph although in difficult diagnostic cases multiple investigations can be complementary (Rogers and Wright, 1987). Whenever there is suspicion of sepsis after an operation involving an anastomosis, the integrity of the suture line should always be assessed by contrast radiology (Krukowski, 1988).

Treatment The principles of treatment of postoperative intra-abdominal sepsis are similar to those of intra-abdominal sepsis from any cause, namely drainage of the septic focus together with removal of any continuing source of infection. However, since postoperative sepsis is frequently poorly localized or is caused by multiple interloop abscesses (Hinsdale and Jaffe, 1984) laparotomy and drainage appears to have several advantages over the percutaneous or the extraperitoneal routes (Rogers and Wright, 1987). Specifically, it is not dependent upon pre-operative localization and, by allowing complete examination of the peritoneal cavity, obviates the risk of overlooking a septic focus.

Anastomotic leakage Postoperative peritonitis due to suture line disruption is associated with a high mortality rate (Bohnen et al, 1983). The diagnosis is frequently delayed, possibly because of its implications of technical failure (Krukowski, 1988), and this may well contribute to the poor outcome associated with non-surgical management in this group of patients. If leakage is confirmed following contrast radiology, laparotomy then drainage alone is inadequate and most surgeons would agree that resection of the septic focus and/or dismantling of the leaking anastomosis is essential if local control is to be achieved. At operation, primary re-anastomosis should be avoided (Schein et al, 1988) and exteriorization practised instead in order to obviate the high incidence of suture line disruption which occurs in the presence of sepsis (Teichmann et al, 1986).

INTRA-ABDOMINAL ABSCESS

Diagnosis

A thorough physical examination is often useful in locating the abscess and should not be overlooked in favour of resorting directly to ultrasound or CT; the patient may be tender over the abscess and a mass may be present on abdominal or rectal examination. Clinical assessment alone may be helpful or diagnostic in up to 70% of patients (Fry et al, 1980; Lurie et al, 1987).

Plain abdominal and chest radiographs are a valuable starting point. The findings of an elevated hemidiaphragm, pleural effusion or the presence of extraluminal gas shadows or a soft tissue mass (present in 50% of patients) point to the need for further investigation either by ultrasound or CT scanning (Connell et al, 1980). Fluoroscopic screening of the diaphragm when a subphrenic abscess is suspected is, however, less useful as the diaphragm is frequently obscured by an associated pleural effusion (Connell et al, 1980).

Ultrasound and CT scanning

Ultrasound and CT are both extremely sensitive and highly specific in the detection of intra-abdominal abscesses and can locate abnormal fluid collections in over 90% of patients (Koehler and Knochel, 1980). Properly executed, false negative scans are rare with a reported specificity of greater than 95% (Taylor et al, 1978; Koehler and Moss, 1980). Ultrasound appears particularly able to localize perihepatic and pelvic collections because the liver and urine-filled bladder both can act as good sonographic windows (Lurie et al, 1987). A further advantage is that unlike CT, ultrasound can be performed using portable machines enabling the investigation to be carried out at the bedside in the critically ill patient. The technique is, however, limited by the presence of stomas, abdominal drains or anything which prevents good contact with the abdominal wall (Lurie et al, 1987).

Although it has been traditionally held that the results of CT scanning are easier to interpret than ultrasound this advantage has become less marked with the advent of real time ultrasound scanning. To prevent false positive CT scans when non-opacified bowel loops are confused with abscess cavities most authorities recommend the investigation be performed after giving oral or rectal contrast medium (Lurie et al, 1987). Although this precludes some patients with a suspected abscess undergoing a useful CT evaluation (e.g. those patients with bowel obstruction), the addition of contrast whenever possible has the added advantage of outlining any anastomotic leakage or fistulous connection.

Radionuclide scanning

Unfortunately, neither CT scanning nor ultrasound can be relied upon to distinguish collections of serous fluid or haematoma from pus (Doust et al, 1977). Radionuclide scanning using [111]indium-labelled autologous leucocytes provides an alternative approach by detecting sequestered labelled leucocytes in inflammatory tissues or abscess cavities. In centres where cell labelling facilities exist, this technique has largely superseded the use of [67]gallium imaging studies, the interpretation of which was limited by non-specific excretion of the isotope into the bowel and kidneys (Thakur et al, 1976). In a recent study, 28 out of 30 abscesses were detected in a cohort of 100 consecutive patients undergoing gamma imaging 24 h after injection of [111]indium-labelled leucocytes. In addition, this study demonstrated that serial scans, performed at 4 and 24 h, led to improved diagnostic accuracy by differentiating those patients with an inflammatory phlegmon from those with a frank abscess cavity (Goldman et al, 1987). Clearly, a major disadvantage to radionuclide scanning is the time required to obtain a positive test result (at least 24 h) leading to an unacceptable delay in the critically ill patient. As a result, the role of radionuclide scans is probably limited to those stable patients in whom intra-abdominal abscess is suspected but in whom CT scanning or abdominal ultrasound examination has been inconclusive.

Treatment—percutaneous catheter drainage or open surgical drainage?

Adequate drainage of an intra-abdominal abscess is the single most important determinant of patient survival and has led to a reduction in the overall mortality rates to 30% (Fry et al, 1980). Early results favoured an extraperitoneal approach wherever possible in order to obviate the risk of intraperitoneal contamination. However, the high mortality rates (55–90%) associated with repeat operations for residual sepsis have led some (Halasz, 1970) to recommend routine formal laparotomy to allow debridement of necrotic tissue and to correct any associated defects, for example anastomotic leaks. Although percutaneous catheter drainage (PCD) was first reported as a means of draining amoebic liver abscesses (Rogers, 1922), it is only since 1970 that the technique has been widely popularized as a means to drain abdominal abscesses. Initially, its use was restricted to single unilocular abscesses without enteric fistulas and with a safe percutaneous access route (Gerzof et al, 1981), but more recently proponents of this technique have extended its use to drain multiple complex abscesses including those with enteric fistulas using transperitoneal, transvisceral or even transpleural routes (Gerzof et al, 1985). What then is the role of either procedure in the management of intra-abdominal abscess? In a recent review comparing open drainage and PCD in the postultrasonography/CT era the overall mortality rate was 22% for 820 patients from 15 studies undergoing open surgical drainage (Landau, 1987). Seventeen per cent of patients required more than one drainage procedure because of recurrent sepsis. In the same review, 727 patients underwent PCD at 15 different centres with an overall recurrence rate of 23% and a 13% mortality rate. Clearly, PCD compares favourably with open drainage although, as pointed out by Landau (1987), those patients undergoing PCD are a preselected group who can usually be managed safely without laparotomy and consequently are at a lower risk. If those studies containing complex abscesses are excluded, the failure rate and mortality rates following PCD fall to 19% and 9%, respectively (Landau, 1987)—clear evidence of the effectiveness of PCD in the treatment of uncomplicated intra-abdominal abscess. However, in studies using PCD to treat complex abscesses (Pruett et al, 1984; Gerzof et al, 1985) recurrence rates (55–86%) and mortality rates (35–62%) were much higher. In particular, patients with complex abscesses associated with fungal infection, malignancy, colonic sepsis or infected pancreatic necrosis do not benefit from PCD (Landau, 1987).

Overall, these results suggest that PCD has a valuable role to play in the management of intra-abdominal abscess and where expertise exists is probably the treatment of choice for the uncomplicated abscess, particularly in the old or debilitated patient. Its use in management of complex abscesses is less clear. The presence of a fistula is not always a contraindication to PCD (Landau, 1987) and the technique may be of value in stable patients with complex abscesses or possibly for moribund patients in an effort to gain time. The decision to abandon or persist with PCD clearly demands careful clinical judgement and close colloboration between surgeons and the interventional radiologist. It is our view that failure to improve within 24–48 h demands open drainage. At present, PCD is contraindicated in abscesses associated with colonic sepsis or infected pancreatic necrosis.

In most patients, a drainage tube is directed into the abscess cavity under local anaesthesia after localization using CT, ultrasound or fluoroscopic control. Large abscesses abutting the anterior abdominal wall can usually be drained by direct insertion of a 12F or 16F trocar catheter (Gerzof et al, 1981). Deeper abscesses are usually localized by fine needle aspiration, a guide wire being introduced into the cavity by the Seldinger technique followed by a series of dilators and finally by a pigtail angiocatheter. Although catheters up to size 24F have been used, most authors prefer to use a size 8–10F in order to minimize the risk of bleeding or fistula formation (Lurie et al, 1987).

The abscess cavity is thoroughly irrigated at the time of insertion in order to remove the initial thick pus and debris. Thereafter, the catheter is flushed with

5–10 ml saline several times a day to prevent blockage. Some centres recommend continuous irrigation or low grade suction (Miller et al, 1982), but under most circumstances, simple dependent drainage appears adequate. Usually, pain, fever and bacteraemia resolve rapidly following PCD because of relief of tension within the abscess cavity (Gerzof et al, 1985). Failure to improve over 2–3 days usually indicates the presence of a second abscess or an undrained loculus and is an indication for urgent repeat ultrasound or CT assessment. Sinography has become less popular because of the risk of septicaemia. Following satisfactory drainage, the abscess cavity is re-evaluated periodically again using CT or ultrasound and the catheter removed when resolution appears complete.

ENTEROCUTANEOUS FISTULAS

The majority of enteric fistulas are caused by surgery and result from either breakdown of an anastomosis or necrosis of an ischaemic segment of bowel. They are a not infrequent complication in patients with post-operative intra-abdominal sepsis. Enteric fistulas are classified as external (enterocutaneous) or internal (enteroenteric) and are either high (greater than 500 ml/24 h) or low output (less than 500 ml/24 h). In a recent series consisting of 114 fistulas in 108 patients 51% were attributable to surgical complications (Rose et al, 1986). The aetiology and distribution of the fistulas in this series are summarized in Tables 4 and 5. Prior to the widespread use of nutritional support, mortality rates in patients with gastrointestinal fistulas varied from 16% to 62% depending upon location and cause (Edmunds et al, 1960). Although controversy still exists as to whether nutritional support alone can reduce the mortality rate in patients with fistulas, there seems little doubt that hyperalimentation along with intensive medical support can improve their rate of spontaneous closure (Rombeau and Rolandelli, 1987).

TABLE 4
Distribution of gastrointestinal fistulas

Location	Type Internal	Type External	No. of patients	
Duodenum		6 ⎫	6	49%
Jejunum/ileum	11	38 ⎭	49	
Colon/rectum	13	17	30	26%
Oesophagus		10	10	8.5%
Biliary		7	7	6.5%
Pancreas		6	6	5%
Gastric		6	6	5%
Total			114	

(After Rose et al, 1986.)

TABLE 5

Aetiology of gastrointestinal fistulas

Aetiology	No. of patients
Surgical complications	58 (51%)
Anastomotic leaks	28
Missed intestinal injury	28
Other	2
Inflammatory diseases	34 (30%)
Crohn's disease	11
Diverticulitis	11
Pancreatitis	3
Other	9
Malignant disease	7 (6%)
Post-irradiation	7 (6%)
Trauma	8 (7%)
Total	108

(After Rose et al, 1986.)

Enteral or parenteral nutrition?

Few studies have examined the comparative impact of enteral and parenteral nutrition on mortality and spontaneous closure rates in patients with fistulas. In an uncontrolled study comparing 41 patients adequately nourished by enteral nutrition with 71 patients who received parenteral nutrition, neither the mortality rate (7% versus 14%) nor the spontaneous closure rate (22% versus 37%) showed any significant difference. It seems far more important that the decision to feed enterally or parenterally should be individualized to meet each patient's needs. Most patients with colocutaneous fistulas or low output ileal fistulas can be treated with enteral nutrition. The ability to feed patients with proximal fistulas obviously depends upon the ability to gain access to the intestine distal to the fistula site either by a nasojejunal tube introduced under radiological control or by means of feeding jejunostomy. It is our practice to use the enteral route whenever possible because of its ease of administration obviating the need for central venous access and the constant risk of sepsis or thromboembolism in an already compromised patient. Generally accepted indications for parenteral nutrition include gastro-intestinal intolerance of enteral feeds, inadequate enteral access and high output fistulas irrespective of site (Rombeau and Rolandelli, 1987).

The role of surgery

Uncontrolled intra-abdominal sepsis is the single most important cause of death in patients with fistulas. In a recent series 11 out of 16 deaths were directly related to septic complications of the fistula (Rose et al, 1986). The importance of early operative intervention to control intra-abdominal sepsis is underlined by the observation that, in the same series, 90% (27 out of 30) fistulas closed spontaneously after surgical control (usually drainage of an abscess) of any ongoing intra-abdominal sepsis. Similarly, in a series of 24 external duodenal fistulas, all of which were the result of surgical procedures, spontaneous closure occurred in 92% (22 patients) once the intra-abdominal sepsis was controlled (Garden et al, 1988). In this series, only two patients required definitive surgical intervention at 5–6 weeks for refractory high output losses. This and other series (Levy et al, 1984) suggest that most postoperative duodenal fistulas can now be effectively managed conservatively, reserving definitive surgical closure for those few cases which do not close spontaneously. Table 6 outlines the most important factors likely to influence spontaneous closure of an enteric fistula. Provided that these basic principles of fistula management are observed, 90–95% of fistulas will undergo spontaneous closure within 4–6 weeks (Rombeau and Rolandelli, 1987), most non-responders being patients who have had radiotherapy or who have inflammatory bowel disease (Rose et al, 1986). From these observations it is clear that the need for definitive surgical intervention in enteric fistulas is becoming increasingly uncommon and when required should be directed at converting an uncontrolled fistula associated with ongoing intra-abdominal sepsis into a controlled fistula. It is preferable to achieve this by exteriorization or resection and stoma formation rather than attempting to perform a difficult and dangerous reanastomosis in a septic abdomen.

Pancreatic fistulas

External pancreatic fistulas are usually the sequel to pancreatic surgery or a bout of acute pancreatitis. High output pancreatic fistulas (> 200 ml/day) are associated with a high rate of infective and metabolic complications and may take months to heal spontaneously (Zinner et al, 1974). Although parenteral nutrition alone will reduce the volume and tryspin content of the output by one-half (Garcia-Puges et al, 1988), recent interest has focused on the use of somatostatin and its analogues as a means to accelerate spontanous closure (Di Constanzo et al, 1982). In one study, the mean time until closure using a combination of total parenteral nutrition (TPN) plus somatostatin infusion in seven out of eight patients was 6 days as compared to 32 days in 17 out of 18 patients treated with TPN alone. One patient in each group required surgical closure (Pederzoli et al, 1986). In a

TABLE 6
Factors influencing spontaneous closure of gastrointestinal fistulas

	Favourable	Unfavourable
Output/day (ml)	< 500 (low)	> 500 (high)
Age (years)	< 40	> 65
Site	Proximal small bowel	Distal small bowel and colon
Aetiology	Anastomotic leak	Complete anastomotic dehiscence, malignancy, inflammatory bowel disease
Anatomy	Long fistulous tract	Distal obstruction epithelialization

(After Rose et al, 1986.)

single case report, a stable long-acting somatostatin analogue (SMS 201-995) was effective within 48 h when administered subcutaneously (Ahren et al, 1988).

Recently, the oral administration of pancreatic proteases has been shown to effectively inhibit exocrin pancretic secretion in patients with external pancreatic fistulas. In a group of five patients all with postoperative pancreatic fistulas, a combination of TPN and oral pancreatic supplements effectively controlled and closed the fistula with 12 days (Garcia-Puges et al, 1988), possibly by exerting an inhibitory feedback control on pancreatic secretion by supplementing the intraduodenal trypsin levels (Ihse et al, 1977).

Wound management

Without adequate drainage, the granulation tissue and skin surrounding an enterocutaneous fistula are continuously bathed with intestinal contents which can lead to a severe excoriation and wound breakdown. Open wound packing or simple tube draining are ineffective and have been replaced by techniques relying on continuous low grade suction appliances together with intensive wound care. Orringer et al (1987) have recently described a technique employing a flat Jackson–Pratt drain placed along the line of the wound but not in direct contact with the stoma (Figure 1). A stomadhesive paste is used to line the skin margin surrounding the granulating wound and the entire site is, in turn, covered with Op-Site to provide an air and watertight seal around the wound. This system eliminates the need for the multiple daily redressings associated with traditional packing techniques and has the advantage that the fistula output can be closely monitored (Orringer et al, 1987).

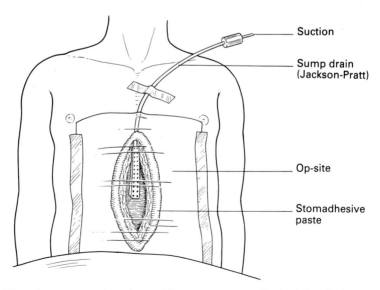

FIGURE I Wound management in patients with enterocutaneous fistulas (after Orringer et al, 1987).

UNCOMMON CAUSES OF INTRA-ABDOMINAL SEPSIS

Peritonitis in continuous ambulatory peritoneal dialysis (CAPD)

Cause and diagnosis

Peritonitis is the main complication of CAPD (Gokal et al, 1982). Its incidence varies, but most of the 2450 patients undergoing CAPD in the UK will on average have an episode once per year (Bint, 1987). The infections are rarely fatal and most episodes can be managed without disruption of the peritoneal dialysis regime. Peritonitis during CAPD is usually caused by contamination when the bag or transfer set is changed and is associated with a cloudy peritoneal dialysate effluent containing more than 100 white blood cells/μl. Clinical peritonitis usually becomes evident 24–48 h after contamination. The commonest infecting organism is *Staphylococcus epidermidis* accounting for 50% of all episodes of confirmed peritonitis (Bint, 1987). The skin also acts as a source for many of the other infecting organisms including *Staphylococcus aureus*, diptheroids and alpha-haemolytic streptococci. Enterobacteria and *Pseudomonas aeruginosa* cause one-fifth of all infections whereas anaerobes are rarely implicated (Bint, 1987).

Positive culture rates can be obtained in 90% of patients if Gram staining and culture techniques are performed on centrifuged samples derived from large volumes of dialysate effluent (Knight et al, 1982).

Treatment

CAPD-associated peritonitis should be treated promptly with antibiotics. Most authors currently recommend the intraperitoneal route (Bint, 1987) as the antibiotics can be delivered directly to the site of infection simply by adding the appropriate antibiotic to the dialysis fluid while CAPD is being continued as usual. A combination of vancomycin and an aminoglycoside is active against most likely pathogens (Gokal et al, 1982) and can be used empirically until specific sensitivities are known. In culture-negative episodes both antibiotics are continued provided the patient is responding (Bint, 1987). Treatment should be continued until at least 5 days after resolution of clinical signs and symptoms and clearing of the dialysate (Gokal et al, 1982). Resistant infections are usually due to *Pseudomonas* or *Staphylococcus aureus* infection and require aggressive treatment with either an anti-pseudomonal penicillin (e.g. ticarcillin) or flucloxacillin as appropriate. Fungal peritonitis is rare but not unknown (1–2% of all cases) and is associated with high morbidity and mortality rates. Intravenous amphotericin B has been effective but most authors recommend early removal of the catheter (Bint, 1987).

Catheter removal

Current evidence suggests that the catheter should be removed in patients with recurrent episodes of peritonitis or those with fulminant attacks caused by *pseudomonas*, *Staphylococcus aureus* or fungi. In addition the catheter should be removed if there is evidence of an associated bowel perforation (i.e. the presence of multiple organisms including anaerobes on culture), or if a catheter tunnel infection develops (Bint, 1987).

Primary or spontaneous bacterial peritonitis (SBP)

Primary or spontaneous bacterial peritonitis implies infection of the peritoneal cavity without a documented source within the abdomen. Pneumococcal peritonitis, which occurs in young girls possibly following entry of organisms into the peritoneal cavity through the fallopian tubes, is extremely uncommon. Of increasing importance, however, is the diagnosis of spontaneous bacterial peritonitis in cirrhotic patients with ascites or in non-cirrhotic diseases such as systemic lupus erythematosis and the nephrotic syndrome (Conn and Fessel, 1971). This infection is now recognized as a common complication of severe liver disease and may affect up to 10–27% of patients (Runyon, 1988). The diagnosis is most reliably made by blood culture inoculation of a fresh sample of ascitic fluid at the bedside (Runyon, 1988). Untreated, the in-hospital mortality rate for SBP approaches 100% (Conn, 1971). Infections are usually caused by Gram-negative organisms and can be effectively treated with beta-lactam antibiotics such as cefotaxime (Runyon, 1988).

CONCLUSIONS AND THE WAY FORWARD

Many of the advances in surgical management outlined above have had little impact on the overall mortality rates in patients with severe intra-abdominal sepsis and it is tempting to suggest that any further improvements in survival are unlikely to be due to refinements in operative technique alone. In the future, enhanced survival may only be achieved by targeting those patients who are at greatest risk and by efforts directed toward preventing the development of intra-abdominal sepsis rather than treatment of the moribund septic patient. In particular, the current interest centred on the role of the gut during surgical stress might well hold the key to the prevention of postoperative sepsis. Optimal support of the gastrointestinal mucosa in the severely ill patient using a combination of hormones and specific nutrients may help preserve the integrity of the intestinal barrier during critical illness and thus prevent host invasion by micro-organisms.

REFERENCES

Ahren B, Tranberg KG & Bengmark S (1988) Treatment of pancreatic fistula with the somatostatin analogue SMS 201-995. *British Journal of Surgery* **75**: 718.
Andrus C, Doering M, Herrmann VM & Kaminski DL (1986) Planned reoperation for generalized intra-abdominal infection. *American Journal of Surgery* **152**: 682–686.
Ayres SM (1985) SCCM's new horizons conference on sepsis and septic shock. *Critical Care Medicine* **13**: 864–866.

Beger HG, Buchler M, Bittner R, Block S, Nevalainen T & Roscher R (1988) Necrosectomy and postoperative local lavage in necrotizing peritonitis. *British Journal of Surgery* **75**: 207–212.

Bint AJ (1987) Diagnosis and management of peritonitis in continuous ambulatory peritoneal dialysis. *Lancet* **i**: 845–847.

Boey JH & Dunphy JE (1985) The peritoneal cavity. In Way LW (ed.) *Current Surgical Diagnosis and Treatment*, pp 401–417. Los Altos, California: Lange.

Bohnen J, Boulanger M, Meakins JL & McLean PH (1983) Prognosis in generalized peritonitis: relation to cause and risk factors. *Archives of Surgery* **118**: 285–290.

Bohnen JMA, Mustard RA, Oxholm SE & Schoulten B (1988) APACHE II. Score and abdominal sepsis. *Archives of Surgery* **123**: 225–229.

Bradley EL (1987) Management of infected pancreatic necrosis by open drainage. *Annals of Surgery* **206**: 542–550.

Butler JA, Huang J & Wilson SE (1987) Repeated laparotomy for postoperative intra-abdominal sepsis. *Archives of Surgery* **122**: 702–706.

Conn HO & Fessel JM (1971) Spontaneous bacterial peritonitis in cirrhosis: variations on a theme. *Medicine* **50**: 161–167.

Connell TR, Stephens DH, Carlson HC & Brown HC (1980) Upper abdominal abscess. A continuing and deadly problem. *American Journal of Roentgenology* **134**: 759–765.

Crepps JT, Welch JP & Orlando R (1987) Management and outcome of retroperitoneal abscess. *Annals of Surgery* **205**: 276–281.

Cuschieri A (1980) Laparoscopy in general surgery and gastroenterology. *British Journal of Hospital Medicine* **24(252)**: 255–258.

Dellinger EP (1988) Use of scoring systems to assess patients with surgical sepsis. *Surgical Clinics of North America* **68**: 123–145.

Di Constanzo J, Cano N & Martin J (1982) Somatostatin in persistent gastrointestinal fistula treated by total parenteral nutrition. *Lancet* **ii**: 338.

Douglas BS (1972) The prevention of residual abscess by peritoneal lavage in experimental peritonitis in dogs. *Australia and New Zealand Journal of Surgery* **42**: 90–93.

Doust BD, Quiroz F & Stewart JM (1977) Ultrasonic distinction of abscesses from other intra-abdominal fluid collections. *American Journal of Surgery* **140**, 675–678.

Edmunds LH, Williams GM & Welch CE (1960) External fistulas arising from the gastrointestinal tract. *Annals of Surgery* **152**: 445–471.

Flint LM (1982) Intra-abdominal sepsis, In Flint LM & Fry DE (eds) *Surgical Infections*, pp 96–124. Contemporary Surgical Management Series. New York: Medical Examination Publishing.

Freischlag J & Busuttil R (1983) The value of postoperative fever evaluation. *Surgery* **94**: 358–363.

Fry DE, Garrison RE, Heitsch RC, Calhoun K & Polk HC (1980) Determinants of death in patients with intra-abdominal abscess. *Surgery* **88**: 517–523.

Garcia-Puges AM, Navarro S, Fernandez-Cruz L, Ros E, Hinojosa L & Pera C (1988) Oral pancreatic enzymes accelerate closure of external pancreatic fistulae. *British Journal of Surgery* **75**: 924–925.

Garcia-Sabrido JL, Tallado JM, Christou NV, Polo JR & Valdecantos E (1988) Treatment of severe intra-abdominal sepsis and/or necrotic foci by an open-abdomen approach. *Archives of Surgery* **123**: 152–156.

Garden JO, Dykes EH & Carter DC (1988) Surgical and nutritional management of post operative duodenal fistulas. *Digestive Disease Science* **33**: 30–35.

Gerzof SG, Robbins AH, Johnson WC, Birkett DH & Nabseth DC (1981) Percutaneous catheter drainage of intraabdominal abscess: a 5 year experience. *New England Journal of Medicine* **305**: 653–657.

Gerzof SG, Johnson WC, Robbins AH & Nabseth DC (1985) Expanded criteria for percutaneous abscess drainage *Archives of Surgery* **120**: 227–232.

Gerzof SG, Banks PA, Robbins AH, Johnson WC, Spechler SJ, Wetzner SM, Sneider JM, Langevin RE & Jay ME (1987) Early diagnosis of pancreatic infection by computed tomography-guided aspiration. *Gastroenterology* **93**: 1315–1320.

Gokal R, Ramos JM, Francis DMA, Ferner RE, Goodship TH, Proud G, Bint AJ, Ward MK & Kerr DN (1982) Peritonitis in continuous ambulatory peritoneal dialysis. Laboratory and clinical studies. *Lancet* **ii**: 1388–1391.

Goldman M, Ambrose NS, Droic Z, Hawker RJ & McCollum C (1987) Indium-111-labelled leucocytes in the diagnosis of abdominal abscess. *British Journal of Surgery* **74**: 184–186.

Halasz NA (1970) Subphrenic abscess, myths and facts. *Journal of the American Medical Association* **214**: 724–726.

Hallerbeck B, Andersson C, Englund N, Glise H, Nihlberg A, Solhaug J & Wahlstrom B (1986) A prospective randomized study of continuous peritoneal lavage postoperatively in the treatment of purulent peritonitis. *Surgery, Gynecology and Obstetrics* **163**: 433–436.

Harbrecht PJ, Garrison H & Fry DE (1984) Early urgent relaparotomy. *Archives of Surgery* **119**: 369–374.

Harris LF & Sparks JE (1980) Retroperitoneal abscess. Case report and review of the literature. *Digestive Disease Science* **25**, 392–394.

Hau T, Hoffman R & Simmonds RL (1978) Mechanisms of the adjuvant effect of hemoglobin in experimental peritonitis: 1. In vivo inhibition of peritoneal leucocytosis. *Surgery* **83**: 223–229.

Hinsdale JG & Jaffe BM (1984) Re-operation for intra-abdominal sepsis. *Annals of Surgery* **199**: 31–36.

Hudspeth AS (1975) Radical surgical debridement in the treatment of advanced generalized peritonitis. *Archives of Surgery* **110**: 1233–1236.

Huizinga WKJ, Baker W, Kadwa T, Van den Ende P, Francis J & Francis M (1988) Management of severe intra-abdominal sepsis: single agent antibiotic therapy with cefotetan versus combination therapy with ampicillin, gentamicin and metronidazole. *British Journal of Surgery* **75**: 1134–1138.

Ihse I, Lilja P & Lundquist I (1977) Feedback regulation of pancreatic enzyme secretion by intestinal trypsin in man. *Digestion* **15**: 303–308.

Kivisaari L, Somer K, Standertskjold-Nordenstam CG, Schroder T, Kivilaasko E & Lempinen M (1984) A new method for the diagnosis of acute haemorrhagic necrotising pancreatitis using contrast enhanced CT. *Gastrointestinal Radiology* **16**: 27–30.

Knaus WA, Zimmermann JE, Wagner DP, Draper EA & Lawrence DE (1981) APACHE-acute physiology and chronic health evaluation: a physiologically based classification system. *Critical Care Medicine* **9**: 591–597.

Knaus WA, Draper EA, Wagner DP & Zimmerman JE (1985) APACHE II: a severity of disease classification system. *Critical Care Medicine* **13**, 818–829.

Knight KR, Polak A, Crump J & Maskell R (1982) Laboratory diagnosis and oral treatment of CAPD peritonitis. *Lancet* **ii**: 1301–1304.

Koehler PR & Knochel JQ (1980) Computed tomography in the evaluation of abdominal abscess. *American Journal of Surgery* **140**: 675–678.

Koehler PR & Moss AA (1980) Diagnosis of intra-abdominal and pelvic abscess by computerized tomography. *Journal of the American Medical Association* **244**: 49–52.

Krukowski ZH (1988) Postoperative abdominal sepsis. *British Journal of Surgery* **75**, 1153–1154.

Krukowski ZH, Koruth NH & Matheson NA (1986) Antibiotic lavage in emergency surgery for peritoneal sepsis. *Journal of the Royal College of Surgeons of Edinburgh* **31**: 1–6.

Lambert ME, Knox RE, Schofield PF & Hancock BD (1986). Management of septic complications of diverticular disease. *British Journal of Surgery* **73**: 576–579.

Landau R (1987). Percutaneous catheter or open surgical drainage of abdominal abscess. *South African Journal of Surgery* **25**: 140–143.

Lavori PW, Louis TA, Bailar JC & Polansky M (1983). Design for experiments: parallel comparisons of treatment. *New England Journal of Medicine* **309**: 1291–1299.

Leaper DJ, Kennedy RH, Sutton A, Johnson E & Roberts N (1987) Treatment of acute bacterial peritonitis: a trial of imipenem/cilistatin against ampicillin-metronidazole-gentamicin. *Scandinavian Journal of Infectious Disease (Supplement)* **52**: 7–10.

Leiboff AR & Soroff HS (1987) The treatment of generalized peritonitis by closed postoperative peritoneal lavage. *Archives of Surgery* **122**: 1005–1010.

Levy E, Cugneuc PH, Frileux P, Hannoun L, Parc R, Huguet C & Loygue J (1984). Postoperative peritonitis due to gastric and duodenal fistulas. Operative management by continuous intraluminal infusion and aspiration. Report of 23 cases. *British Journal of Surgery* **71**: 543–546.

Lurie K, Plzak L & Deveney CW (1987) Intra-abdominal abscess in the 1980s. *Surgical Clinics of North America* **67**: 621–632.

Lygidakis NJ (1986) Risk factors in peritonitis. *British Journal of Clinical Practice* **40**: 181–186.

Miller MH, Frederick PR, Tocino I & Bahr AL (1982). Percutaneous catheter drainage of intra-abdominal fluid collections including infected biliary ducts and gallbladders. *American Journal of Surgery* **144**: 660–667.

Mustard R, Bohnen J, Haseeb S & Kasina R (1987) C-reactive protein levels predict postoperative septic complications. *Archives of Surgery* **122**: 69–73.

Nicholson ML, McC Mortensen NJ & Espiner HJ (1988) Pancreatic abscess: results of prolonged irrigation of the pancreatic bed after surgery. *British Journal of Surgery* **75**: 88–91.

O'Dwyer ST, Michie H, Ziegler TR, Revhaug A, Smith RJ & Wilmore DW (1988) A single dose of endotoxin increases intestinal permeability in healthy humans. *Archives of Surgery* **123**: 1459–1464.

O'Quinn R & Marini JJ (1983) Pulmonary artery occlusion pressure: clinical physiology, measurement, and interpretation. *American Review of Respiratory Disease* **128**: 319–326.

Orringer JS, Mendeloff NE & Eckhauser FE (1987). Management of wounds in patients with complex enterocutaneous fistulas. *Surgery, Gynecology and Obstetrics* **165**: 79–81.

Paterson-Brown S, Eckersley JRT, Sim AJW & Dudley HAF (1986) Laparoscopy as an adjunct to decision making in the 'acute abdomen'. *British Journal of Surgery* **73**: 1022–1024.

Pederzoli P, Bassi C, Falconi M, Albrigo R, Vantini I & Micciolo R (1986). Conservative treatment of external pancreatic fistulas with parenteral nutrition alone or in combination with continuous intravenous infusion of somatostatin, glucagon or calcitonin. *Surgery, Gynecology and Obstetrics* **163**: 428–432.

Polk HC & Fry DE (1980) Radical peritoneal debridement for established peritonitis. *Annals of Surgery* **192**: 350–355.

Pruett TL, Rotstein OD, Crass J, Frick MP, Flohr A & Simmons RL (1984) Percutaneous aspiration and drainage for suspected intra-abdominal infection. *Surgery* **96**: 731–737.

Richards WO, Scovill W, Shin B & Reed W (1983). Acute renal failure associated with increased intra-abdominal pressure. *Annals of Surgery* **197**: 183–187.

Richardson J, Flint L & Polk H (1983) Peritoneal lavage: a useful diagnostic adjunct for peritonitis. *Surgery* **94**: 826–829.

Rogers L (1922) Lettersonian lectures on amoebic abscess. *Lancet* i: 677–684.

Rogers PN & Wright IH (1987) Post-operative intra-abdominal sepsis. *British Journal of Surgery* **74**: 973–975.

Rombeau JL & Rolandelli RH (1987) Enteral and parenteral nutrition in patients with enteric fistulas and short bowel syndrome. *Surgical Clinics of North America* **66**: 551–571.

Rosato EF, Chu WH & Mullen JL (1972) Peritoneal lavage treatment of experimental peritonitis. *Journal of Surgical Research* **12**: 138–140.

Rose D, Yarborough MF, Canizaro PC & Lowry SF (1986) One hundred and fourteen fistulas of the gastrointestinal tract treated with total parenteral nutrition. *Surgery, Gynecology and Obstetrics* **163**: 345–350.

Runyon BA (1988) Spontaneous bacterial peritonitis: an explosion of information. *Hepatology* **8**: 171–175.

Sakai L, Daake J & Kaminski DL (1981) Acute perforation of sigmoid diverticuli. *American Journal of Surgery* **42**: 12–16.

Schein M, Saadia R, Freinkel Z & Decker DE (1988) Aggressive treatment of severe diffuse peritonitis: a prospective study. *British Journal of Surgery* **75**: 173–176.

Sheinfield J, Ertuk E, Spataro RF & Cockett ATK (1987) Perinephric abscess: current concepts. *Journal of Urology* **137**: 191–194.

Solomkin JS (1988) Use of new beta-lactam antibiotics for surgical infections. *Surgical Clinics of North America* **68**: 1–24.

Taylor KJ, Sullivan DC, Wasson JF & Rosefield AT (1978) Ultrasound and gallium scanning for the diagnosis of abdominal and pelvic abscess. *Gastrointestinal Radiology* **3**: 281–286.

Teichmann W, Wittman DH & Andreone PA (1986) Scheduled re-operation for diffuse peritonitis. *Archives of Surgery* **121**: 147–152.

Thakur ML, Coleman RE, Mayhall CG & Welch MJ (1976) Preparation and evaluation of [111]Indium-labelled leucocytes as an abscess imaging agent in dogs. *Radiology* **119**: 731–739.

Walsh GL, Chiasson P, Hedderich G, Wexler MJ & Meakins JL (1988) The open abdomen. The marlex mesh and Zipper technique. *Surgical Clinics of North America* **68**: 25–40.

Wilmore DW, Smith RJ, O'Dwyer ST, Jacobs DO, Ziegler TR & Wang X-D (1988) The gut: a central organ after surgical stress. *Surgery* **104**: 917–923.

Wouters DB, Krom RF, Slooff MH, Koostra G & Kuitjer PJ (1983) The use of marlex mesh in patients with generalized peritonitis and multiple organ failure. *Surgery, Gynecology and Obstetrics* **156**: 609–617.

Zinner MJ, Baker RR & Cameron JL (1974) Pancreatic cutaneous fistulas. *Surgery, Gynecology and Obstetrics* **138**: 710–712.

14

TRAUMATIC AND IATROGENIC EMERGENCIES

A. N. Kingsnorth and I. T. Gilmore

MANAGEMENT OF BLUNT AND PENETRATING INJURIES OF THE ABDOMINAL VISCERA

Initial management and assessment

Blunt injuries of the abdomen generally occur in severely injured patients as a result of deceleration, crush and shear sustained in road traffic accidents. Such injuries are often recognized at a late stage because priority has been given to more obvious cerebral, thoracic or skeletal injuries, with the result that neglected abdominal injuries contribute to 25% of death from multiple trauma. An awareness of the high probability of abdominal visceral injury in such patients, a knowledge of the mechanism of the injury and the early application of minimally invasive diagnostic techniques such as peritoneal lavage can improve the outcome in patients who have sustained a visceral injury from which death may be eminently avoidable (Trunkey, 1984; Rowlands, 1988).

Penetrating injuries, usually seen in the assault victim, are often multiple and entry wounds caused by a knife may not be obvious (Oreskovich and Carrico, 1983; Lambrianides and Rosin, 1984). Low velocity bullets cause a similar type of injury by incising tissues along the track of entry with the added complication of richochet injury should the parts of the bullet strike bone.

The immediate management of an injured patient in the accident and emergency department will give priority to cardiorespiratory and neurological status and the exclusion of major vascular, airway and chest trauma. When a patent airway, adequate ventilation and peripheral perfusion have been established, a thorough examination can be undertaken which will include assessment of the abdomen.

Historical features indicating a high index of suspicion for abdominal visceral injury include multiple injuries, rapid deceleration injury, a fall from more than 15 feet, extensive soft tissue or crush injury, penetrating injuries between nipple and thigh and traffic accidents involving prolonged entrapment. Shoulder-tip pain should not necessarily be taken to indicate subdiaphragmatic trauma as there may be a primary skeletal injury.

Clinical examination of the abdomen may give the first indication of visceral injury but the physical signs are non-specific unless there is obvious bowel evisceration, massive distension, marked peritonism or the injury is due to gunshot wounds or bomb blast. Under these circumstances operation should be undertaken without delay. Investigation should include full blood count with haematocrit, urea, electrolytes, and blood gas analysis. X-ray of chest, abdomen and pelvis is rarely diagnostic unless subphrenic gas is seen when again laparotomy is mandatory. Although serum amylase may rise sharply following pancreatic injury, raised levels are also seen following small bowel injury, head injury and in the presence of high blood alcohol. Urgent laparatomy is recommended in persistently hypotensive patients not responding to fluid replacement or where there is inability to assess adequately the patient because of unresponsiveness due to alcohol, drugs or a neurological injury.

Penetrating stab wounds in stable patients may be managed safely by a conservative policy in the absence of clinical or radiological evidence of bowel perforation, major haemorrhage or evisceration (Thompson et al, 1980; Goldberger et al, 1982). Close monitoring of vital signs and interval examination of the abdomen must be carried out (Huizinga et al, 1987). Tachycardia, pyrexia, hypotension or signs of peritonism will indicate the need for prompt exploration (Demetriades and Rabinowitz, 1987).

When history or physical examination is not diagnostic and doubt remains about the presence or absence of an abdominal visceral injury the next investigation will depend on the availability of CT scanning of the abdomen. The alternative is diagnostic peritoneal lavage (DPL) which carries a small risk (5% complication rate including bowel or bladder perforation, trauma to the iliac vessels and instillation of fluid into extraperitoneal tissues) and will not detect retroperitoneal injuries (Fischer et al, 1978). DPL should be performed by the surgeon intending to carry out an operation if the test proves positive. An open minilaparotomy is safer than the closed method. One litre infusion of warm saline (15 ml/kg in children) should be allowed to distribute in the peritoneal cavity for 10 min before the infusion bag is lowered in order to observe the nature of the return fluid; if the test is equivocal (i.e. no gross evidence of blood, bile or faeces) a sample should be sent to the laboratory for red cell count (positive tests > 100 000/μl), white cell count (positive test > 500/μl) and amylase (positive test > 175 U/ml). Laparoscopy is an alternative diagnostic test only for those with the necessary expertise in patients who can be safely anaesthetized, e.g. a child, haemodynamically stable for whom arrangements have been made to proceed to full laparotomy if necessary.

Other radiological investigations for assessing abdominal visceral injury which could be employed in less urgent clinical situations include ultrasound scanning (for detection of free fluid or diaphragmatic rupture), contrast studies (leakage from upper gastrointestinal viscera or diaphragmatic rupture), retrograde pancreatography or angiography (mesenteric vascular injury).

Unless the vital signs suggest that haemorrhage can be controlled only by immediate surgical intervention, once a diagnosis of significant visceral injury has been made the priority is to stabilize the patient as quickly as possible, administer broad spectrum antibiotics, and to make the necessary preparation for surgery. Minimum preoperative preparation includes a urinary catheter, nasogastric tube and blood pressure monitoring.

Place of CT scanning

The threshold for performing this procedure will depend on availability. CT scanning is especially useful in the assessment of patients in whom the severity of the signs of shock are accompanied by a minimum of physical signs. In this situation, injury to the liver or retroperitoneal organs may be present but not easily detectable. Haematomas, laceration and disruption of the capsule of the liver or injury of any retroperitoneal structure can be clearly outlined by sequential cuts of the abdomen. In the USA all trauma centres are required by law to have a CT scanner available throughout the day and night. A similar recommendation has been put forward by the Royal College of Surgeons for all district general hospitals in the United Kingdom. Not only may a CT scan be helpful in the early management of abdominal injury but should a patient's condition deteriorate, a follow-up CT scan will be the quickest way to an early diagnosis.

Operative strategies

At operation, a generous mildline incision provides rapid access and wide exposure with the option to extend the incision onto either the right or left lateral chest wall or across the lower sternum. If a massive haemoperitoneum is present, injury to liver, spleen or major vessels is likely. The small bowel should be lifted out, clot rapidly evacuated (with two large bore suckers) and the quadrants of the abdomen packed. The site of blood loss will usually be revealed as successive packs are removed. Pressure will help to control venous bleeding, Pringle's manoeuvre (digital compression of the free edge of the lesser omentum) will control liver haemorrhage and aortic cross-clamping may control arterial mesenteric haemorrhage. The lesser sac and retroperitoneal viscera (second and third part of duodenum, pancreas) must not be overlooked and may require extensive mobilization to exclude major injury.

Once discovered, the management of specific injuries should follow well-established principles. Diaphragmatic rupture is nearly always the result of blunt trauma, affects the left side in 90% of cases and is accompanied by other visceral injuries which have priority. Repair via the abdomen with non-absorbable sutures is generally effective although large defects may require prosthetic repair.

Gastrointestinal injuries

Gastric injuries are invariably the result of penetrating trauma and rarely require more than debridement and suture. The posterior wall of the stomach and structures behind it should be carefully examined to exclude deeper penetration. Small bowel is frequently damaged because of its length. Injuries range from small bruises to complex lacerations resulting from blast and ischaemia resulting from mesenteric vascular damage. Bruises affecting less than the diameter of the bowel require no treatment; simple lacerations with minimal contamination can be sutured; all other injuries (serosal defect, palpable mural defect, complex lacerations, ischaemic bowel) should be resected. Disrupted mesenteric vessels should be exposed to gain proximal control and repair carried out by suture, patch graft or tube graft. Prosthetic grafts should be avoided for vein repair.

Liver injury

Liver injury carries with it a reputation for high morbidity and mortality (Lewis and Trunkey, 1981). In reality this is not the case; only a minority of patients have complex injuries which require specialist attention and these cases occur more commonly as a result of blast trauma resulting in multiple injuries to other organs (Cogbill et al, 1988; Sheldon and Rutledge, 1989). Bleeding which has stopped with overlying clot formation should be left undisturbed and a drain placed near to the site of injury (Cox et al, 1988). This includes subcapsular haematomas of whatever size (Figure 1). Simple lacerations that continue to ooze can be treated by simple suture; if stitches are placed without tension, it is rare for these lacerations to result in intrahepatic haematoma, necrosis or haemobilia. Coagulation disorders often complicate liver injury and should be monitored and corrected if necessary. When bleeding is massive, parenchymal blood loss can be controlled by packing with large gauze swabs and consideration given to specialist transfer. Survival is rare if the hepatic veins have been sheared from the vena cava because control of haemorrhage by the alert surgeon is only possible once clamps and slings have been applied to portal vein, hepatic artery and inferior vena cava (IVC) (double balloon catheters introduced into the IVC to straddle the ruptured hepatic veins are useless). Hepatic artery ligation should be avoided. Except where there are extensive macerated injuries, there has been a move in specialist centres away from formal resection to hepatotomy with suture ligation of individual

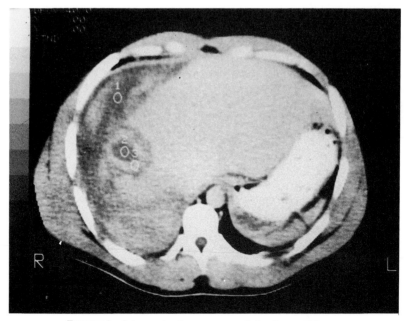

FIGURE I Subcapsular haematoma of the liver—CT scan.

bleeding vessels and bile duct radicles with good results. Preliminary results in dogs suggest fibrin glue may replace suturing and limited debridement in simple, penetrating liver injuries (Hauser, 1989)

Pancreatic injury

Pancreatic injury can be notoriously difficult to detect both radiologically and at laparotomy (Feliciano et al, 1987). Suspicious signs include peripancreatic oedema or haematoma, especially around the region of the second part of the duodenum or the prerenal fascia on either side. In these circumstances, formal exposure of the head, body and tail, including exposure of the entire length of the duodenum, is essential. If an injury is discovered an assessment of ductal integrity by on-table pancreatography is the next priority. Ductal rupture is treated by distal pancreatectomy (injury in the body or tail) anastomosis to a Roux loop (injury in the head) or pancreaticoduodenectomy (injury to pancreatic duct in the head combined with significant duodenal or bile duct injury). Sump suction drains are advisable.

Colorectal injury

The approach to colorectal injuries has recently undergone revision because the complications associated with colostomy formation and closure can exceed those associated with a carefully considered primary closure (Birch et al, 1986). Primary repair of colonic injuries is considered sufficient unless other abdominal findings suggest an additional risk requiring resection. Such risk factors include complex lacerations, gross faecal contamination, delay in operating for more than 8 h and major injury of neighbouring viscera, particularly urinary tract and abdominal wall. Resection of the right colon can safely be completed with ileotransverse anastomosis; resection of the left colon should be completed with end colostomy and a mucous fistula (or closed rectal stump). The addition of a time-consuming on-table colonic lavage in an attempt to perform primary anastomosis is not warranted in this emergency situation. Rectal injuries caused by blast frequently coexist with complex injuries of the lower urinary tract, pelvic vasculature and pripheral nerves. Proctectomy is frequently necessary and may return the patient more rapidly to a better quality of life than attempts at faecal diversion followed by reconstruction and sphincter repair. Penetrating injuries of the rectum require preoperative assessment with proctoscopy, sigmoidoscopy with minimal insufflation and intravenus urogram. Injuries of the upper rectum caused by wounding via the abdomen can generally be closed primarily and covered by an end colostomy. Injuries of the lower rectum caused by wounding via the perineum are complicated by a high rate of sepsis and therefore vigorous efforts should be made to eliminate all faecal residue and other contamination. This can be done with rectal washouts, presacral drainage and broad spectrum antibiotics. In this situation, primary sphincter repair will also stand the best chance of success. No attempt should be made to close the colostomy unless there is radiological evidence of integrity of the repair, there is no pelvic sepsis and sphincter function is adequate to maintain continence.

Conclusion

Without the development of specialized trauma centres, potentially preventable deaths in severely injured patients will continue to occur. In California, Trunkey found that where trauma services are relatively poorly organized 40–73% of deaths from trauma are potentially preventable. In neighbouring counties with an organized system of trauma centres, preventable deaths from trauma were reduced to 9% (Trunkey, 1985). Similar schemes exist in France, West Germany and Japan and since their introduction, similar reductions in deaths from road traffic accidents have been observed. Perhaps the most important element of a trauma centre is the concentration of medical expertise with the result that the severely injured patient is managed by specially trained staff, even before arrival in the hospital. Priorities on admission are clearly recognized as there is no delay in identifying specific visceral injuries. This is of paramount importance in the abdomen where the potential for life-threatening haemorrhage or sepsis is high if injuries are missed for any length of time.

COMPLICATIONS OF UPPER GASTROINTESTINAL ENDOSCOPY

A number of comprehensive surveys have established that complications resulting from fibre optic gastroscopy are uncommon. A survey of 101 units who replied to a questionnaire circulated by the British Society of Gastroenterology (BSG) revealed that one in 5474 examinations is complicated by perforation (Dawson and Cockel, 1981). Among 211 410 examinations reported in a survey of members of the American Society of Gastroenterology the overall rate of complications was 1.32 per 1000 and the perforation rate was 1 per 3330 examinations (Mandelstam et al, 1976). The complication rate is increased at least fourfold when a therapeutic manoeuvre such as stricture dilatation is carried out and rises even further if the stricture is malignant and the patient medically unfit; in such circumstances approximately one in 100 procedures may result in perforation. Finally, the BSG survey showed that palliative intubation for a carcinoma of the mid or lower oesophagus caused perforation in one in 13 procedures; all these patients were treated conservatively and there was no resulting mortality. In fact overall mortality is extremely low, figures being quoted at between 1.4 and 3.0 deaths per 10 000 procedures which includes diagnostic and therapeutic examinations (Mandelstam et al, 1976; Shahmir and Schuman, 1980; Dawson and Cockel, 1981; Reiertsen et al, 1987).

The major complications are perforation, bleeding, aspiration and respiratory problems arising from topical or intravenous anaesthesia.

Perforation

The hypopharynx and upper oesophagus are the most vulnerable to perforation, accounting for approximately two-thirds of cases. The lower oesophagus, although perforated less frequently (about 20% of cases), is the most dangerous site, carrying a high mortality. The cause of perforation in the upper oesophagus tends to be anatomical due to exertion of force in attempting to negotiate the endoscope over the bony projections of osteoarthritis of the cervical spine or through an unexpected high stricture, or rarely through intubation of a Zenkers diverticulum or pharyngeal pouch. The cause in the mid and lower oesophagus is more usually disease when acute inflammation or carcinoma are the complicating factor. Perforations of the stomach or duodenum are rare and are seen when incipient perforation of a penetrating ulcer is precipitated by air insufflation or biopsy. Because the stomach is larger and entirely intraperitoneal, perforation of this organ is considerably more frequent than the duodenum.

Recognition of extraluminal structures by the endoscopist, excessive pain, abdominal distension or the appearance of subcutaneous emphysema give rise to the suspicion that perforation has occurred. An erect chest X-ray may show mediastinal emphysema or gas below the diaphragm (Figure 2) and a prompt X-ray with water-soluble contrast should be performed to localize the leak (Figure 3). In spite of free gas or other overt clinical signs a contrast study may not be helpful and further management will have to be based on clinical grounds. A perforation of the mild or lower oesophagus may be silent and if the patient is then discharged home the early warning signs may be missed and presentation will occur when sepsis has spread and multiorgan failure is incipient.

Management of perforation depends on the site, size and the underlying pathological condition. Clearly, those with advanced cancer should be treated conservatively after discussion with the patient's relatives. Recognized perforations treated actively carry a mortality of between 10% and 20%. As most perforations are small tears and not large rents caused by excessive force, those

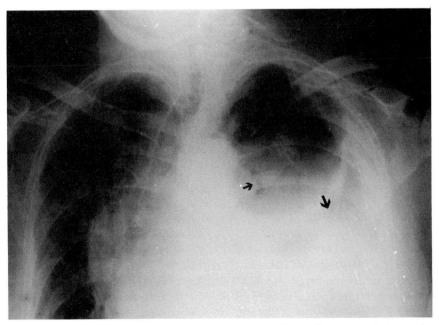

FIGURE 2 Mediastinal emphysema (small arrow) and pleural effusion (large arrow) after endoscopic oesophageal perforation.

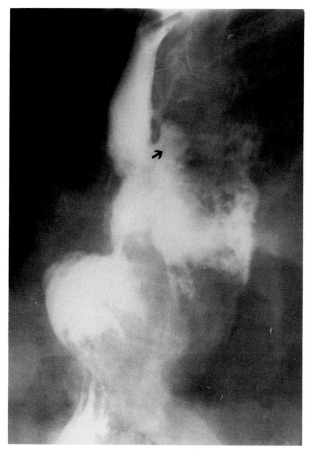

FIGURE 3 Gastrografin swallow after endoscopic oesophageal perforation (leak shown by arrow).

of the mid-oesophagus, generally splits in a stricture or carcinoma, are nearly always managed successfully by conservative treatment with nasogastric suction, intravenous fluids and antibiotics. A similar course and management will suffice for small perforations in the upper oesophagus. A tear in the lower oesophagus or a large rent higher up is more likely to require surgical repair and the decision to operate should be taken within 12 h of the incident because established local sepsis will compromise the success of any repair. Within this time period a direct suture of a clean tear has a good chance of success, but large ragged tears and those older than 12 h are best treated by local flaps or resection. Thoracotomy under these circumstances carries a 50% mortality, but alternatives such as chest drain insertion and pleural irrigation are inadequate and carry a higher mortality.

Precautions can be taken to minimize the risks of perforation: modern fibre optic forward viewing endoscopes can and should be passed through the pharynx and cricopharynx under direct vision, and in the elderly the hypopharynx should be negotiated with special care, to avoid friction posteriorly on prominent osteophytes. If the endoscope becomes obstructed and the way forward not visible, a diverticulum or upper end of a stricture may have been entered. At this point it is prudent to terminate the examination and send the patient for a barium swallow. Strictures at any level should be negotiated with caution and a clear view obtained at all levels. Inexperience plays a large part in all iatrogenic injuries and trainees should have adequate training against the pitfalls. Further training will be necessary in therapeutic manoeuvres because in inexperienced hands dilatation and stricture intubation carry a high risk.

Bleeding

Although occurring with approximately the same frequency as perforation, i.e. one case per 3500 examinations, the outcome is much more benign, overall mortality being less than 5%. In two-thirds of diagnostic cases the source is the stomach and has been initiated by biopsy of an ulcer which continues to bleed. Occasional bleeding from duodenal ulcer occurs in this way. The oesophagus accounts for nearly all the remainder of cases, the source being varices in approximately half, and bleeding after variceal sclerotherapy is the commonest cause in interventional endoscopy. It usually settles with vasoactive drugs and/or tamponade. The majority of other bleeds settle after blood transfusion; in Mandelstam's series only four out of 30 postendoscopic haemorrhages required surgical intervention; two of these were fatal, both patients having impaired coagulation. The operation performed should be the minimum to arrest bleeding avoiding resection and lengthy procedures.

Haemorrhage can be avoided by recognition and careful negotiation of oesophageal varices, judicious biopsy of ulcerating lesions and avoidance of biopsy and trauma in patients with coagulation disorders.

COMPLICATIONS OF ERCP

In a survey of 10 435 diagnostic examinations, the overall incidence of complications was 3% and the mortality 0.2%. Of the 15 deaths in this series, 13 were due to sepsis arising in the biliary tree (8) or the pancreas (5); two other deaths were from intestinal perforation and variceal haemorrhage (Bilbao et al, 1976). Sphincterotomy for retrieval of common duct stones increases the complication rate to between 6% and 10% and mortality directly related to the procedure rises to 1%, although the 30-day mortality is nearer 4% because this assessment takes into account cardiovascular-related deaths (Cotton, 1980; Leese et al, 1985; Leuschner, 1986).

Pancreatitis

There is a wide variation in the reported incidence of acute pancreatitis following ERCP. A prospective study with serial amylase measurements found hyper-amylasaemia (> 3000 IU/l) in 75% of patients and acute pancreatitis in 11.3% (LaFerla et al, 1986). Retrospective series tend to report a much lower incidence with figures ranging from 0.6% to 3% (Hamilton et al, 1983). Sphincterotomy increases the risk, and although it has been suggested that this risk is only present when a pancreatogram has been obtained simultaneously, this is not always the case.

The major factor in the aetiology of acute pancreatitis after ERCP is repeated injection of contrast into the duct, even in the absence of pancreatic acinar opacification. There is an increased incidence of sepsis associated with injection into an obstructed duct or into a pseudocyst. Under these circumstances there is a considerable risk of abscess formation (Figure 4).

Fortunately the course of post-ERCP acute pancreatitis is relatively benign, few deaths having been recorded, nor have there been many reports of progression to necrosis, abscess or pseudocyst formation. Treatment can therefore be limited to nasogastric suction and intravenous fluids. Although the value of antibiotics in acute pancreatitis is doubtful, in this situation because of the suspicion that the cause could be related to ductal contamination (from the endoscope or the duodenum) a course of broad spectrum antibiotics is advisable. Routine antibiotic prophylaxis is not indicated for diagnostic pancreatography, but many patients will be jaundiced and be prescribed antibiotics prior to endoscopic manipulation of the biliary tree. The possibility that acute pancreatitis has followed ERCP will be raised in patients with abdominal pain, fever and leucocytosis, and following confirmation by serum amylase estimation, computed tomographic (CT) scanning may help in assessing the severity and extent of the inflammation (Kuhlman et al, 1989; Lambiase et al, 1989). Following a prolonged course serial CT is the most effective means of monitoring and detecting the rare occurrence of pseudocyst formation or retroperitoneal abscess.

The incidence of acute pancreatitis can be reduced by taking care to avoid acinar filling, which can be achieved by having the assistance of a radiologist, accurately collimating the X-ray beam for good definition, stopping ductal injection once

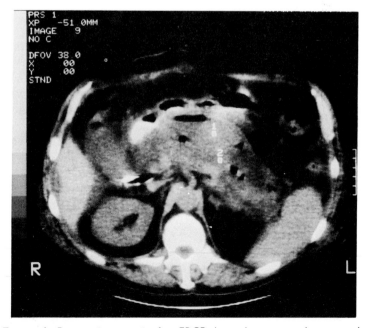

FIGURE 4 Pancreatic necrosis after ERCP shown by computed tomography.

main branch filling is recognized and avoiding repeated injections. Modern non-ionic contrast media are also less likely to cause pancreatitis, but they are more expensive. In addition if ERCP is carried out for definition of ductal anatomy associated with a pseudocyst then elective surgical intrevention should be prepared for shortly after the procedure.

Cholangitis

Biliary sepsis is generally a complication of failure to remove common duct stones after sphincterotomy, although there is a small incidence (less than 1%) after diagnostic ERCP which is nearly always associated with injection of contrast into an obstructed duct (Habr-Gama and Waye, 1989). After sphincterotomy for biliary calculi, stone clearance will not be achieved in about 6–8% of patients and up to a quarter of these patients will develop cholangitis in spite of antibiotic prophylaxis (Cotton, 1980; Leese et al, 1985; Martin and Tweedle, 1987; Tanaka et al, 1987).

Recognition is based on the classical clinical triad, i.e. abdominal pain, fever and jaundice and immediate therapy should begin with broad spectrum antibiotics, intravenous fluid and restriction of oral intake. Because of the high risk of cholangitis when duct clearance is not achieved, a strong case can be made for passing a nasobiliary tube into the upper duct for drainage and this manoeuvre can minimize the septic sequelae. *Pseudomonas*, as well as other Gram-negative bacilli, is quite a common organism. Piperacillin or mezlocillin have been recently recommended for the treatment of cholangitis (Editorial, 1989). Nevertheless, these prophylactic measures and antibiotics will fail in 20–40% of patients and surgical drainage of the duct will be necessary. Choledochoduodenostomy or transduodenal sphincteroplasty are the surgical options and both, in the elective situation, carry a mortality of 5% (Baker et al, 1987; Sellner et al, 1988). The mortality more than doubles in post-sphincterotomy patients with cholangitis because most had been preselected for non-surgical treatment on account of age or medical unfitness. Nevertheless, surgery should not be delayed more than 24–48 h in those not responding to medical treatment.

The incidence of cholangitis can be reduced by avoiding overfilling or repeated contrast injection into an obstructed duct. When large stones are present an adequate sphincterotomy should be performed up to what is considered safe in that patient. If the facility for immediate transduodenal lithotripsy exists then stones that fail to pass through an adequate sphincterotomy can be fragmented during the same procedure with the extraction of the resulting stone particles.

Impacted stones (Figure 5)

This problem is closely related to and is managed in an almost identical manner to cholangitis because it so often leads to biliary sepsis. If the stone is impacted within a Dormia basket is is usually possible to release it by advancing the basket and stone as far into the biliary tree as possible until the basket curls back on itself

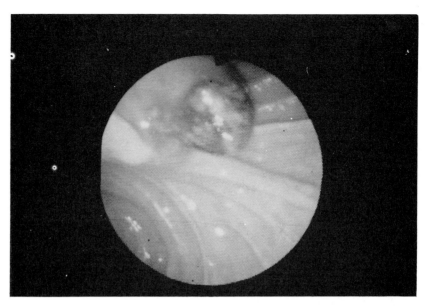

FIGURE 5 Gallstone impacted in the papilla of Vater, seen endoscopically.

and drops the stone. If the stone and basket are firmly lodged at the papilla the basket handle can be cut off and the endoscope removed and reinserted alongside the basket. It is then usually possible to enlarge the sphincterotomy with a needle knife. If this fails, it is sometimes possible to pass a nasobiliary tube beyond the stone which will then pass spontaneously within 48 h in about 50% of patients. The remainder will require surgical intervention by transduodenal sphinctero-plasty with the consequent hazards outlined above. If a patient is known in advance to have common duct stones larger than 2.5 cm and is not an undue anaesthetic risk then it may be wiser to plan elective surgery rather than risk stone impaction, cholangitis and the greater hazards of surgery under these conditions.

Perforation

This is apparent clinically in about 1% of patients who have had endoscopic sphincterotomy. It is probably more frequent but asymptomatic, as sometimes retroperitoneal air is seen by chance on subsequent X-rays. Free perforation into the peritoneal cavity is rare and the clinical features are usually those of retroperitoneal perforation—pain, fever and tenderness. An ileus may develop as may a palpable mass. Pancreatitis should be excluded by estimation of the serum amylase, and ultrasound or CT scanning will demonstrate any significant collection retroperitoneally. Management is initially conservative—intravenous fluids and broad spectrum antibiotics—and surgical drainage is rarely required. The risks of perforation can be minimized by tailoring the length of sphincterotomy to the size of stone and to the intramural portion of the bile duct (this is much shorter in a flat, effaced papilla, making perforation more likely).

COMPLICATIONS OF COLONOSCOPY

Analysis of several colonoscopy series confirms the relative safety of this procedure in a diagnostic or therapeutic setting when compared with the surgical alternative (Habr-Gama and Waye, 1989). The overall complication rate, of which perforation and haemorrhage account for the majority, is between 1% and 2.1% (Ghazi and Grossman, 1982; Macrae et al, 1983). Deaths however are uncommon, ranging from 0.02% to 0.15%, and there is no mortality in some published series. Deaths are rarely due to perforation or bleeding but result more often from cardiorespiratory causes consequent upon oversedation.

Perforation

The incidence of perforation is reported to be between 0.2% and 0.6% following diagnostic examination and up 1.2% with the addition of polypectomy (Rogers et al, 1975; Brynitz et al, 1986; Nivatvongs, 1988). The causes are largely due to two factors, the inappropriate use of mechanical force, generally in a difficult anatomical situation, and the misapplication of equipment used for polypectomy. Perforation may be incomplete with a tear occurring in the serosa alone which is benign, generally caused by traction or overdistension and probably much under-diagnosed, or occurring in the mucosa alone which can lead to emphysema of the colonic wall, retroperitoneal gas and rarely to pneumoperitoneum by a process of tracking. A confidently diagnosed incomplete tear can be treated conservatively with nasogastric suction, intravenous fluids and antibiotics. Forceful introduction of the endoscope results in perforation occurring in a number of well-defined anatomical sites; the sigmoid colon especially if a large loop develops, the site of strictures or adhesions or in segments of severe diverticular disease. Inappropriate electrocoagulation causes perforation by transmural coagulation necrosis or an accidental burn on the opposite wall of the bowel.

Most complete perforations are recognized instantly due to direct visualization of extracolonic structures by the endoscopist, pneumoperitoneum or peritonism. For this reason prompt surgical intervention is highly successful, death being exceptional except for the rare cardiorespiratory complication. The reason for this outcome is the lack of sepsis and a clean colon, because preparation for colonoscopy is similar to preparation for colonic surgery. A segmental resection may be necessary if a long tear or a large diathermy burn is present, but many perforations can be safely dealt with by suture alone if the bowel has been well prepared and there is no local peritoneal contamination. A stoma will be necessary when contamination is present, and if there is associated carcinoma, diverticular disease or inflammatory bowel disease a resection may be indicated.

Prevention depends on adequate training and a thorough knowledge of electrocoagulation techniques used for polypectomy. It has been stated that a colonoscopist in training should be carefully supervised for 50 examinations and perform not less than six examinations per week to maintain and improve expertise (Hunt, 1983). Perforations during polypectomy can be minimized by not tackling lesions with a broad base, applying the snare on the pedicle a few millimetres away from the bowel wall and ensuring that the snare does not touch or burn the opposite wall.

Bleeding

Although haemorrhage accounts for more than half of all complications following colonoscopic polypectomy, the majority of bleeds are classified as minor. Occasional haemorrhages occur extrinsic to the colonic lumen as a result of mesenteric tears or occasionally laceration of the liver or spleen caused by excessive force or adhesions. Approximately one in 400 polypectomies are complicated by a haemorrhage requiring transfusion. Nearly all such events occur during polypectomies over 2 cm in size. Approximately 80% of major bleeds will stop spontaneously after blood transfusion and the remainder are resolved with straightforward open surgical colostomy and suture ligation of the bleeding vessel. As in perforations requiring surgery the operation carries virtually no mortality because intervention can be planned and the bowel has been prepared. Secondary haemorrhage is an unpredictable complication presenting at 7–14 days but which is rarely significant enough to require surgery. Informed consent must include an explanation of this complication so that should it occur patients will seek prompt medical attention, supervised monitoring and appropriate treatment if required.

Measures to avoid this complication are similar to those that should be adopted to avoid perforation, especially adequate training and skilful use of diathermy snares for polypectomy, i.e. low power, slow transection and if immediate haemorrhage is seen the stalk should be resnared and held for 10 min.

OTHER COMPLICATIONS OF ENDOSCOPY

These are mostly common to the different fibre optic endoscopic procedures, and particularly relate to the use of intravenous sedation and analgesia. While infrequent, they are in part preventable by awareness of the risk and attention to detail. They are predisposed to by:

(1) an increasing percentage of elderly and infirm patients undergoing endoscopic investigations, often with coexisting cardiac or pulmonary disease;
(2) a tendency for the endoscopist to administer the sedation himself, often in more liberal dosage than customarily used by anaesthetists, and for his attention thereafter to be concentrated on the procedure rather than on the patient;
(3) an unawareness of the precipitate fall in pO_2 that may occur silently.

Cardiac

Transient and asymptomatic electrocardiogram changes are quite common when Holter monitoring is used throughout endoscopy, either changes in ST segments or arrhythmias. The rhythm changes are usually isolated supraventricular or ventricular beats, occasionally coming in sustained runs (Levy and Abinader, 1977). They have been reported in 29 of 63 patients undergoing colonoscopy, and were more frequent in those with pre-existing cardiac disease (Alam et al, 1976). In a series of more than 25 000 colonoscopies, there were three instances of myocardial infarction, a frequency of about 0.01%. Rogers (1981) and Macrae et al (1983) report one death from myocardial ischaemia in 5000 cases.

Vasovagal symptoms including faintness, sweating, hypotension and bradycardia may occur, especially with excessive air insufflation or painful instrumentation during colonoscopy (Hunt, 1983). It is likely that atropine would afford protection from this but it is not so commonly administered routinely with sedation as some years ago. Hypotension and hypovolaemia may result from the use of mannitol for whole gut irrigation prior to colonoscopy, particularly in the elderly, as there is a net loss of fluid into the gut (Gilmore et al, 1981). On the other hand, whole gut irrigation with saline results in salt and water absorption, with the associated risk of heart failure in the elderly.

A final cardiac complication to be borne in mind in both lower and upper gastrointestinal endoscopy is that of infective endocarditis, although it must be exceedingly rare. Bacteraemia has been reported in 3–8% patients undergoing gastroscopy (Schull et al, 1975) and is also a transient event during colonoscopy (Rogers, 1981). Current recommendations in the UK are for prophylaxis only in those with prosthetic heart valves or a history of infective endocarditis where amoxycillin 1 g + gentamicin 120 mg are given intramuscularly just before endoscopy followed by 0.5 g amoxycillin by mouth 6 h later. In those patients with genuine allergy to penicillin an alternative is vancomycin 1 g intravenously over the 60 min prior to endoscopy with gentamicin 120 mg 15 min before.

Pulmonary

Respiratory depression is the commonest significant complication, especially in the elderly. Although there is a trend towards performing routine gastroscopy with topical anaesthesia only, in the UK intravenous sedation is still used in 80–90% of examinations. Diazepam is the commonest agent used, and the incidence of thrombophlebitis, initially very troublesome, has been reduced by dissolving it in an oily medium. A more potent benzodiazepine, midazolam, is gaining in popularity and is probably no more prone to produce respiratory depression or apnoea when used in equipotent doses, but is more effective than diazepam in producing amnesia for the procedure. The important steps in minimizing the risk of respiratory depression are to give the sedation slowly, over several minutes and to give the minimum necessary. The dose required in the elderly may be only one-half to one-quarter of the usual adult dose by weight. Modern, small diameter gastroscopes have less influence in reducing the effective upper airway, and a rapid, skilled examination is likely to be safer than a prolonged and difficult one. Patients with known lung disease may benefit from oxygen administered by nasal spectacles and should be examined without sedation if the procedure is otherwise well tolerated. It seems likely that in the next few years there will be increasing pressure to use pulse oximeters routinely, as is becoming normal practice in anaesthesia.

If respiratory depression is recognized in time, it can usually be reversed by the use of an appropriate antagonist, naloxone in the case of opiate analgesia and flumazanil for benzodiazapine sedation. Both antagonists provide prompt and spectacular reversal, but they should be rarely required if premedication is cautiously used. There is no indication for their routine use, and there may be rebound sedation because the half-life of the antagonist is shorter.

Pulmonary aspiration and subsequent chest infection is extremely rare as a clinical problem after upper gastrointestinal endoscopy, although radiographic evidence of aspiration of contrast medium instilled into the stomach has been reported to occur in up to 25% of examinations (Prout and Metreweli, 1972). The frequency is unlikely to be as high with the modern slimline instruments.

Infection

Transmission of infections such as *Salmonella* is very well documented (O'Connor and Axon, 1983), and infection in the form of cholangitis is a particularly serious and potentially fatal complication of ERCP. It has been shown that *Pseudomonas* cholangitis and septicaemia has been the result of instrument contamination (Low et al, 1980). There is also a case of hepatitis B transmission by endoscopy (Birnie et al, 1983). Current anxieties about HIV infection have been crucial in establishing guidelines about disinfection of instruments both between patients and at the beginning and end of lists (Working Party of the BSG, 1988).

Miscellaneous

Other complications are rare and may be the consequence of an adverse reaction to a drug used before or during the procedure. No account would be complete without reference to colonic explosion during diathermy procedures after mannitol bowel preparation (Bigard et al, 1979), which has now been reported on at least three occasions.

COMPLICATIONS OF LIVER BIOPSY

Detailed analysis of large numbers of liver biopsies has confirmed the safety of this procedure and the rarity of complications. Nevertheless this has been achieved by careful technique, awareness of the potential hazards and patient selection (Perrault et al, 1978; Hegarty and Williams, 1984). The complication rate, which includes moderate to severe pain or hypotension or both, is of the order of 6% mortality is so low it is difficult to quantify but in a large series death occurred at a rate of nine per 100 000 biopsies and only in patients with malignancy or cirrhosis (Piccinino et al, 1986). Two-thirds of complications are diagnosed within 2 h of biopsy and 96% within 24 h.

Bleeding

This is generally unpredictable and is due to arterial puncture or perforation of a distended portal vein radicle in patients with cirrhosis. Patients with impaired coagulation will continue to bleed for longer after such a mishap because of prolonged haemostasis. Symptoms are apparent almost immediately heralded by pain and subsequently with signs of shock if bleeding is massive. Haemorrhage is rarely catastrophic, leaving time for natural haemodilution and allowing for monitoring of blood loss by measurement of haematocrit or haemoglobin estimation. In Piccinino's series, of the 22 patients (from a total of 68 276 biopsies) who developed haemoperitoneum, eight required an operation (three of whom died), three died from massive bleeding before operation could be performed and 11 recovered with blood transfusion. Thus in suspected cases of postbiopsy bleeding it is sufficient to observe vital signs closely and site an intravenous cannula for blood transfusion should it be required. The need for transfusion will be based on the patient's prebiopsy haemoglobin, stability of vital signs or decrease in haemoglobin level below 10 g/dl. Adopting a similar strategy for 1000 patients undergoing liver biopsy only five required transfusion and none required laparotomy to stem the bleeding (Perrault et al, 1978). Alternatively the transjugular approach can be used (Gilmore et al, 1977) although even then the liver capsule can be transgressed from within and haemoperitoneum result (Bull et al, 1983). Haemorrhage after percutaneous biopsy is commoner using the Tru-cut than Menghini needle (Piccinino et al, 1986) but the former obtains superior samples for histological assessment, especially in cirrhosis (Littlewood et al, 1982; Colombo et al, 1988). Multiple passes increase the risk of complications, but a second core should be taken when seeking confirmation of metastatic disease if the first is macroscopically normal. Deep jaundice and/or ascites also increase the risks of the procedure.

The most obvious measure in reducing the incidence of bleeding is to avoid biopsy in patients with a low platelet count (below 80×10^9/l) or a prolonged prothrombin time (greater than 3 s despite vitamin K). If a biopsy is vital for further management in such patients then 6 units of platelets and/or 2 units of fresh frozen plasma can be given, to begin half an hour before the procedure and finish 1 h afterwards. In addition the track can be plugged with absorbable gelatin sponge on withdrawal of the biopsy needle (Riley et al, 1984; Tobin et al, 1989). Biopsy should also be avoided in uncooperative patients and comatose or anaesthetized patients because of uncontrollable movements and greatly increased liability to laceration of liver parenchyma. The training and experience of the operator is directly related to complication rate.

Haemobilia is a rare and special type of postbiopsy bleeding. It occurs immediately or a few weeks after the procedure and results from a communicating puncture between adjacent arterial and biliary channels within the liver resulting in sudden and dramatic effluxes of blood into the bile ducts. The presenting symptoms are biliary pain, jaundice, melaena and shock. Angiography is both diagnostic and therapeutic, the damaged arteriole being plugged with gelfoam or coils after selective catheterization. Very rarely a liver resection may be necessary which should be undertaken under controlled conditions in a specialist unit.

Bile peritonitis

Intraperitoneal leakage of bile after percutaneous biopsy is extremely unlikely unless the biliary tree is distended due to obstruction or the gallbladder is inadvertently punctured. Since the development of reliable ultrasonography liver biopsy is rarely performed in extrahepatic obstruction, but in a study of 100 cases (Morris et al, 1975) few complications were seen. When biliary peritonitis occurs, pain and signs of peritonism are the principle feature, and conservative management with nasogastric aspiration, intravenous fluids and analgesics is usually sufficient. However, gallbladder perforation carries a high mortality if left untreated and early surgery should be considered. With increasing use of ultrasound guided liver biopsy this particular complication should not occur and prebiopsy scanning is particularly important when the liver is small.

CONCLUSIONS AND THE WAY AHEAD

As medical audit becomes more widely practised, further and more accurate data on outcome of these procedures will become available, and it may be that in the UK the therapeutic endoscopic procedures should be covered under the Confidential Enquiry into Perioperative Deaths. With greater attention to monitoring of sedated patients for endoscopic procedures and the increasing trend to perform diagnostic gastroscopy without sedation, one anticipates a significant reduction in anaesthetic-related complications, but this may be more than offset by an increasing proportion of therapeutic and hence more risky procedures, such as endoscopic laser and biliary therapy.

REFERENCES

Alam M, Schuman BM, Duvernoy WFC & Madrazo AC (1976) Continuous electrocardiographic monitoring during colonoscopy. *Gastroinestinal Endoscopy* **22**: 203–205.

Baker AR, Neoptolemos JP, Leese T & Fossard DP (1987) Choledochoduodenostomy, transduodenal sphincteroplasty and sphincterotomy for calculi of the common bile duct. *British Journal of Surgery* **164**: 245–251.

Bigard MA, Gaucher P & Lassale C (1979) Fatal colonic explosions during colonoscopic polypectomy. *Gastroenterology* **77**: 1307–1310.

Bilbao MK, Dotter CT, Lee TG & Katon RM (1976). Complications of endoscopic retrograde cholangiopancreatography (ERCP): a study of 10 000 cases. *Gastroenterology* **70**: 314–320.

Birch JM, Gevirtzman L, Jordan GL et al (1986) The injured colon. *Annals of Surgery* **201**: 701–711.

Birnie GC, Quigley EM, Clements GB, Follet EAC & Watkinson G (1983) Endoscopic transmission of hepatitis B virus. *Gut* **24**: 171–174.

Brynitz S, Kjaergard H & Struckmann J (1986) Perforations from colonoscopy during diagnosis and treatment of polyps. *Ann. Chir. Gynaecol.* **75**: 142–145.

Bull HJ, Gilmore IT, Bradley RD, Marigold JH & Thompson RPH (1983) Experience with transjugular liver biopsy. *Gut* **24**: 1057–1060.

Cogbill RH, Moore EE, Jurkovich GJ, Feliciano DV, Morris JA & Mucha P (1988) Severe hepatic injury: a multi-center experience with 1,335 liver injuries. *Journal of Trauma* **28**, 1433–1438.

Colombo M, Ninno ED, DeFranchis R, DeFazio C, Festorazzi S, Ronchi G & Tommasini MA (1988) Ultrasound-assisted percutaneous liver biopsy: superiority of the Tru-cut over the Menghini needle for diagnosis of cirrhosis. *Gastroenterology* **95**: 487–489.

Cotton PB (1980) Non-operative removal of bile duct stones by duodenoscopic sphincterotomy. *British Journal of Surgery* **67**: 1–5.

Cox EF, Flancbaum I, Dauterive AH & Paulson RL (1988) Blunt trauma of the liver: analysis of management and mortality in 323 consecutive patients. *Annals of Surgery* **207**: 126–134.

Dawson J & Cockel R (1981) Oesophageal perforation at fibreoptic gastroscopy. *British Medical Journal* **283**: 583.

Demetriades D & Rabinowitz B (1987) Indications for operation in abdominal stab wounds. *Annals of Surgery* **205**: 129–132.

Editorial (1989) Antibiotics for cholangitis. *Lancet* **2**: 781–782.

Feliciano DV, Martin TD, Cruse, PA et al (1987) Management of combined pancreaticoduodenal injuries. *Annals of Surgery* **205**: 673–679.

Fischer RP, Beverlin BC, Engrav LH et al (1978) Diagnostic peritoneal lavage, fourteen years and 2586 patients later. *American Journal of Surgery* **136**: 701–704.

Ghazi A & Grossman M (1982) Complications of colonoscopy and polypectomy. *Surgical Clinics of North America* **62**: 889–896.

Gilmore IT, Bradley RD & Thompson RPH (1977) Transjugular liver biopsy. *British Medical Journal* **2**: 100–101.

Gilmore IT, Ellis WR, Barrett GW, Pendower JEH & Parkins RA (1981) A comparison of two preparations for gut lavage prior to colonoscopy. *British Journal of Surgery* **68**: 388–389.

Goldberger JH, Bernstein DM, Rodman GD & Suarez CA (1982) Selection of patients with abdominal stab wounds for laparotomy. *Journal of Trauma* **20**: 476–480.

Habr-Gama A & Waye JD (1989) Complications and hazards of gastrointestinal endoscopy. *World Journal of Surgery* **13**: 193–201.

Hamilton I, Lintott DJ, Rothwell J & Axon ATR (1983) Acute pancreatitis following endoscopic retrograde cholangiopancreatography. *Clinical Radiology* **34**: 543–546.

Hauser CJ (1989) Hemostasis of solid viscus trauma by intraparenchymal injection of fibrin glue. *Archives of Surgery* **124**: 291–293.

Hegarty JE & Williams R (1984) Liver biopsy: techniques, clinical applications and complications. *British Medical Journal* **288**: 1254–1256.

Huizinga WK, Baker LW & Mtshali ZW (1987) Selective management of abdominal and thoracic stab wounds with established peritoneal penetration: the eviscerated omentum. *American Journal of Surgery* **153**: 564–568.

Hunt RH (1983) Towards safer colonoscopy. *Gut* **24**: 371–375.

Kuhlman JE, Fishman EK, Milligan FD & Siegelman SS (1989) Complications of endoscopic retrograde sphincterotomy: computed tomographic evaluation. *Gastrointestinal Radiology* **14**: 127–132.

LaFerla G, Gordon S, Archibald M & Murray WR (1986) Hyperamylasemia and acute pancreatitis following endoscopic retrograde cholangiopancreatography. *Pancreas* **1**: 160–164.

Lambiase RE, Cronan JJ & Ridlen M (1989) Perforation of the common bile duct during endoscopic sphincterotomy: recognition on computed tomography and successful percutaneous treatment. *Gastrointestinal Radiology* **14**: 133–136.

Lambrianides AL & Rosin RD (1984) Penetrating stab injuries of the chest and abdomen. *Injury* **15**: 300–303.

Leese T, Neoptolomos JP & Carr-Locke DL (1985) Successes, failures, early complications and their management following endoscopic sphincterotomy: results in 394 consecutive patients from a single centre. *British Journal of Surgery* **72**: 215–219.

Leuschner U (1986) Endoscopic therapy in biliary calculi. *Clinics in Gastroenterology* **15**: 333–359.

Levy N & Abinader E (1977) Continuous electrocardiographic monitoring with Holter electrocardiorecorder throughout all stages of gastroscopy. *American Journal of Digestive Disease* **22**: 1091–1096.

Lewis FR & Trunkey DD (1981) Management of major liver trauma. In Carter DC & Polk HC (eds) *Trauma*, pp 99–109. London: Butterworth.

Littlewood ER, Gilmore IT, Murray-Lyon IM, Stephens KR & Paradinas FJ (1982) Comparison of the Tru-cut and shure-cut liver biopsy needles. *Journal of Clinical Pathology* **35**: 761–763.

Low DE, Micflikier AB, Kennedy JK & Stiver HG (1980) Infectious complications of endoscopic retrograde cholangiopancreatography. *Archives of Internal Medicine* **140**: 1076–1077.

Macrae FA, Tan KG & Williams CB (1983) Towards safer colonoscopy: a report on the complications of 5,000 diagnostic or therapeutic colonoscopies. *Gut* **24**: 376–383.

Mandelstam P, Sugawa C, Silvas SE, Nebel OT & Rogers BHG (1976) Complications associated with esophagogastroduodenoscopy and with esophageal dilation. *Gastrointest. Endoscopy* **23**: 16–19.

Martin DF & Tweedle DEF (1987) Endoscopic management of common duct stones without cholecystectomy. *British Journal of Surgery* **74**: 209–211.

Morris JS, Gallo GA, Scheuer PJ & Sherlock S (1975) Percutaneous liver biopsy in patients with large bile duct obstruction. *Gastroenterology* **68**: 750–754.

Nivatvongs S (1988) Complications in colonoscopic polypectomy: Lessons to learn from an experience with 1576 polyps. *American Surgeon* **57**: 61–63.

O'Connor HJ & Axon ATR (1983) Gastrointestinal endoscopy: infection and disinfection. *Gut* **24**: 1067–1077.

Oreskovich MR & Carrico CJ (1983) Stab wounds of the anterior abdomen. *Annals of Surgery* **198**: 411–419.

Perrault J, McGill DB, Ott BJ & Taylor WF (1978) Liver biopsy: complications in 1000 inpatients and outpatients. *Gastroenterology* **74**: 103–106.

Piccinino F, Sagnelli E, Pasquale G & Giusti G (1986) Complications following percutaneous liver biopsy: a multicentre retrospective study on 68,276 biopsies. *Journal of Hepatology* **2**: 165–173.

Prout BJ & Metreweli C (1972) Pulmonary aspiration after fibre-endoscopy of the upper gastrointestinal tract. *British Medical Journal* **4**: 269–271.

Reiertsen O, Skjoto J, Jacobsen CD & Rosseland AR (1987) Complications of fiberoptic gastrointestinal endoscopy—five years' experience in a central hospital. *Endoscopy* **19**: 1–6.

Riley SA, Ellis WR, Irving HC, Lintott DJ, Axon ATR & Losowsky MS (1984) Percutaneous liver biopsy with plugging of needle track: a safe method for use in patients with impaired coagulation. *Lancet* **ii**: 436.

Rogers BHG (1981) Complications and hazards of colonoscopy. In Hunt RH & Waye JD (eds) *Colonoscopy: Techniques, Clinical Practice and Colour Atlas*, pp 237–264. London: Chapman and Hall.

Rogers BHG, Silvas SE, Nebel OT, Sugawa C & Mandelstam P (1975) Complications of flexible fiberoptic colonoscopy and polypectomy. *Gastroinestinal Endoscopy* **22**: 73–77.

Rowlands BJ (1988) Management of abdominal trauma. In Taylor I (ed) *Progress in Surgery*, vol. 3. Edinburgh: Churchill Livingstone.

Schull HJ, Greene BM, Allen SD, Dunn DG & Schenker S (1975) Bacteremia with upper gastrointestinal endoscopy. *Annals of Internal Medicine* **83**: 212–214.

Shahmir M & Schuman BM (1980) Complications of fiberoptic endoscopy. *Gastrointestinal Endoscopy* **26**: 86–91.

Sellner FJ, Wimberger M & Jelinek R (1988) Factors affecting mortality in transduodenal sphincteroplasty. *Surgery, Gynecology and Obstetrics* **167**: 23–27.

Sheldon GF & Rutledge R (1989) Hepatic trauma. *Advances in Surgery* **22**: 179–194.

Tanaka M, Ikeda S, Yoshimoto H & Matsumoto S (1987) The long-term fate of the gallbladder after endoscopic sphincterotomy: complete follow-up study of 122 patients. *American Journal of Surgery* **154**: 505–509.

Thompson JS, Moore JE, Duzer-Moore S et al (1980) The evolution of abdominal stab wound management. *Journal of Trauma* **20**: 478–484.

Tobin MV & Gilmore IT (1989) Plugged liver biopsy in patients with impaired coagulation. *Digestive Disease Science* **34**: 13–15.

Trunkey DD (1984) Abdominal trauma. In Trunkey DD & Lewis FR (eds) *Current Therapy in Trauma 1984–1985*. St Louis: CV Mosby.

Trunkey DD (1985) Towards optimal trauma care. *Archives of Emergency Medicine* **2**: 181–195.

Working Party of the British Society of Gastroenterology (1988) Cleaning and disinfection of equipment for gastrointestinal flexible endoscopy: interim recommendations. *Gut* **29**: 1134–1151.

15

CHILDHOOD GASTROENTEROLOGICAL EMERGENCIES

I. R. Sanderson and J. A. Walker-Smith

INTRODUCTION

Acute problems related to the gastrointestinal tract are a common reason for children to attend accident and emergency units. The doctor on duty must be able to distinguish the genuine emergency from the background of non-urgent, albeit troubling, symptoms for which parents seek advice. For example, the acute onset of vomiting due to gastroenteritis or acute intestinal obstruction is an emergency, whereas vomiting due to gastro-oesophageal reflux is not. A careful history from the parents is needed to make this distinction. Gastrointestinal emergencies in children can be considered under the following headings: gastrointestinal bleeding; gastroenteritis; jaundice; emergencies associated with chronic gastrointestinal problems.

GASTROINTESTINAL BLEEDING

Acute loss of blood can cause rapid hypovolaemia leading to poor perfusion of essential organs; the life of a young infant may be threatened very quickly. Gastrointestinal bleeding can be the result of blood loss from damaged or abnormal blood vessels, coagulation defects or inflammation of the gastrointestinal mucosa. Loss of blood from damaged vessels is the most important reason for significant bleeding. The main causes are given in Table 1. Secondly, bleeding can also occur into a normal gastrointestinal tract when there are significant derangements of coagulability of the blood, for example disseminated intravascular coagulation. Prothrombin time, partial thromboplastin time and platelet count must therefore be measured. A history of ingestion of drugs that affect platelet function should also be sought. Aspirin, although now rarely used in children, affects platelet adhesiveness as well as being a cause of gastric erosions. Finally, on rare occasions, inflammation of the gastrointestinal mucosa may produce sufficient leakage of blood to cause hypovolaemia.

TABLE I

Causes of gastrointestinal
blood loss due to damaged
or abnormal blood vessels

Oesophageal varices
Mallory–Weiss tear
Gastric erosions
Gastric ulcer
Duodenal ulcer
Meckel's diverticulum
Diffuse haemangioma
Vascular telengiectasia
Polyps
Trauma
Henoch–Schönlein purpura

Resuscitation

Assessment

The severity of blood loss is assessed by seeking clinical evidence of shock. Poor peripheral perfusion is detected by low skin temperature which can be noted on palpation and, if available, quantified by a thermocouple whose reference lead measures body core temperature. Reduction in blood pressure and compensatory tachycardia may be apparent. It is important to be aware of the normal blood pressure and heart rate in children, as these can differ significantly from adults (Table 2). The most direct assessment of intravascular volume is measurement of central venous pressure. However, insertion of a catheter into the central veins of a hypovolaemic child is difficult and wastes time that is better directed toward resuscitation. Nevertheless, it is useful to monitor central venous pressure in a child who is adequately transfused but is likely to have a further episode of bleeding, as the clinician may be alerted by a fall in pressure before other clinical signs are evident.

TABLE 2

Blood pressure (BP) and heart rate in children of different ages

Age	Systolic BP (± SD)	Diastolic BP (± SD)	Heart rate (range)
I day	70 (± 7)	40 (± 5)	70 to 120
I month	99 (± 11)	57 (± 8)	80 to 160
3 years	99 (± 10)	57 (± 8)	75 to 120
10 years	114 (± 10)	65 (± 9)	70 to 110
16 years (boys)	125 (± 10)	67 (± 8)	70 to 110
16 years (girls)	115 (± 11)		

From Linde (1968).

Therapy

Rapid replacement of fluid is needed before diagnostic steps are undertaken. Plasma is given while blood is being cross-matched, and then whole blood is infused to replace the assessed loss.

Postresuscitation assessment

Once resuscitatory measures are underway, further investigation is directed towards determining the cause and effects of hypovolaemia. Renal function is assessed by monitoring hourly urine output, which may necessitate catheterization of the urinary bladder, by regular weighing and by the measurement of plasma urea, creatinine and electrolytes. Measurement of urinary osmolality, urea and sodium will help the clinician to decide whether oliguria is due to renal hypoperfusion or acute tubular necrosis. A full neurological examination is required to discover any residual damage to brain or spinal cord. This examination may need repeating during the course of the casualty attendance. The detection of the cause of gastrointestinal blood loss has improved greatly as a result of the wider use of endoscopy in children (Hyams et al, 1985). However, radiological techniques may still be required.

In children with haematemesis, oesophagogastroduodenoscopy is sufficient, but with melaena or the presence of fresh blood in the stools, both colonoscopy and upper gastrointestinal endoscopy are required. Gastroscopy cannot be avoided in children with rectal bleeding, as active haemorrhage in the upper gastrointestinal tract can cause hyperperistalsis, leading to the appearance of fresh blood in the stools (Fellows and Nebesar, 1974).

Bleeding from the jejunum and ileum cannot be detected endoscopically in most cases. A Meckel's diverticulum of the ileum is diagnosed by using ^{99m}Tc pertechnetate which is concentrated by ectopic gastric mucosa which is usually present in diverticula that bleed. Rutherford and Akers (1966) found gastric mucosa in 42 of 43 Meckel's diverticula removed because of bleeding. The detection of gastric mucosa by radionuclide scanning can be made more sensitive by prior treatment with H_2 receptor antagonists.

For active bleeding that has escaped detection by these techniques, further radionuclide studies should be undertaken before angiography is attempted. Two techniques are now available. ^{99m}Tc sulphur colloid is the easier to prepare, and after intravenous administration may detect bleeding at rates as low as 0.1 ml/min (Alavi, 1980). The tracer will accumulate at bleeding points, because circulating tracer is otherwise quickly cleared by the liver and spleen. However, bleeding may be missed if the scan is carried out at a time of low blood loss. This problem can be overcome by the use of ^{99m}Tc-labelled red cells. Although more difficult to prepare, infusion of red cells will allow discovery of bleeding at any time within the next 24 h (Winzelberg et al, 1981).

Occasionally angiography is helpful, particularly in assessing the size and extent of vascular malformations.

Definitive treatment

Once the child is stable and the source of the bleeding has been found, appropriate definitive treatment is undertaken. Oesophageal varices are managed by injection sclerotherapy (Howard et al, 1984), which is continued at regular intervals after control of bleeding. Duodenal ulceration and gastric erosions are managed with antacids and H_2 receptor antagonists. Polyps are ensnared and removed at endoscopy. Meckel's diverticulum is excised at operation. Vascular abnormalities may be resected if they do not involve surrounding soft tissue structures.

GASTROENTERITIS

Acute gastroenteritis is the clinical syndrome of diarrhoea and/or vomiting of acute onset, often accompanied by fever and constitutional disturbance. It is infective in origin and is not secondary to a disease process outside the gastrointestinal tract (Walker-Smith, 1988). Its importance as an emergency is underlined by the associated high mortality of this condition in developing countries. In 1980 there were 4.6 million deaths due to diarrhoea in children under 5 years of age in Africa, Asia (excluding China) and Latin America (Snyder and Merson, 1982).

TABLE 3
Infectious agents that cause gastroenteritis

Viruses
Rotavirus
Adenovirus
Astrovirus
Calicivirus
Norwalk agent
Coronavirus
Small round virus

Bacteria
Shigella
Salmonella
Campylobacter
E. coli
   Enterotoxic
   Enteropathogenic
   Enteroinvasive
   Enterohaemorrhagic
Aeromonas
Protozoa
Giardia
Amoeba
Cryptosporidia

The reason that gastroenteritis is of such severity in young children is their high fluid turnover as a proportion of their total body water. A net fluid loss of 500 ml in a 3-month-old infant (about 10 heavily soaked napkins or diapers) is around 10% of its body weight, and enough to cause circulatory collapse. This degree of dehydration causes metabolic, osmotic and structural changes in the central nervous system, eventually leading to death. The essence of management is replacement with fluid of appropriate volume and electrolyte content.

Causes and differential diagnosis of gastroenteritis

Within the definition of gastroenteritis, the illness may be caused by viral, bacterial or protozoal organisms (Table 3). Extensive microbiological investigations of stool, including direct electron microscopy, are needed to detect these. The clinical features of gastroenteritis may be mimicked by conditions outside the gastrointestinal tract (Table 4). These require detection and appropriate early treatment, and it is therefore important that medical staff involved in the management of these children should have a thorough experience of paediatric disease.

Assessment of the child with gastroenteritis

Characterization of the clinical picture

Important clues about the cause of the vomiting and diarrhoea can be obtained

TABLE 4
Illnesses that cause acute onset of clinical features similar
to gastroenteritis

Infections
Upper respiratory tract infection including otitis media
Pneumonia
Septicaemia
Meningitis
Urinary tract infection
Measles
Malaria
Haemolytic uraemic syndrome

Surgical disorders
Acute appendicitis
Intussusception
Pyloric stenosis
Intestinal obstruction

Acute food intolerance
Coeliac disease

Inflammatory bowel disease
Other conditions
Diabetic ketoacidosis
Inherited organic acidaemias

from the clinical features of the case. Certain features are more common in particular infections (Table 5), but there is a wide overlap between them. If a child has recently returned from abroad, a serious pathogen is more likely.

Assessment of degree of dehydration

The simplest and most direct way of assessing the degree of dehydration is to compare the weight of an ill child with its weight measured just before the onset of diarrhoea or vomiting, but usually this premorbid weight has not been measured, or its accuracy is open to question. Thus, assessment is one of clinical acumen. In fact, it is one of the few areas in medicine where a purely clinical assessment has to be translated into quantifiable terms. Moreover, the clinician's assessment is easily checked by the child's increase in weight following successful therapy. The guidelines for assessment of the degree of dehydration, related to percentage of loss of body weight, are well established (Table 6). They are indispensible to the management of gastroenteritis because not only the amount of fluid, but also its composition and mode of delivery, depend on the degree of dehydration.

There are areas in which the guidelines may be misleading. Skin turgor is often not reduced in infants with hypernatraemia (see below). Such infants present with a fontanelle depressed to a degree which seems out of proportion to other physical signs, and sometimes their skin feels doughy. Skin turgor is also difficult to assess in children with chronic malnutrition, and the degree of dehydration is sometimes overestimated by doctors inexperienced in their management. Moistness of the mucous membranes of the mouth may be falsely interpreted as a sign of good hydration in children who have recently vomited or taken a drink. Severe dehydration is less common in children over 2 years of age, but when it does occur it is easily underestimated, because greater levels of dehydration occur before clinically obvious changes.

Exclusion of other conditions causing vomiting and diarrhoea

Infections outside the gastrointestinal tract may be detected by clinical examination, but confirmation may require special investigations, such as chest X-ray or lumbar puncture. Urinary tract infection can be excluded only by urine cultures, however. Some infections can cause both a primary gastroenteritis and also affect other organs. For instance, bacterial gastroenteritis can be associated with septicaemia following intestinal invasion. Diabetes mellitus can be diagnosed by testing for glycosuria. Haemolytic uraemic syndrome is detected by examination of the blood film for red cell fragments and thrombocytopaenia, as well as by assessing renal function.

Acid–base status of the blood should be assessed in children with peripheral vasoconstriction. Often acidosis is a consequence of poor peripheral perfusion leading to anaerobic respiration, but if there is a large base deficit then organic acids should be sought in the urine as this may imply an inherited enzyme defect.

Assessment of plasma electrolytes and renal function

Gastroenteritis can lead to a profound change in plasma electrolyte concentrations.

TABLE 5

Clinical features of different aetiological agents

	Rotavirus	Other viruses	Salmonella	Shigella	Campylobacter	Cryptosporidia	Amoeba
Age	Any age	Any age	Any age	Any age	Any age	Any age	Any age
Foreign travel	Rare	Rare	Rare	Common	Rare	Rare	Common
Vomiting present	Common	Sometimes	Common	Rare	Rare	Rare	Rare
Fever	Common	Rare	Rare	Common	Rare	Rare	Rare
Abdominal pain	Rare	Rare	Variable	Common	Common	Unusual	Common
Convulsions	Febrile convulsion	Rare	Rare	Well recognized	Rare	Rare	Rare
Blood in stools	Rare	Rare	Rare	Common	Common	Rare	Common
Reducing substances	Common	Rare	Rare	Variable	Rare	Rare	Rare

TABLE 6

Clinical features of dehydration according to percentage loss of body weight

Degree of dehydration	Associated clinical features
2–3%	Thirst, mild oliguria
5%	Discernible alteration in skin tone, slightly sunken eyes, thirst, oliguria, dry mucous membrane, sunken fontanelle
7–8%	Very obvious loss of skin turgor, sunken eyes, dry mucous membrane, restlessness or apathy, sunken fontanelle
10% (and over)	All the above, but also peripheral vasoconstriction, hypotension, cyanosis and occasionally hyperpyrexia

Sodium A child with gastroenteritis can be hypernatraemic (sodium > 150 mmol/l), isonatraemic (sodium 130–150 mmol/l) or hyponatraemic (sodium < 130 mmol/l). These terms apply to the concentration of sodium in the circulation and are not a measure of total body sodium, for even in hypernatraemic dehydration there can be total body sodium depletion. Hyponatraemia occurs when sodium loss exceeds water loss. This is particularly marked in conditions where there is intestinal secretion of sodium, for example in diarrhoea caused by bacterial enterotoxins, such as cholera and enterotoxogenic strains of *E. coli*, but this may also be seen with enteropathogenic *E. coli*, and rotavirus infections.

Hypernatraemia is a dangerous complication of gastroenteritis. Not only is the degree of dehydration easily underestimated, but also it is associated with a higher mortality. The hypernatraemia can be caused by an increased solute load in the lumen of the intestine, but the introduction of low solute infant milk formulae in the 1970s has made this complication less common in recent years (Manuel and Walker-Smith, 1980).

Potassium Loose stools contain significant amounts of potassium. Cardiac complications secondary to hypokalaemia are fortunately rare. Hyperkalaemia may be seen secondary to hypovalaemic renal failure.

Detection of renal failure

Blood urea levels increase secondary to dehydration, but as long as renal function is not impaired, then creatinine levels will remain normal. Prerenal failure, secondary to circulatory collapse, can be distinguished by its high associated urinary urea concentration, from the acute tubular necrosis which occurs following prolonged renal hypoperfusion.

Determination of causative organism

Stool microbiology is helpful because: (a) it can help to distinguish gastroenteritis from other causes of vomiting and diarrhoea; (b) it can be helpful in predicting future events (for instance, the discovery of *Cryptosporidia* or *Shigella* indicates a more chronic cause); (c) it is important for reasons of public health (*Salmonella* and *Shigella* are notifiable diseases); (d) it sometimes indicates that antimicrobial therapy is appropriate.

Stool is sent for the following investigations:

(1) Light microscopy. Examination under the light microscope is necessary to detect protozoal causes of diarrhoea. *Giardia* and *Amoeba* can be detected in fresh stool without special stains; the detection of *Cryptosporidia* requires staining by a modified Ziel Nielson stain.

(2) Bacterial culture. This is the basis of confirming bacterial causes of diarrhoea. Serotyping of *E.coli* is important to detect the presence of enteropathogenic strains.

(3) Electron microscopy. Electron microscopy of negatively stained stools will reveal the presence of viruses. Rotavirus is the commonest viral agent found, and there is an ELISA method for its detection in centres that do not possess electron microscopy facilities.

Treatment of gastroenteritis

Fluid and electrolyte therapy

The danger of gastroenteritis lies in the associated fluid and electrolyte imbalance. Management is directed towards correcting this. Treatment is not given to reduce the amount of vomiting or diarrhoea. It is important that parents realize this, otherwise it will be thought that the recommended treatment is ineffective. The diarrhoea and vomiting will be self-limiting and should settle within 2 weeks. If it does not settle, the child is described as having the postenteritis syndrome.

The initial management of the child depends on the degree of dehydration. Subsequent management is concerned with restoring the rehydrated child to a normal diet. Babies who are breast fed should continue to receive their mother's milk, but otherwise milk and diet should be stopped.

Table 7 summarizes the different forms of treatment for each level of dehydration. In every case, children will require the amount of fluid that a well child of similar age would need—the maintenance requirement. This varies according to the age and weight of the child. An infant will require 150–180 ml/kg per day, whereas a school child will require 60 ml/kg per day. In addition, dehydrated children will require replacement fluid. Except in severely dehydrated children with hypernatraemia, this extra fluid should be replaced over 24 h. Thus an infant weighing W kg whose maintenance requirement is V ml/kg/24 h and who is y % dehydrated will require

$$WV \text{ (maintenance)} + 1000\, W\, \frac{y}{100} \text{ (replacement) ml}$$

$$= W(V + 10y) \text{ ml in 24 hours.}$$

In the second 24 h if the child is fully hydrated he will be able to return to WV ml per day.

TABLE 7
Management of children according to degree of dehydration

Degree of Dehydration	Day 1	Day 2	Day 3
(1) Not dehydrated (below 1 year)	Oral rehydration solution (ORS)	Full strength milk	Full strength milk (and solids if taken)
(2) Not dehydrated (over 1 year)	Oral rehydration solution	ORS and solids	Full strength milk and solids
(3) Up to 7% dehydrated	Oral rehydration solution, maintenance and replacement	As for hydrated children with gastroenteritis	
(4) 7–9% dehydrated (iso-, hyponatraemia)	i.v. rehydration (0.18% saline + 4% dextrose), maintenance and replacement	ORS	As day 2 not dehydrated children
(5) 7–9% hyponatraemia dehydration	i.v. rehydration (0.45% saline + 5% dextrose), maintenance + $\frac{1}{2}$ replacement	i.v. rehydration (0.18% saline + 5% dextrose), maintenance + $\frac{1}{2}$	ORS
(6) 10% dehydrated	Resuscitation with 4.5% albumin (20 ml/kg) over 30 min then as in groups 4 or 5		

This simple formula has to be modified if losses continue to be large. For instance, if a secretory diarrhoea is present, an additional daily replacement of fluid, equal in volume and in electrolyte concentrations to that of the stool, should be given.

In children who have a level of dehydration less than 7% oral rehydration with a commercial solution such as Rehydrat, Dioralyte or Dextralyte is recommended; this regime can be given irrespective of the initial plasma sodium concentration.

In children with dehydration of 7% or greater, the fluid should be given intravenously. It is recommended that 0.45% saline/5% dextrose is given until plasma electrolyte assays are available. Thereafter children who are not hypernatraemic can be changed to 0.18% saline + 4.3% dextrose. Those with hypernatraemia should continue with the higher concentration of saline. At this stage potassium should be added to the solutions if the child is not in renal failure.

Children with dehydration of 10% or more are clinically shocked. They require emergency intravenous resuscitation with plasma (20 ml of fluid per kg over half an hour) and then should be changed to an electrolyte solution. It is important to subtract the plasma that has been given intravenously from the required replacement over the next 24 h.

Untreated hypernatraemic dehydration can lead to brain shrinkage with consequent intracranial haemorrhage and ultimately death. Treatment of this condition can in itself cause morbidity, as a new equilibrium will have been established between the intracellular and extracellular compartments. Rapid reduction in plasma osmolality will cause cerebral oedema and convulsions. The aim is to restore fluid volume while correcting the sodium concentration slowly.

Wherever possible this should be done by the enteral route. It is now becoming increasingly accepted that if a child with hypernatraemic dehydration does not need emergency resuscitation, then the intravenous route should be avoided. Absorption through the gut is a gentler process and allows plasma membrane osmotic forces to re-equilibrate, thus avoiding intracellular oedema.

The fluid deficit should be replaced over 48 h rather than 24 h. Monitoring of serum sodium concentrations are important, and a fall of greater than 5 mmol/l per day should be avoided.

Admission of children with gastroenteritis

Most children with gastroenteritis do not require admission. Those who do are: (1) dehydrated children; (2) children with vomiting of such magnitude that oral rehydration may be insufficient; (3) children whose parents lack the ability or confidence to look after the child at home.

Children who are managed as out-patients should always be weighed at presentation and medically reviewed to check that their recovery is satisfactory.

Return to a normal diet

The time required to return to a normal diet depends on the initial management. For instance, a 3-month-old baby who is not dehydrated can return to a normal diet of milk after 24 h. A baby with hypernatraemia who has lost 10% of its body weight will require 48 h of intravenous fluid replacement, followed by 24 h oral rehydration, before returning to bottle milk.

It has become widely recognized that the majority of children with gastroenteritis can return to full strength cow's milk; however, a certain number will exhibit reducing substances in their stools once full strength milk is used. These children will require a further 24 h oral rehydration solution and then a 4 day period during which the concentration of milk is increased to full strength.

Specific therapy

Specific antimicrobial treatment is not recommended usually, except in *Shigella* and protozoal infections (Table 8). Severe *Campylobacter* infections may warrant

TABLE 8
Agents in which antimicrobial therapy is advised

Shigella dysenteria	Antimicrobial agent according to sensitivity, but nalidixic acid is often effective
(Other *Shigella* spp. do not require specific treatment)	
(*Campylobacter*	Erythromycin, only if symptoms severe)
Entamoeba histolytica	Metronidazole and diloxamide furoate
Giardia lamblia	Metronidazole
Enteropathogenic *E. coli*	Intravenous gentamicin

antibiotic therapy. The use of intravenous antibiotics in enteropathogenic *E. coli* infections is recommended by some when the infection is demonstrated to cause small intestinal enteropathy on biopsy with the presence of adherent organisms (Hill et al, 1988).

Postenteritis syndrome

The development of chronic diarrhoea is outside the scope of this chapter, but a few words should be said. The first is that if diarrhoea has persisted for more than 14 days, it is important to question the original diagnosis of gastroenteritis. This is, of course, much easier to do if adequate stool microbiology has been undertaken at presentation. If reducing substances are present in the stool, it is likely that the child has developed a cow's milk protein postenteritis enteropathy, which can be diagnosed by small bowel biopsy and treated by a cow's milk-free diet. Another possibility is that the child has developed a second, later, infection, thus extending the time course of the diarrhoea. Some organisms, such as *Cryptosporidia*, *Shigella* and *Giardia* can lead to a more chronic diarrhoea.

JAUNDICE

The appearance of jaundice in a child is dramatic and usually leads parents to seek immediate medical advice. It is clinically apparent when plasma bilirubin levels exceed 80 μmol/l in neonates or 30 μmol/l in older children. Not every case of jaundice constitutes a paediatric emergency, but some do. It is important for the physician to recognize those children who require immediate admission and treatment.

It is useful to classify jaundice into unconjugated or conjugated hyperbilirubinaemia. The conjugated form can readily be distinguished by the detection of bilirubin in the urine with bilistix or multistix, as well as by laboratory assay of the plasma.

Unconjugated hyperbilirubinaemia

Unconjugated hyperbilirubinaemia is important not only because it may indicate an underlying disorder, but also because high levels may cause damage to the central nervous system. Kernicterus results from the deposition of unconjugated bilirubin in the brain, leading to death or brain damage, the latter usually presenting as a form of athetoid cerebral palsy. Unconjugated bilirubin is bound to albumin in the blood, but at levels of around 350 μmol/l significant amounts of this insoluble compound remain unbound and are deposited in the brain. The susceptibility of the brain to such damage lessens with age and so this is a problem of the neonatal period, except in the Crigler–Najjar syndrome, where very high levels of unconjugated bilirubin occur, because of the absence of bilirubin UDP glucuronyl transferase. While the neonate is being investigated, it is crucial also to control the level of unconjugated bilirubin once it rises above the critical level.

Causes of unconjugated hyperbilirubinaemia in the newborn

Plasma bilirubin levels are at their highest in the neonatal period. At this time jaundice may be clinically evident without any important sequelae. This physiological jaundice relates to several factors, including shorter lifespan of erythrocytes in the newborn, decreased hepatic uptake of bilirubin and some reabsorption of bilirubin by the small intestine. Jaundice cannot be considered physiological if it occurs in the first 24 h of life, rise above 100 μmol/l in a full-term baby, or is still present after 7 days. Babies who have jaundice in the first 24 h or beyond 3 weeks should be admitted for investigation and treatment. Similarly, infants with plasma levels greater than 240 μmol/l at any time need admission, as a pathological cause is likely (Table 9). The appropriate investigations that need to be undertaken are shown in Table 10. It is important to remember that

TABLE 9
Causes of unconjugated hyperbilirubinaemia

Haemolysis
  (1) Immune mediated
    (a) Rhesus disease
    (b) ABO incompatibility
  (2) Red cell defects
    (a) Membrane defects, e.g. spherocytosis, stomatocytosis
    (b) Enzyme defects, e.g. G6PD deficiency, pyruvate kinase deficiency
Polycythaemia
  Twin–twin transfusion
  Late cord clamping
Infection
  Septicaemia
  Urinary tract infection
Hypothyroidism
Galactosaemia
Fructosaemia
Hypoxia
Hypoglycaemia
Meconium retention

TABLE 10
Investigation of unconjugated hyperbilirubinaemia in the neonate

Haemoglobin
Reticulocyte count
Maternal blood group and antibodies
Infant blood group
Coombs test
G6PD level
Blood culture
Urine culture
Urine tested by glucose oxidase stick
Urine tested for reducing substances (sent for chromatography if positive)
Thyroid function tests

galactosaemia or fructosaemia can only be detected by sugar in the urine if the baby is receiving oral feeding.

Management of unconjugated hyperbilirubinaemia in the neonate

Prevention

Much has been accomplished in the past 20 years to prevent undesirable haemolysis. The most important innovation has been the use of anti-D in rhesus-negative mothers following obstetric procedures. The early clamping of the umbilical cord by midwives and obstetricians following the second stage of labour reduces the risk of transfusion from the placenta. Babies with a haematocrit of greater than 70% usually have plasma exchanged for blood.

Reduction of bilirubin levels by phototherapy

The avoidance of kernicterus is the prime objective in the treatment of babies with high levels of unconjugated bilirubin. Exposing infants to light with a wavelength of 400–500 nm leads to the production of photoisomers of bilirubin (Stoll et al, 1979). These molecules have terminal pyrrole rings which have rotated through 180° and are thus not able to form intramolecular hydrogen bonds. The result is a more polar structure which can be excreted into bile without conjugation. The bilirubin level at which phototherapy is commenced depends on the size of the child. If the weight of the child is W g, phototherapy should be commenced when the bilirubin level is has reached $W/10$ μmol/l (Mowatt, 1987). For term babies it is commenced when the level is 215 μmol/l. Complications include a large increase in insensible water loss, increased frequency of stools, possibly due to lactose intolerance, and possible retinal damage if the eyes are not suitably covered. Phototherapy does not need to be continuous throughout the day, and it is important that there are periods of feeding and close maternal contact away from the phototherapy lamps.

Reduction of bilirubin levels by exchange transfusion

Exchange transfusion is necessary for plasma bilirubin levels greater than 340 μmol/l (or $W/5$ in preterm infants) or a level rising by 8 μmol/l/h or more. This is best performed with an umbilical venous catheter with its tip in the inferior vena cava after introduction through the patent ductus venosus. In babies more than 2 days old, other sites of entry will be needed. Fresh blood should be cross-matched against serum from both mother and child. Twice the circulatory blood volume of the child should be exchanged in small increments. Care should be taken to avoid electrolyte changes, particularly in plasma calcium concentration. Hypothermia will be induced if the blood is not satisfactorily warmed before infusion. When there is immune haemolysis, this procedure has the advantage of reducing the maternal antibody level in the child as well as reducing the bilirubin level. Phototherapy can be continued whilst the exchange transfusion is taking place. Once it is complete, further monitoring of the plasma bilirubin level is necessary to establish whether further exchange is required.

Unconjugated hyperbilirubinaemia in the older child

Unconjugated hyperbilirubinaemia, acholuric jaundice, is almost always due to haemolysis in the older child. Haemoglobinopathies such as sickle cell disease or thalassaemia may present with jaundice, and children with G6PD deficiency can become acutely jaundiced following the ingestion of beans or oxidizing drugs. Malaria may also cause haemolytic anaemia. Transfusion is often required for correction of the anaemia.

Conjugated hyperbilirubinaemia

The presence of bilirubin in the urine, resulting from conjugated hyperbilirubinaemia, always indicates a pathological process, and is usually due to either hepatitis or biliary obstruction.

Infancy

The need for urgent admission is dictated by the coagulability of the blood. A child with prolonged prothrombin time requires intravenous vitamin K_1, administered slowly under medical supervision because of possible anaphylaxis. As infections such as septicaemia and urinary tract infection may also present with jaundice, any ill-looking child should be admitted for bacteriological investigation. Even if the child is well and has normal coagulation, admission will be usually required to determine the cause of the jaundice (Table 11). Speedy diagnosis is needed, as the prognosis for biliary atresia is particularly dependent on early surgery. Some causes of jaundice can be suspected from clinical examination. For instance, hypoplasia of the bile ducts is often associated with a systolic murmer and abnormal fascies (Alagille's syndrome); galactosaemia can lead to cataract formation, and septo-optic dysplasia is associated with hypopituitrism. Intensive investigation may be needed to make a definitive diagnosis (Mowat, 1987), and even then about half of cases of infantile jaundice will have no recognized aetiology (Dick and Mowat, 1985).

Conjugated hyperbilirubinaemia in the older child

Provided that clotting studies are normal, this is rarely a paediatric emergency. Table 12 lists some of the causes. Hepatitis A is the most common, but rapid referral is advisable to determine a more serious cause. Gallstones are rare in childhood, but may be seen in chronic haemolytic anaemias such as sickle cell disease. In particularly ill children with these conditions, drainage of the gallbladder by cholecystostomy followed by definitive cholecystectomy when the child is fitter may be preferable to immediate cholecystectomy.

TABLE 11

Causes of conjugated hyperbilirubinaemia in infancy

General
Septicaemia
Urinary tract infection
Chromosomal disorders (e.g. trisomy 13, 18)
Total parenteral nutrition

Liver disorders
Congenital infections
α_1-Antitrypsin deficiency
Biliary hypoplasia
Galactosaemia
Tyrosinaemia
Drugs
Septo-optic dysplasia
Cystic fibrosis
Idiopathic

Bile duct problems
Biliary atresia
Choledochal cyst

TABLE 12

Reasons for conjugated hyperbilirubinaemia in the older child

Infective
Viral
  Hepatitis A
  Hepatitis B
  Hepatitis C
  Cytomegalavirus
  Infectious mononucleosis
Bacterial
  Weil's disease
Protozoal
  Toxoplasmosis

Non-infective
Chronic persistent hepatitis
Chronic active hepatitis
Wilson's disease
Drug therapy
Sclerosing cholangitis
Gallstones

TABLE 13

Gastrointestinal conditions that have complications requiring emergency treatment

Inflammatory bowel disease	
Ulcerative colitis ⎱	Toxic megacolon (Sanderson, 1986)
Crohn's disease ⎰	Sclerosing cholangitis (Mowat, 1987)
Crohn's disease	Subacute obstruction (Sharb, 1989)
Liver disease	
Cirrhosis	Bleeding oesophageal varices (Rikkers, 1988)
	Hepatic encephalopathy
Biliary atresia (post-Kasai operation)	Ascending cholangitis

EMERGENCIES ASSOCIATED WITH CHRONIC GASTROINTESTINAL DISORDERS OF CHILDHOOD

Certain diseases of the liver and gastrointestinal tract which do not ordinarily require emergency treatment may occasionally need urgent management because of complications. These are described in Table 13. If possible, the emergency management of these patients should be discussed with the clinicians responsible for the overall care of their gastrointestinal disease.

CONCLUSIONS AND THE WAY FORWARD

The future of paediatric gastroenterology depends upon the development of simple diagnostic tests and the application of simple technology to therapy. Also doctors and parents need to be made aware of these developments.

In the case of therapy, the development of oral rehydration therapy (ORT) for acute diarrhoea has been a remarkable success. Further refinement is required, especially to develop formulations most appropriate to the needs of developed as well as developing communities (Guandalini, 1989; Walker-Smith, 1989). There is also a need to reduce stool volume and frequency as well as correcting dehydration. ORT is effective therapy in preventing death from dehydration, but does not significantly alter stool volume, a major anxiety for most mothers of babies with acute diarrhoea.

Education of parents concerning the prevention of dehydration due to acute gastroenteritis is possible. The medical profession, especially general practitioners, need to be better informed about the diagnosis and management of paediatric gastroenterological emergencies. Such emergencies tend to be relatively rare events for individual general practitioners. Clearly access to expert paediatric gastroenterological opinion is essential.

REFERENCES

Alavai A, Dann RW, Baum & Biery DN (1985) Scintigraphic detection of acute gastrointestinal bleeding. *Radiology* **124**: 753–756.

Dick AC & Mowat AP (1985) Hepatitis syndrome in infancy—an epidemiological survey with 10 yr follow up. *Archives of Disease in Childhood* **60**: 512–516.

Fellows KE & Nebesar RA (1974) Abdominal hepatic and visceral angiography. In Gyepes MT (ed.) *Angiography of Infants and Children*, pp 193–232. New York: Grune and Stratton.

Guandalini S (1989) Overview of childhood acute diarrhoea in Europe: Implications for oral rehydration therapy. *Acta Paediatrica Scandinavica* **Supplement 364**: 5–13.

Hill SM, Phillips AD, Walker-Smith JA, Sanderson IR & Milla PJ (1988) Antibiotics for *Escherichia coli* gastroenteritis. *Lancet* **1**: 701.

Howard ER, & Mowat AP (1984) Hepato biliary disorders in infancy: Hepatitis; extra hepatic biliary atresia; intrahepatic biliary hypoplasia. In Thomas HC & McSween RNM (eds) *Recent Advances in Hepatology*, pp 153–169. London: Churchill-Livingston.

Howard ER, Stomatkis JD & Mowat AP (1984) Management of esophageal varices in children by injection sclerotherapy. *Journal of Pediatric Surgery* **19**: 2–5.

Hyams JS, Leichtner AM & Schwartz AN (1985) Recent advances in diagnosis and treatment of gastrointestinal hemorrhage in infants and children. *Journal of Pediatrics* **106**: 1–9.

Linde SMD (1968) Blood pressure standards for normal children as determined under office conditions. *Clinics in Pediatrics (Philadelphia)* **7**: 401–403.

Manuel PD & Walker-Smith JA (1980) Decline of hypernatraemia as a problem in gastroenteritis. *Archives of Disease in Childhood* **55**: 124–127.

Mowat AP (1987) *Liver Disorders in Childhood*. London: Butterworths.

Rikkers LF (1988) Variceal hemorrhage.*Gastroenterology Clinics of North America* **17**: 289–302.

Rutherford RB & Akers DR (1966) Meckel's diverticulum. A review of 148 pediatric patients with special reference to the pattern of bleeding and to mesodiverticular vascular bands. *Surgery* **59**: 618–626.

Sanderson IR (1986) Chronic inflammatory bowel disease in childhood. *Clinics in Gastroenterology* **15**: 71–87.

Sharb PE (1989) Surgical therapy for Crohn's disease. *Gastroenterology Clinics of North America* **18**: 111–128.

Snyder JD & Merson MH (1982) The magnitude of the global problem of acute diarrhoeal disease: a review of actual surveillance data. *Bulletin of the World Health Organization* **60**: 605–613.

Stoll MS, Zenove EA, Ostrow JD & Zarembo JE (1979) Preparation and properties of bilirubin photoisomers. *Biochemical Journal* **183**: 139–146.

Walker-Smith JA (1988) Gastroenteritis. In *Diseases of Small Intestine in Childhood*, 3rd edn, Chap. 6, pp 185–285. London: Butterworths.

Walker-Smith JA (1989) The role of oral rehydration solutions in the children of Europe: Implications of oral rehydration therapy. *Acta Paediatrica Scandinavica* **Supplement 364**: 13–17.

Winzelberg GG, Froelich JW, McKusick KA, Walkman AC, Greenfield AJ, Athanasoulis CA & Strauss HW (1981) Radio nuclide localization of lower gastrointestinal haemorrhage. *Radiology* **139**: 465–469.

16

PAEDIATRIC SURGICAL EMERGENCIES

D. P. Drake

INTRODUCTION

Children of all ages present with surgical emergencies relating to the gastrointestinal tract. This chapter deals only with those conditions which are peculiar to the newborn and young infants, and are rarely, if ever, encountered in adults. Other disorders which commonly present in adult practice, such as peptic ulceration, pancreatitis and acute appendicitis, also occur in childhood but are not discussed in this section. The acute abdomen in children presents a particular challenge to paediatricians and surgeons. This important topic has been reviewed in detail by two experienced paediatric surgeons (O'Donnell, 1985; Jones, 1987). Although the presenting features of the acute abdomen are very different in young children, the principles of management are similar to those established in adult practice.

PRINCIPLES OF DIAGNOSIS AND TREATMENT

Neonatal surgical emergencies are uncommon and constant vigilance is required on the part of the medical and nursing staff in maternity units to recognize the presenting symptoms and signs. Delay in diagnosis of intestinal obstruction will often lead to fluid and electrolyte imbalance and aspiration pneumonia, thus complicating the management of the patient and the results of surgical treatment. Inability to swallow saliva, abdominal distension, delay in passing meconium and bilious vomiting are the four cardinal features suggesting that a newborn may have a surgical emergency.

Transfer to a regional unit is advised so that the infant can benefit from the expertise of all members of staff who are experienced in treating a large number of patients with varied surgical problems. Anaesthetic specialist skills are vital and nursing skills are of the utmost importance. Transport of neonates for operation can be achieved without detriment (Spitz et al, 1984).

Antenatal ultrasound scanning may detect anomalies of the gastro-intestinal tract in the mid or third trimester. Polyhydramnios may point to an obstruction of the oesophagus or proximal small bowel. A consistently empty stomach indicates an oesophageal atresia without a distal fistula lower. Meconium ileus can be detected as bright echogenic meconium and dilated loops of small bowel. A dilated first part of duodenum with an empty small intestine indicates a duodenal atresia. However, a distal large bowel obstruction will not cause antenatal intestinal dilatation, so most cases of Hirschsprung's disease and anorectal anomalies will remain undetected. *In utero* intervention or premature delivery is not indicated for antenatally diagnosed gastrointestinal obstruction. However, prior warning leading to delivery in a unit with appropriate paediatric skills and early surgical assessment facilitates the postnatal management and improves outcome.

Priorities in perioperative care are control of temperature and regulation of fluid and electrolyte balance. Intravenous fluids should be based on 10% glucose solution with physiological requirements of sodium and potassium added. Hypoglycaemia, hypocalcaemia or hypomagnesaemia may cause convulsions and serum levels of these substances must be monitored. Fluid restriction is recommended in the first 48 h of life with only 50 ml/kg/24 h being given as maintenance fluids. Abnormal losses, usually gastric aspirates, are replaced with intravenous isotonic saline with added potassium. Intravenous colloid as 4.5% albumin, 10–20 ml/kg, is recommended for infants who have a poor peripheral circulation, hypotension or signs of sepsis.

Prophylactic antibiotics are recommended at the time of surgery as wound infection rates following neonatal operations are over 10%, being especially high in small-for-dates babies who have immature immune systems (Madden et al, 1989).

Associated anomalies often affect the outcome of surgical treatment and malformations occurring in the first 6 weeks after conception have a particularly high incidence of associated anomalies. The VACTERL association links together anomalies of the *v*ertebrae, *a*norectum, *c*ardiovascular system, *t*rachea and *oe*sophagus, *r*enal system and the upper *l*imbs (Boocock and Donnai, 1987; Chittimittrapap et al, 1989). By contrast, a small bowel atresia occurring in the last trimester is most often an isolated anomaly.

OESOPHAGEAL ATRESIA

Oesophageal atresia occurs in one in 3000 deliveries, the majority having a fistula between the posterior wall of the trachea and the lower oesophagus (see Figure 1). Fifty per cent of the pregnancies are complicated by polyhydramnios and the babies are often of low birthweight. Following birth, the babies are unable to swallow saliva or mucus and characteristically blow bubbles at the mouth ('mucousy babies'). Cyanotic episodes occur if the upper airway becomes blocked with secretions. The diagnosis is confirmed by passing a size 8 or 10 F naso-oesophageal tube and taking a chest radiograph (see Figure 2) to confirm the level of the atresia, usually between the second and fourth thoracic vertebrae, or 10–12 cm from the nares. A fine-bore tube should not be used because it will become curled in the upper oesophagus, may not show up clearly on X-ray and will lead to confusion and delay in making the diagnosis. Air in the stomach will indicate the presence of a distal tracheo-oesophageal fistula.

The first priority of management is to keep the upper airway clear with continuous or frequent intermittent suction of the pharynx and upper oesophageal

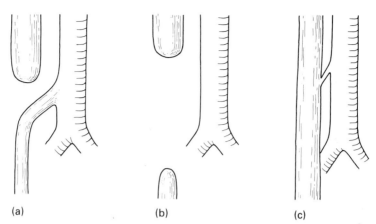

FIGURE 1 (a) Oesophageal atresia with distal tracheo-oesophageal fistula. (b) Isolated oesophageal atresia. (c) H-type tracheo-oesophageal fistula.

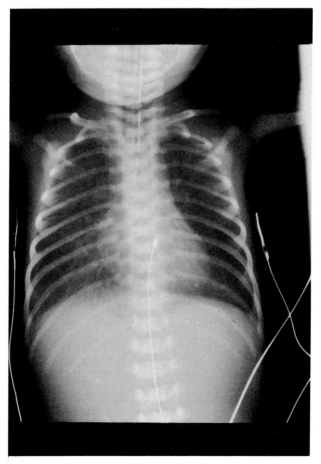

FIGURE 2 Chest radiograph with Replogle tube in upper oesophageal pouch and an umbilical arterial catheter confirming a left descending aorta. The lack of gas in the stomach suggests an oesophageal atresia with no distal tracheo-oesophageal fistula.

pouch. This is best achieved with a double lumen Replogle naso-oesophageal tube on continuous low suction. Reflux of gastric acid up through the fistula into the lungs is minimized by nursing the patient prone. The patient must not be offered an oral feed as this will predispose to aspiration and pneumonia. A solution of 10% dextrose with 0.18% saline (50 ml/kg) should be given intravenously on the first day and is sufficient to maintain fluid balance.

If there is clinical evidence of congenital cardiac disease the opinion of a cardiologist should be sought and an echocardiogram would be helpful. The anus should be checked to ensure it is normal, and blood sent for karyotyping if there are dysmorphic features.

The surgical priority is to repair the tracheo-oesophageal fistula within 24 h of birth even if the infant is premature, has severe respiratory distress, aspiration pneumonia or associated severe anomalies. Assisted positive pressure ventilation, if required, may be complicated by the tracheo-oesophageal fistula leading not only to overinflation and often perforation of the stomach but also to ineffective inflation of stiff lungs.

The operative approach is a right thoractomy performed under general anaesthesia with ventilation via an endotracheal tube. The chest is opened via the fourth intercostal space and the structures of the mediastinum approached extrapleurally. The fistula is isolated, divided and the posterior wall of the trachea repaired. If the infant's condition is stable the surgeon proceeds to mobilize the upper oesophageal pouch and perform an oesophageal anastomosis. If the atresia is too long to allow a primary repair there are a number of options after closing the lower oesophagus and establishing a gastrostomy feeding tube to nourish the infant.

(1) Leave the upper oesophagus *in situ* on continuous suction for 2–3 months and perform a delayed primary anastomosis.
(2) Bring out the upper oesophagus to the left side of the neck as a drainage cervical oesophagostomy. This allows sham feeding and the infant can be cared for at home. At approximately 6 months of age an oesophageal replacement is carried out and may be achieved by using a colonic interposition (Freeman and Cass, 1982) or drawing the mobilized stomach into the mediastinum and performing an oesophagogastric anastomosis in the neck (Valente et al, 1987).

The results of treatment depend on the associated anomalies and the length of the atresia. Very few infants die from complications of the oesophageal surgery and over 70% of those with significant associated anomalies may survive (Spitz et al, 1987).

Complications following repair include:

(1) Anastomotic strictures requiring dilatation.
(2) Anastomotic leakage. A 'radiological' leak may be managed with antibiotics, drainage and intravenous feeding. A disruption of the anastomosis usually requires sacrificing the oesophagus and bringing out a cervical oesophagostomy.
(3) Refistulation from the oesophageal repair to the posterior wall of the trachea requiring formal repair at a second thoractomy.

(4) Gastro-oesophageal reflux, which may be severe and justify surgical repair such as a Nissen fundoplication.

(5) Tracheomalacia. All patients born with a tracheo-oesophageal fistula have a degree of tracheomalacia with narrowing of the trachea on expiration. This produces the characteristically brassy cough which persists throughout childhood. In severe cases, the trachea collapses in expiration causing severe stridor and cyanotic episodes. These 'dying spells' are best managed with an aortopexy through a left thoracotomy, approximating the arch of the aorta to the sternum (Benjamin et al, 1976).

Normal development and weight gain can be expected following an uncomplicated primary oesophageal repair. After replacement surgery, the children often progress along or near to the 3rd centile.

Tracheo-oesophageal fistula

This fistula, usually in association with oesophageal atresia, joins trachea and lower oesophagus. An uncommon variant, a fistula to the upper pouch, may be detected on endoscopy. Occasionally an isolated tracheo-oesophageal fistula will occur with no atresia (see Figure 1).

A large fistula will present in the young infant or neonate with aspiration pneumonia and an abdomen distended with excessive air swallowed through the fistula. Diagnosis may be difficult. Radiological examination is best attempted with the patient prone and small volumes of barium introduced via a naso-oesophageal tube, which is slowly withdrawn. At oesophagoscopy it is usually impossible to visualize the fistula which is more easily seen on bronchoscopy, at which a fine catheter may be passed through the fistula to aid identification at open operation. Repair is usually performed through a right cervical approach, great care being required to protect the recurrent laryngeal nerve.

A smaller tracheo-oesophageal fistula may present much later in childhood or even in adult life.

HIATUS HERNIA

Gastro-oesophageal reflux in infants is very common and usually self-limiting in the first year of life. Frequent regurgitation at the end of a milk feed is managed by thickening the feeds with cornflour and positioning the infant in an upright posture. Severe reflux, which may cause oesophagitis and ulceration, presents with blood-stained vomitus or anaemia. The baby may be reluctant to complete a feed. These symptoms may be controlled medically with H_2 antagonists, but severe reflux may cause respiratory symptoms from recurrent aspiration.

The reflux may be assessed with a barium swallow, a 24 h pH monitor and endoscopically. If medical management fails to control the symptoms, an antireflux operation, such as a Nissen fundoplication, should be considered before the oesophagitis progresses to a stricture or before there is impairment of lung function from recurrent aspiration.

The Nissen fundoplication gives excellent control of the reflux but is associated with significant postoperative complications (Leape and Ramenofsky, 1980) including gas bloat and adhesion obstruction. The latter can be difficult to diagnose clinically as the patient is unable to vomit and presents only with abdominal pain. If the obstruction is high, there is very little abdominal distension, and the complication may pass unrecognized until perforation of the bowel occurs.

A large, fixed hiatus hernia rarely occurs in infants, but may present as an air fluid level in the inferior mediastinum on a chest radiograph. Medical treatment is not indicated and surgical repair should be performed as soon as the patient is fit.

PYLORIC STENOSIS

This condition has been widely recognized since Hirschsprung's description of two cases at autopsy in 1888. Ramstedt's successful pyloromyotomy in 1911 encouraged surgeons to operate on those infants, even when intraveous fluids and general anaesthesia were not available. In a recent series (Zeidan et al, 1988) mortality was related only to severe associated anomalies.

The disorder is an acquired hypertrophy of the smooth muscle of the pylorus but its cause remains obscure. It is more common in boys with a sex ratio of 5 : 1 and the incidence in northern Europe is 2–3 cases per 1000 births; however, the condition has only half the incidence in North America and in the Middle East it is as low as one case per 2000 births. There is a hereditary factor with the sons of affected mothers having an incidence of 20% (Carter and Evans, 1969).

Most infants are seen between the ages of 2 and 6 weeks with forceful non-bilious vomiting and failure to gain weight. The vomiting occurs during or after a feed and the infant is again soon hungry. The diagnosis is confirmed clinically by performing a test feed, the stomach being first emptied by aspirating a nasogastric tube and the infant is offered a milk feed. The examiner sits on the left side of the infant and palpates the right hypochondrium with the fingers of the left hand placed flat on the abdominal wall. The pyloric tumour is hard, the size of a small olive and characteristically is felt intermittently, depending on the relaxation of the rectus abdominis muscle and peristalsis passing down the antrum. Visible gastric peristalsis is a non-specific sign. Alternatively, the empty stomach may be inflated with 20–40 ml of air instilled down the nasogastric tube to facilitate palpation of the abnormal pylorus.

The test feed may need to be repeated over a period of several days, allowing time to consider a differential diagnosis, which includes overfeeding, gastro-oesophageal reflux, urinary tract infection, meningitis and the salt-losing congenital adrenal hyperplasia. If the diagnosis of pyloric stenosis cannot be confirmed on test feeding, imaging is helpful. An ultrasound scan will provide measurements of the muscle thickness and length of the pyloric canal. These simple measurements do not always differentiate the hypertrophic pylorus from the normal and it is more accurate to calculate the pyloric muscle index (Carver et al, 1987). Many radiologists prefer a barium study to demonstrate the pyloric canal, to assess gastric emptying and to diagnose rarer abnormalities such as hiatus hernia, malrotation or duodenal stenosis.

The loss of gastric juice may result in hypochloraemic alkalosis, which is assessed by measuring the serum chloride and bicarbonate. If present, this should be corrected with intravenous isotonic saline with added potassium chloride. Pyloromyotomy is not an emergency procedure and should be undertaken only when the infant is well hydrated, has an adequate urine output and is in electrolyte balance.

The operation is best performed under a general anaesthetic with the stomach previously irrigated with isotonic saline and emptied of retained milk and mucus. The incision is transverse in the right hypochondrium, dividing the rectus abdominis muscle and entering the peritoneal cavity over the liver, which is retracted upwards.The antrum of the stomach is delivered, followed by the pylorus. The muscle is incised down to the mucosa, especial care being taken at the duodenal fornix. The pyloric muscle is then spread to ensure an adequate myotomy, with the mucosa bulging to the level of the serosa and the two halves of the pylorus moving independently. Air is milked through the pylorus to check for any breach in the mucosa, which must be carefully repaired with an omental patch.

Postoperatively feeds are introduced after 12 h and strengthened to full feeds by 48 h. Postoperative wound infections are reported in up to 10% of cases, usually due to *Staphylococcus aureus* and can be minimized by careful skin preparation and the use of an adhesive skin drape to exclude the umbilicus from the operative field. Undetected mucosal breaches can cause fatal peritonitis. An inadequate myotomy will lead to recurrent vomiting and requires a second operation after a delay of a few weeks. Wound dehiscence is caused by poor surgical technique. The long-term prognosis is excellent with no increased incidence of gastrointestinal disease later in life.

DUODENAL ATRESIA

The incidence of duodenal atresia is one in 10 000 births. A third of the infants have Down's syndrome and 20% have associated cardiovascular anomalies. In a minority polyhydramnios complicates the pregnancy but the dilated first part of duodenum is being increasingly detected on antenatal ultrasound scans. The anomaly occurs in the first 6 weeks after conception at the junction of the foregut and midgut. Usually between the blind ends there is a gap containing pancreatic tissue and the bile duct has two openings, one above and one below (see Figure 3). Less often, the atresia takes the form of a membrane or 'wind sock' across the lumen of the duodenum, with a small opening not allowing the free passage of milk.

These infants present in the first 12 h of life with vomiting, which is usually bile stained. A plain abdominal radiograph demonstrates the 'double bubble' with air in the stomach and first part of duodenum but no air beyond the site of obstruction. The clarity of the radiograph is much improved by injecting 15 ml of air down the nasogastric tube immediately prior to the exposure.

The stomach should be kept empty by aspirating on a nasogastric tube, to prevent persistent vomiting and aspiration. Surgical repair is best performed early while the patient is well nourished. When the infant has Down's syndrome and

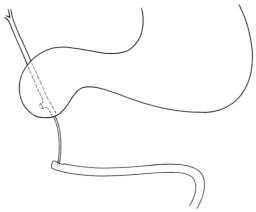

FIGURE 3 Duodenal atresia. The common bile duct opens into both the cranial and the caudal duodenum.

associated anomalies, intravenous feeding may be required if surgery is delayed by the need for investigations and discussion with the parents.

The operation is performed through an upper abdominal transverse incision. The hepatic flexure and right transverse colon are mobilized off the duodenum and the anomaly defined. Saline should be injected into the caudal lumen of the duodenum to exclude a second atresia. The repair is an anterior duodenoduodenostomy taking care to avoid damage to the bile duct lying posterior to the duodenum. A single layer of interrupted sutures is satisfactory. Gastrostomy and transanastomotic tubes probably confer no advantages and are associated with complications of perforation and dislodgement (Rangecroft and Courtney, 1980), and the postoperative course can be well managed with a nasogastric tube, feeds being introduced within 5–7 days.

A duodenojejunostomy may be required if the duodenum beyond is poorly developed. For a membranous 'wind sock', the duodenum is opened longitudinally on its antimesenteric border. Care is taken to avoid the bile duct which opens onto the membrane, but the anterolateral segment of the obstruction is resected. The duodenum is then closed transversely. Attempts to deal with these membranes endoscopically have usually not been successful.

EXTRINSIC DUODENAL OBSTRUCTION

Malrotation of the duodenal loop, leaving the duodenojejunal junction in the midline or to the right of the midline, predisposes to volvulus of the midgut on its unstable mesentery. Midgut rotation fails at the end of the first trimester and the caecum remains in the upper abdomen. Malrotation is seen in association with Down's syndrome, congenital diaphragmatic hernia, exomphalos major, and congenital heart disease with atrial isomerism; however, in the majority the malrotation is an isolated anomaly.

The obstruction of the duodenum is usually intermittent and presents in the first 3 months of life with bilious vomiting, which is aggravated by feeding but resolves when the stomach is aspirated. This intermittent pattern causes delay in diagnosis, which can be fatal. Should the midgut volvulus tighten around its mesentery, the blood supply and venous drainage of the small bowel will be impaired with first engorgement and then ischaemia. Irreversible gangrene can occur within 12 h of the first bilious vomit and, for this reason, all infants with green vomitus must be investigated immediately (Millar et al, 1987).

A plain abdominal radiograph may be entirely normal but may show all the small bowel on the right of the abdomen or a dilated first part of duodenum. A barium meal is indicated to demonstrate the abnormal duodenal loop with the first loop of jejunum to the right of the midline.

If there is passage of bloody stools or signs of hypovolaemic shock, there must be no delay in resuscitation with intravenous fluids and blood transfusion followed by immediate laparotomy. The absence of the transverse colon in its normal position is the first indication of a volvulus. On delivering the entire small bowel from the abdomen, the volvulus can be visualized and untwisted in a clockwise direction. The duodenum is then freed from under a number of flimsy peritoneal bands (Ladd's bands) to achieve free drainage of the duodenum into the jejunum well to the right of the midline. Adhesions in the base of the mesentery are divided to allow the caecum to take up a position well to the left of the abdominal cavity. This exaggeration of the failure of normal rotation stabilizes the midgut mesentery and prevents a further volvulus. The appendix is either removed or inverted after dividing its mesentery, to avoid an atypical appendicitis later in life.

If the small bowel is ischaemic over its entire length, simply untwisting the volvulus and performing a second laparotomy after 24 h may be indicated. The condition still carries an unacceptably high mortality because of delay in diagnosis; survivors may be left with the problems of a short bowel following massive resection at the second laparotomy.

SMALL BOWEL ATRESIAS

Most atresias in the jejunum and ileum are isolated anomalies, caused by vascular accidents of the mesentery late in pregnancy. Some atresias are multiple and the lower ileum may be supplied by a single branch of the ileocolic artery, allowing the ileum to spiral around its abnormal mesentery and present as an 'apple peel'. Atresias may be classified as in Figure 4.

The infant presents with bilious vomiting and abdominal distension. A small volume of meconium may be passed initially and in a low ileal atresia vomiting may be delayed several days. Plain abdominal radiographs will demonstrate dilated loops of bowel with fluid levels. Jejunal atresias give a characteristic appearance with only one or two loops of dilated bowel but ileal atresia may be difficult to distinguish from Hirschsprung's disease. However, a barium enema will demonstrate a microcolon in cases of atresia. If the dilated bowel was perforated *in utero*, speckled calcification will be seen on the radiograph indicating the presence of meconium peritonitis. At laparotomy, the grossly distended upper bowel should be resected or tapered (Howard and Othersen, 1973) so that bowel of reasonable size may be anastomosed end-to-back to the narrow distal ileum

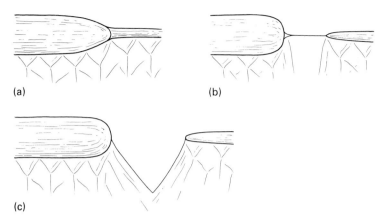

(a)   (b)

(c)

FIGURE 4   Small bowel atresia. (a) Type I — serosa and muscle in continuity. (b) Type II — a fibrous
band. (c) Type III — segments of intestine separated with mesenteric gap.

(Nixon and Tawes, 1971). The bowel beyond must be irrigated with saline to
exclude multiple membranous atresias (Type I).

The prognosis is related to the length of small bowel preserved (Patrapinyokul
et al, 1989); small bowel as short as 20 cm is compatible with full enteral feeding
if the ileocaecal valve is intact. Associated abnormalities, such as biliary atresia or
cystic fibrosis, are uncommon, but must be considered if there is prolonged
jaundice or failure to thrive with pulmonary infections.

MECKEL'S DIVERTICULUM

Meckel's diverticulum is the commonest congenital anomoly of the gastrointestinal tract but is most often a chance finding of no clinical significance and
excision is not always recommended (Soltero and Bill, 1976). A Meckel's diverticulum represents the remnant of the connection between the yolk sac and the midgut. A patent vitellointestinal tract is the most primitive form of this anomaly;
some diverticula are attached to the umbilicus with a fibrous cord and others are
isolated subumbilical cysts (see Figure 5). The Meckel's diverticulum is attached
to the antimesenteric border of the ileus, has an independent blood supply but is
often adherent to the lateral wall of the ileum and its mesentery. Ectopic gastric
mucosa is found in up to 40% of diverticula; less commonly pancreatic tissue is
present.

A persistent vitellointestinal tract will leak small bowel contents from the
umbilicus, may prolapse with several centimetres of inverted ileum exposed or
cause a mid-gut volvulus. A Meckel's diverticulum may give rise to an internal
hernia by adhering to the ileal mesentery. Acute inflammation may mimic
appendicitis and perforation is described. Acute peptic ulceration of adjacent small
bowel mucosa may present as a brisk haemorrhage with 'brick red' blood at
the rectum or less commonly as anaemia with occult blood in the faeces.
Intussusceptions after the age of 18 months may have a diverticulum as the lead
point.

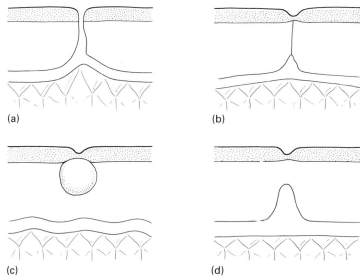

(a)   (b)

(c)   (d)

FIGURE 5 (a) Patent vitellointestinal tract. (b) Fibrous cord from umbilicus to Meckel's diverticulum.
(c) Enteric cyst beneath umbilicus. (d) Meckel's diverticulum.

Barium studies are generally unhelpful in the diagnosis of a Meckel's diverticulum, but the ectopic gastric mucosa may be demonstrated on a technetium pertechnetate isotope scan, enhanced by predosing the patient with cimetidine to suppress gastric uptake.

If a Meckel's diverticulum is an incidental finding at a laparotomy, excision should be considered if there is thickening of the wall suggesting ectopic mucosa, adhesions predisposing to a volvulus or internal hernia, or if there has been unexplained recurrent abdominal pain. In the presence of an acutely inflamed appendix, it is unwise to deliver three feet of ileum to look for an incidental diverticulum, which will be present in 2% of patients. However, for unexplained abdominal pain or peritonitis, Meckel's diverticulum is one of many causes that should be sought.

The technique for performing a diverticulectomy depends on the circumstances. For large diverticula and those with a peptic ulcer of the adjacent small bowel mucosa, a T-shaped resection of the diverticulum with a short length of ileum is recommended, repaired by a primary end-to-end anastomosis. For small diverticula, a wedge-shaped excision at the base of the diverticulum is adequate. The incision is closed transversely to avoid a stenosis. Care should always be taken to secure the blood vessels passing to the Meckel's diverticulum.

The surgeon must be aware of the risks to the patient following a diverticulectomy, which include a 5% reoperation rate for obstruction or leakage and a 0.5% mortality related to peritonitis (Leizomarck et al, 1986).

DUPLICATION CYSTS

These are all rare and may occur in the mediastinum or in the abdomen associated with the small bowel or the colon. Some contain ectopic gastric mucosa and present as gastrointestinal haemorrhage; others present as an abdominal mass and cause partial obstruction of the adjacent bowel. Duplications of the foregut and hindgut are usually associated with vertebral anomalies. Small duplication cysts in the wall of the small bowel may form the apex of an intussusception or predispose to a volvulus of the mid-gut (Ravitch, 1986).

Operative management depends on the situation of the duplication. Small abdominal and all mediastinal duplications should be excised, but long tubular duplications may be drained distally into the bowel or managed by a mucosal dissection. This preserves the muscle tube and the blood supply which is often shared with the adjacent intestine.

MECONIUM ILEUS

One in 15 000 infants is born with bulky viscid meconium obstructing the ileum. The underlying cause is most often cystic fibrosis, although only 15% of patients with cystic fibrosis have this complication. Meconium obstruction is also described in 'small-for-dates' babies, who do not have cystic fibrosis. The abnormally bright echogenic meconium and dilated loops of intestine can be detected on ultrasound scanning in the third trimester.

Abdominal distension may be noted at birth before the first feed and the bulky meconium can be palpated in distended loops of ileum. There will be delay in passing meconium and bilious vomiting following feeds. Abdominal radiographs (Figure 6) confirm the dilated loops of intestine without gas fluid levels. The abnormal meconium has a characteristically foamy appearance; intraperitoneal calcification indicates meconium peritonitis related to an intra-uterine perforation.

Uncomplicated meconium ileus may be successfully managed with a gastro-grafin® enema (Noblett, 1969). This will demonstrate a small unused 'micro-colon', and reflux of gastrografin® into dilated loops of ileum should relieve the obstruction, as gastrografin® acts as a detergent and an irritant. Partial relief of the obstruction is an indication for a repeat enema, but, if gastrografin does not fill dilated loops containing meconium, a complication such as an atresia or volvulus should be suspected.

A laparotomy is indicated if the infant has evidence of meconium peritonitis or a failed gastrografin® enema. At operation the site of the obstruction in the terminal ileum is confirmed, and, after opening the distended ileum, the viscid 'rubbery' meconium is removed by saline irrigation until the lumen of the intestine is cleared down to the sigmoid colon. A grossly distended segment of ileum may need to be resected and continuity of the intestine re-established, but often a simple closure of the enterostomy is sufficient. Only rarely will a temporary double-barrelled ileostomy be indicated.

Postoperatively the patient is best managed jointly with a paediatrician who has a special interest in cystic fibrosis. The underlying diagnosis may be confirmed with a sweat test to demonstrate raised levels of sodium or chloride. As it is difficult to collect a sufficient volume of sweat in the first few weeks of life, alternative tests are helpful and it is now possible to identify an abnormal cystic fibrosis gene on the short arm of chromosome seven (Rommens et al, 1989) in 70% of infants with cystic fibrosis. When milk feeds are introduced pancreatic enzymes

(a)

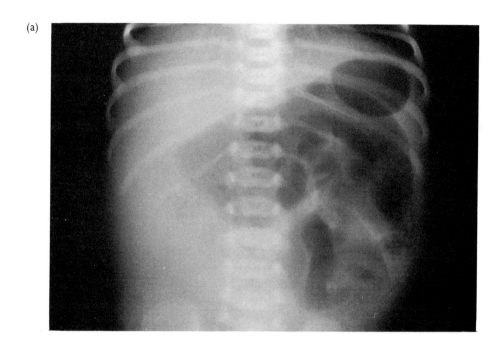

(b)

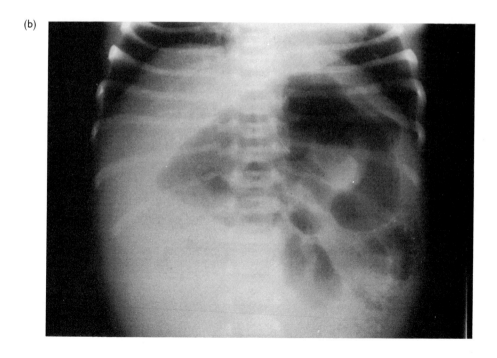

Figure 6 (a) Supine and (b) erect abdominal radiographs — small bowel obstruction with foamy meconium and only a single gas fluid level in stomach.

will be required to aid absorption. Regular prophylactic chest physiotherapy is indicated.

The short-term prognosis is now excellent, several units reporting 100% survival after both radiological and operative management of full-term infants with meconium ileus. The 'small-for-dates' babies still have a significant mortality related to the complications of prematurity.

INTUSSUSCEPTION

Intussusception occurs in approximately two per 1000 infants and there is evidence that it is becoming less common (Hutchison et al, 1980). Two-thirds of cases occur in the first year of life, usually soon after the infant is weaned. Boys are affected more often than girls. The condition is uncommon after the second birthday, when there is an increased chance of an anatomical lead point such as a Meckel's diverticulum, a polyp or even a lymphoma.

The commonest aetiology is lymphoid hyperplasia of a Peyer's patch in the terminal ileum, related to a viral infection, most often an adenovirus. Although the typical presentation in an infant aged 4–8 months can be easily diagnosed, delays occur with atypical cases, especially those in the postoperative period after a laparotomy for another indication, such as a hiatus hernia or renal pathology. Children with Henoch–Schönlein purpura have a higher than expected incidence of intussusception, which may be difficult to distinguish from the commoner submucosal haematomas that resolve spontaneously. Delay in making the diagnosis is the cause of the small but persistent mortality from intussusception.

The history is usually an acute onset of colicky pain associated with vomiting, facial pallor and flexing the hips. Rectal bleeding occurs after 12–24 h and is mixed with mucus, giving a 'redcurrant jelly stool'. There may be a pre-existing upper respiratory tract infection or gastroenteritis, but most of these infants have been well and thriving until this acute illness.

On examination, there may be a sausage-shaped mass across the epigastrium. This may be obscured by abdominal tenderness and is more easily felt in a sedated child. A rectal examination to detect blood or the apex of the intussusception must never be omitted. If the patient has a cold poorly perfused periphery, the presentation is late and there is probably ischaemia or gangrene of the intussusceptum.

A plain abdominal radiograph suggests the diagnosis if there is a soft tissue shadow corresponding to the intussusception or evidence of a small bowel obstruction. However, a contrast enema is more reliable in confirming the diagnosis in a doubtful case.

The initial management is to resuscitate the patient with intravenous fluids if there are signs of hypovolaemia or a history of prolonged vomiting. A nasogastric tube is passed to empty the stomach and appropriate analgesia administered. Hydrostatic reduction of the intussusception is indicated if there is no suspicion of ischaemia or perforation, and may be achieved with a barium enema using the pressure of a three foot column of barium. A surgeon and operating theatre must be available for the rare colonic perforation which requires an immediate laparotomy. Better success has been achieved with reduction by oxygen delivered intermittently via a rectal tube with a flow of 2 l/ min at a pressure of 80 mmHg.

Reduction rates of over 70% have been reported (de Campo and Phelan, 1989). The best results are reported in China where there is experience with many thousands of cases. Gas reduction is quicker, less painful and can be achieved on out-patients with no sedation. The criteria for successful radiological reduction are twofold; first, filling the terminal ileum with contrast and second, relief of symptoms with a contented infant. Both criteria are of the utmost importance.

Laparotomy is indicated for those patients presenting with signs of ischaemia or peritonitis and in those failures of contrast or oxygen reduction. Cross-matched blood must be available and broad spectrum antibiotics are indicated. The incision is right transverse, above the umbilicus, if there is a large mass, or in the right iliac fossa, if the intussusception has been partially reduced. The intussusception should be reduced by pressure from the distal end and initially can be performed within the abdomen. The final reduction is usually best performed after delivering the mass out of the abdomen and supporting it in warm saline packs. When reduction is complete, a careful inspection is required, checking for viability of the bowel and for a specific lead point, which should be resected. If viability is doubtful, the bowel should be returned to the abdomen for 10 min and then reinspected. This is a convenient time to perform an incidental appendicectomy.

If the intussusception will not reduce or the intestine is not viable, a resection must be carried out preserving as much bowel as possible. The ileocaecal valve should be preserved whenever possible. Following resection an end-to-end anastomosis is recommended unless the infant is 'in extremis'. Overall there is a 4% recurrence rate following reduction of intussusception but the rate is higher after hydrostatic than operative reduction (Ein and Stephens, 1971). This large series, with most cases presenting in the first 24 h of the illness, demonstrates how one children's hospital can achieve zero mortality. Prompt diagnosis and adequate resuscitation are essential to minimize the morbidity and mortality following an intussusception.

The first recurrence should be managed using the same guidelines as for an initial intussusception. A patient having a second recurrence should be considered for a laparotomy to identify a specific lead point or to undergo a resection to prevent further recurrences by resecting the intussuscepting bowel.

NECROTIZING ENTEROCOLITIS

Previously uncommon, necrotizing enterocolitis has been the commonest indication for admission to a neonatal surgical unit since the late 1970s. It was originally described in association with umbilical vein catheterization (Corkery et al, 1968). Up to 5% of all admissions to neonatal units will develop necrotizing enterocolitis (Kliegman and Fanaroff, 1981). Most affected newborns are premature with the respiratory distress syndrome, but enterocolitis may also occur rarely in full-term babies with no associated disorder. The intestinal mucosa may be damaged by hypoxia, invasive bacteria or hyperosmolar feeds (Pearse and Roberton, 1986). Babies with respiratory distress and cyanotic heart disease are at increased risk. Epidemics have been reported in neonatal intensive care wards (Howard et al, 1977) but many different microorganisms have been identified.

Clostridial infection with septicaemia may also cause haemolysis and is associated with a very aggressive illness and a high mortality. Delaying the introduction of enteral feeding and the administration of prophylactic oral vancomycin may reduce the incidence in babies at risk (Ng et al, 1988). Prenatal hypoxia related to placental insufficiency and perinatal stress and asphyxia may be aetiological factors; also overloading a newborn with fluid has been shown to increase the incidence of necrotizing enterocolitis (Bell et al, 1980). Necrotizing enterocolitis may affect small or large bowel, the terminal ileum and right colon being the commonest sites. Histologically there are microthromboses, haemorrhage, inflammatory change, intramural gas and frank necrosis. Resolving necrotic areas may fibrose and stricture.

The clinical presentation includes abdominal distension, bilious vomiting and bloody diarrhoea. The infant will be lethargic and unwilling to feed; erythema of the anterior abdominal wall suggests full thickness necrosis of the bowel wall with peritonitis. When the disease is suspected, all gastric feeds must be stopped and the stomach aspirated. Broad spectrum intravenous antibiotics, usually benzyl-penicillin, gentamicin and metronidazole, are administered with intravenous fluids. Plasma is infused to maintain the circulating volume, blood may be transfused if indicated and total parenteral nutrition established. Positive pressure ventilation will be required in many patients who develop bradycardia, apnoeic spells or become acidotic. Thrombocytopenia suggests extensive disease.

The diagnosis is confirmed on plain abdominal radiographs, which show intra-mural gas (Figure 7). A lateral decubitus view, right side up, is required to demonstrate the presence or absence of free gas above the liver. Gas in the portal vein radicles indicates severe necrosis with a poor prognosis.

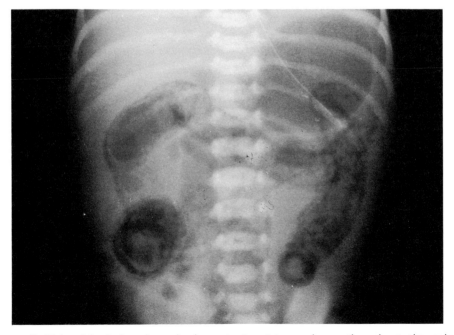

FIGURE 7 Plain abdominal radiograph demonstrating intramural gas throughout the colon—necrotizing enterocolitis.

Many patients will respond to intensive medical treatment and gastric feeding may be reintroduced after 10 days. There is a late stricture rate of approximately 10% (Beasley et al, 1986), often presenting as a feeding problem with poor weight gain. Therefore a barium enema is indicated to investigate gastrointestinal symptoms following necrotizing enterocolitis.

The indications for an urgent laparotomy are radiological evidence of a perforation or failure to make progress on medical treatment. At operation, necrotic bowel must be excised and a primary anastomosis is recommended in most cases (Sparnon and Kiely, 1987). If there is extensive small bowel disease, a proximal loop jejunostomy may allow healing of defunctioned bowel left *in situ*. Before elective closure of any stoma, distal contrast studies must be performed to exclude strictures.

The mortality for these infants referred to surgical units remains around 25% (Jackman et al, 1990). An associated congenital anomaly, thrombocytopenia or acidosis at presentation indicate a poor prognosis (Dykes et al, 1985). Amongst the survivors there is a 50% incidence of a significant handicap, including developmental delay, chronic respiratory disease and the short bowel syndrome. Prevention is of paramount importance for this acquired condition. Stopping gastric feeds at the first suspicion of disease should also limit the progression of the necrotic process. Recommendations to reduce the incidence of necrotizing enterocolitis would include cautious introduction of enteral feeding, delayed in patients at risk, and avoidance of overhydration.

HIRSCHSPRUNG'S DISEASE

Hirschsprung's disease is the commonest cause of intestinal obstruction in the newborn, affecting one in 5000 children. There is a lack of ganglion cells in the bowel wall affecting the rectum and a variable length of colon above. In 10% of cases the entire colon is aganglionic (Bodian et al, 1949). There is an increased incidence in near relatives of affected patients and in Down's syndrome, but most babies with Hirschsprung's disease are born at term with no associated anomalies. The typical short segment affecting the rectum and distal sigmoid colon is more common in boys.

The clinical presentation is delay beyond the first 24 h in passing meconium, with abdominal distension following feeds and bilious vomiting. A plain abdominal radiograph will show dilated loops of bowel with fluid levels on an erect film (Figure 8). The rectum is empty of gas if the film is taken before performing a rectal examination, which may be followed by an explosive passage of flatus and meconium. Delay in confirming the diagnosis predisposes to enterocolitis, which can be fatal. After the initial delay in passing meconium, the infant may develop diarrhoea with abdominal distension and failure to thrive. The management of this complication includes enteral vancomycin and colonic irrigations with saline (Thomas et al, 1982).

The investigation of an infant with suspected Hirschsprung's disease must include a rectal biopsy, best performed using a suction technique (Campbell and Noblett, 1969) without anaesthesia. Specimens of mucosa with submucosa can be examined histologically for the presence of ganglion cells and histochemically for acetylcholinesterase-positive nerve fibres (Barr et al, 1985). An absence of ganglion cells with an increase in nerve fibres is diagnostic of Hirschsprung's disease, but an adequate biopsy with submucosa must be examined by an experienced pathologist to achieve reliable results. A barium enema may indicate the length of segment involved by demonstrating a 'cone' with proximal dilatation of the normally innervated bowel. However, contrast studies may be misleading, especially in patients with total colonic aganglionosis, and the diagnosis should never be made on radiological evidence alone.

The treatment of the patient is to establish a stoma in bowel that has ganglion cells, whose presence is confirmed by frozen section histological examination. A right transverse colostomy is satisfactory for the majority of cases and acts as a defunctioning stoma for the definitive operation 6 months later. Alternatively, a stoma just above the 'cone' may be established, using this level for the pull through operation without a defunctioning stoma. Definitive operations in the neonate are recommended only by a small minority of surgeons and generally carry a higher complication rate.

The definitive pull-through operation can be planned when the infant is 6

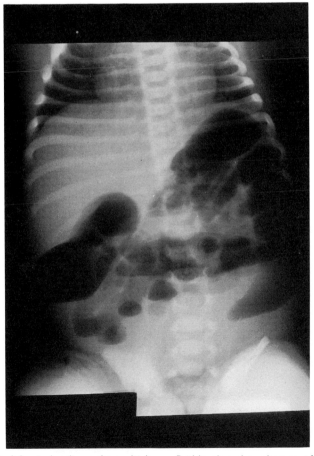

FIGURE 8 Erect abdominal radiograph—multiple gas fluid levels and an absence of gas in the rectum and distal sigmoid colon. Hirschsprung's disease.

months old. Three techniques, first described by Swenson, Duhamel and Soave, have been modified and give good results in experienced hands (Nixon, 1988).

The mortality associated with Hirschsprung's disease is related to delay in making the diagnosis. Many newborns with aganglionosis will pass normal stools for a few days following a rectal examination or saline washout. After being discharged home, they develop severe constipation or enterocolitis and diarrhoea. Should the colon perforate at this stage resuscitation with emergency laparotomy will often fail to save the child's life. The definitive operation carries a very low mortality but anastomotic leaks can lead to pelvic cellulitis and destruction of nerve endings. This will severely compromise bowel training and faecal continence.

ANORECTAL ANOMALIES

Congenital anomalies of the anal canal and rectum affect one in 4000 newborns. The rectum and urogenital sinus develop from the primitive cloaca 4–6 weeks after conception and, when abnormalities occur, there are associated anomalies in half the infants, affecting especially the cardiovascular and renal systems. If the three lower segments of the sacrum are missing, development and innervation of the pelvic floor muscles will be deficient. There are many variations of these anomalies but they may be grouped into low, intermediate and high.

Low anomalies are represented by the covered anus with an anocutaeous fistula in the male or an anterior ectopic stenotic anus in the female. These can be recognized on inspection of the perineum at the age of 18–24 h and are managed with an anoplasty, often performed under a caudal anaesthetic. Apart from a tendency to constipation, the long-term results are excellent.

Intermediate anomalies present with a rectourethral fistula in a boy or a vulval opening in a girl. These are best managed with an initial colostomy of the proximal sigmoid colon. When the infant is thriving, between 6 weeks and 6 months, a posterior sagittal anorectoplasty may be performed (Pena and de Vries, 1982). The covering colostomy should be closed only when the neoanus has been dilated to a suitable size (Hegar 10–12) without bleeding.

High anomalies include a rectovesical fistula in a boy or high rectovaginal fistula or a cloacal anomaly in a girl. After an initial colostomy, the definitive operation may involve a laparotomy in addition to a pelvic operation. Most intermediate anomalies will have a good prognosis for faecal continence, but the high anomalies, especially those with a sacral anomaly, may have life-long difficulties with soiling. The success of the reconstruction depends on the preoperative definition of the anatomy of the pelvic organs with a combined distal loopogram and micturating cystogram. A midline dissection then allows full mobilization of the rectal pouch and repair of the fistula but preservation of the pelvic floor muscles and innervation.

Mortality is related to associated anomalies, particularly of the cardiovascular and renal systems. Some will require correction of complex cardiac anomalies and others will be at risk of developing chronic renal failure from a combination of dysplastic kidneys and vesicoureteric reflux. All these patients must be treated and followed up in specialist units.

CONCLUSIONS AND THE WAY FORWARD

An improved understanding of neonatal physiology has resulted in shorter lengths of stay in hospital, less morbidity and a lower mortality. However, prematurity complicates all aspects of surgical management and mortality rates of 30% are reported (Zamir et al, 1989) for patients weighing less than 1500 g who undergo major operations. The prevention of acquired disorders would be of enormous benefit, particularly necrotizing enterocolitis, as this condition carries a high mortality and a high rate of long-term handicap in the survivors.

The short bowel syndrome may follow the management of volvulus, multiple atresias or necrotizing enterocolitis. Total parenteral nutrition allows for growth of the patient and the remaining small bowel, but is often complicated by septicaemia or cholestatic jaundice. The latter is less common in infants who can tolerate some gastric feeding but may progress to liver failure in patients with no gastrointestinal absorption. The adaptive response to a short bowel involves a compensatory increase in the mucosal surface by villous hyperplasia. Enteral feeding stimulates this growth and infants with only 15 cm of small bowel but an intact ileocaecal valve can be weaned on to a full oral diet. Long-term survivors are also reported with only 25 cm of small bowel and no ileocaecal valve (Dorney et al, 1985). Operations to lengthen the bowel or interpose antiperistalsis segments are still of unproven value (Bianchi, 1984) and small bowel transplantation has not yet been established for infants.

Long-term follow up for all patients undergoing a bowel resection is recommended. Not only do some patients develop a vitamin B_{12} deficiency after excision of the terminal ileum, but anastomotic ulcers have been described (Parashar et al, 1988) presenting with bleeding and anaemia.

REFERENCES

Barr LC, Booth J, Filipe MI & Lawson LON (1985) Clinical valuation of the histochemical diagnosis of Hirschsprung's Disease. *Gut* **26**: 393–399.

Beasley SW, Auldist AW, Ramanujan TM & Campbell NT (1986) Surgical management of necrotising enterocolitis. 1965–1984. *Pediatric Surgery International* **1**: 210–217.

Bell EF, Warburton D, Stonestreet BS & Oh W (1980) The effect of fluid administration on premature infants. *New England Journal of Medicine* **302**: 598–603.

Benjamin B, Cohen D & Glasson M (1976) Tracheomalacia in association with congenital tracheo-oesophageal fistula. *Surgery* **79**: 504–508.

Bianchi A (1984) Intestinal lengthening: an experimental and clinical review. *Journal of the Royal Society of Medicine* **77**: (supplement 3): 35–41.

Bodian M, Stephens FD & Ward BCH (1949) Hirschsprung's disease and idiopathic megacolon. *Lancet* i: 6–11.

Boocock GR & Donnai D (1987) Ano-rectal malformations: familial aspects and associated anomalies. *Archives of Disease in Childhood* **62**: 576–579.

Campbell PE & Noblett H (1969) Rectal suction biopsy in the diagnosis of Hirschsprung's disease. *Journal of Pediatric Surgery* **4**: 410–414.

Carter CO & Evans KA (1969) Inheritance of congenital pyloric stenosis. *Journal of Medical Genetics* **6**: 223–254.

Carver RA, Okorie NM, Steiner GM & Dickson JAS (1987) Infantile hypertrophic pyloric stenosis—diagnosis from the pyloric muscle index. *Clinical Radiology* **138**: 625–627.

Chittimittrapap S, Spitz L, Kiely EM & Brereton RJ (1989) Oesophageal atresia and associated anomalies. *Archives of Disease in Childhood* **64**: 364–368.

Corkery JJ, Dubowitz V, Lister J & Moossa A (1968) Colonic perforation after exchange transfusion. *British Medical Journal* **4**: 345–349.

De Campo JF & Phelan E (1989) Gas reduction of intussusception. *Pediatric Radiology* **19**: 297–298.

Dorney SFA, Ament ME, Berquist WE, Vargas JH & Hassall E (1985) Improved survival in very short bowel of infancy with use of long-term parenteral nutrition. *Journal of Pediatrics* **107**: 521–525.

Dykes EH, Gilmour WH & Azmy AF (1985) Prediction of outcome following necrotising enterocolitis in a neonatal surgical unit. *Journal of Pediatric Surgery* **20**: 3–5.

Ein SH & Stephens CA (1971) Intussusception, 354 cases in 10 years. *Journal of Pediatric Surgery* **6**: 16–27.

Freeman NV & Cass DT (1982) Colon interposition, a modification of the Waterston technique. *Journal of Pediatric Surgery* **17**: 17–21.

Howard ET & Othersen HB (1973) Proximal jejunoplasty in the treatment of jejunal atresia. *Journal of Pediatric Surgery* **8**: 685–690.

Howard FM, Flynn DM, Bradley JM, Noone P & Szawarkowski M (1977) Outbreak of nectrotising enterocolitis caused by clostridium butyricum. *Lancet* **ii**: 1099–1102.

Hutchison IF, Olayiwola B & Young DG (1980) Intussusception in infancy and childhood. *British Journal of Surgery* **67**: 209–212.

Jackman S, Brereton RJ & Wright VM (1990) Results of surgical correction of neonatal necrotising enterocolitis. *British Journal of Surgery* **77**: 146–148.

Jones PF (1987) *Emergency Abdominal Surgery*, chap. 3. Oxford: Blackwell Scientific Publications.

Kliegman RM & Fanaroff AA (1981) Neonatal necrotising enterocolitis: a nine year experience. *American Journal of Diseases in Children* **135**: 603–607.

Leape LL & Ramenofsky ML (1980) Surgical treatment of gastro-esophageal reflux in children. *American Journal of Diseases in Children* **134**: 935–938.

Leizomarck CE, Bonman-Sandelin K, Frisell J & Raf L (1986) Meckel's diverticulum in the adult. *British Journal of Surgery* **73**: 146–149.

Madden NP, Levinsky RJ, Bayston R, Harvey B, Turner MW & Spitz L (1989) Surgery sepsis and non-specific immune function in neonates. *Journal of Pediatric Surgery* **24**: 562–566.

Millar AJW, Rode H, Brown RA & Cywes S (1987) The deadly vomit—malrotation and midgut volvulus. *Pediatric Surgery International* **2**: 172–176.

Ng PC, Dear PRF & Thomas DFM (1988) Oral vancomycin in prevention of necrotising enterocolitis. *Archives of Disease in Childhood* **63**: 1390–1393.

Nixon HH (1988) Hirschsprung's disease. In *Rob and Smith's Operative Surgery*, 4th edn, pp 375–391. London: Butterworths.

Nixon HH & Tawes R (1971) Etiology and treatment of small bowel atresia. *Surgery* **69**: 41–51.

Noblett HR (1969) Treatment of meconium ileus by gastrografin enema: a preliminary report. *Journal of Pediatric Surgery* **4**: 190–197.

O'Donnell B (1985) *Abdominal Pain in Children*, chaps 1–11. Oxford: Blackwell Scientific Publications.

Parashar K, Kyawhla S, Booth IW, Buick RG & Corkery JJ (1988) Ileocolic ulceration: a long-term complication following ileo-colic anastomosis. *Journal of Pediatric Surgery* **23**: 226–228.

Patrapinyokul S, Brereton RJ, Spitz L, Kiely EM & Agrawal M (1989) Small bowel atresia and stenosis. *Pediatric Surgery International* **4**: 390–395.

Pearse RG & Roberton NRC (1986) Infection in the newborn. In *Textbook of Neonatology*, chap 28. London: Churchill Livingstone.

Pena A & de Varies PA (1982) Posterior sagittal anorectoplasty. *Journal of Pediatric Surgery* **17:** 796–811.

Rangecroft L & Courtney DF (1980) The use of transanastomotic feeding tubes in neonatal duodenal obstruction. *Zeitschrift Kinderchirugie.* **29**: 268–270.

Ravitch MM (1986) Duplications of the gastro-intestinal tract. *Pediatric Surgery*, 4th edn, pp 911–920. Chicago: Year Book Medical Publishers Inc.

Rommens JM, Iannuzzi MC, Karem B et al (1989) Identification of the cystic fibrosis gene. *Science* **245**: 1059–1065.

Soltero MJ & Bill AM (1976) The natural history of Meckel's diverticulum and its relation to incidental removal. *American Journal of Surgery* **132**: 168–173.

Sparnon AL & Kiely EM (1987) Resection and primary anastomosis for necrotising enterocolitis. *Pediatric Surgery International* **2**: 101–104.

Spitz L, Kiely EM & Brereton RJ (1987) Esophageal atresia: five year experience with 148 cases. *Journal of Pediatric Surgery* **22**: 103–108.

Spitz L, Wallis M & Graves HF (1984) Transport of the surgical neonate. *Archives of Disease in Childhood* **59**: 284–288.

Thomas DFM, Fermie DS, Malone M, Bayston R & Spitz L (1982) Association between clostridium difficile and enterocolitis in Hirschsprung's disease. *Lancet* **i**: 78–79.

Valente A, Brereton RJ & Mackersie A (1987) Esophageal replacement with whole stomach in infants and children. *Journal of Pediatric Surgery* **22**: 913–917.

Zamir O, Udassin R, Anad I et al (1989) The prognosis of low birth weight infants undergoing major surgery. *Pediatric Surgery International* **4**: 16–20.

Zeidan B, Wyatt J, Mackersie A & Brereton RJ (1988) Recent results of treatment of infantile hypertrophic pyloric stenosis. *Archives of Diseases in Childhood* **63**: 1060–1064.

17

TROPICAL AND INFECTIVE EMERGENCIES

Dion R. Bell

CHOLERA

In its classical form, cholera, caused by *Vibrio cholerae* of classical or El Tor types, causes severe watery diarrhoea rapidly leading to dehydration. Severe cholera presents a genuine medical emergency (Barua and Burrows, 1974; Manson Bahr and Bell, 1987).

The current pandemic of cholera, the seventh, began in the Celebes in 1961. It spread inexorably westward in the following years and is now distributed world-wide in places where environmental and personal hygiene are poor and water supplies are inadequate. It was long believed that the reservoir of cholera was confined to man, but there is now increasing evidence that there might well be a natural reservoir of cholera in marine life in coastal or estuarine waters. Infection has frequently been associated with the ingestion of inadequately cooked seafood.

Pathogenesis

Infection is acquired by ingesting the organism, a small actively motile Gram-negative organism of characteristic 'c' shape, but an effective barrier to infection is presented by gastric acid. There is a definitely enhanced risk of clinical infection in those with hypochlorhydria, or under circumstances when gastric acid is diluted or neutralized by food.

If sufficient organisms manage to pass through from the stomach to the small intestine without being destroyed, then subsequent events depend on various biological characteristics of the organism. Strains of the organism which secrete cholera toxin (choleragen), probably enhanced by adherence of the organism to the enterocytes via pili, produce diarrhoea by a purely biochemical means. The organisms are not invasive and do not cause inflammatory changes in the mucosa.

Choleragen, via a complex biochemical mechanism, enhances the intracellular level of cyclic adenosine monophosphate (cAMP) which results in a net flow of water and electrolytes across the mucosa into the lumen of the gut. This protein-free filtrate of the plasma is produced along the length of the small intestine. The volume swamps the absorptive capacity of the colon, and the net result is the passage of the typical watery stools. After the first stool or two has been passed, faecal contents are washed out of the gut and bile secretion is inhibited. The typical stool is now described as 'the rice water stool' and has a similar composition in electrolytes to that of plasma although the loss of potassium and bicarbonate is relatively enhanced.

The duration of the diarrhoea produced by cholera is a matter of 5–10 days, and to that extent the disease is self-limiting. However, the disease may be limited by the demise of the patient from profound dehydration and hypovolaemic shock. The situation is aggravated by the development of vomiting, especially as acidosis develops. The hypoperfusion of the kidneys associated with hypotension may result in renal failure. Tubular necrosis may occur, and so prerenal failure is followed by true renal failure.

Blood changes in cholera

Rapid loss of water leads to haemoconcentration and an increase in the concentration of plasma proteins. Both these factors combine to cause an increase in blood viscosity, and also lead to a rise in the specific gravity of the blood, a simple test used in cholera outbreaks to assess the severity of the patient's dehydration.

The clinical picture of cholera

The clinical picture is one of profound dehydration. There is loss of tissue turgor, the eyes are sunken, and there may be wrinkling of the skin of the fingers ('washerwomens hands'). Respiration is often sighing because of acidosis, and the patient may be semiconscious or even unconscious when he presents. Except in children, in whom there may be slight pyrexia, the temperature is normal or subnormal. Muscle cramps are a very distinctive feature of cholera, and may affect the limb muscles and also the abdomen. They result from a reduced concentration of calcium and chloride ions in the blood. A clinical observation that increases the likelihood of cholera as the cause of the diarrhoea is the passage of watery stools from a patient who is apparently oblivious of it. In children the loss of water is relatively more than the loss of electrolyte leading to hypertonic dehydration as a result.

The clinical spectrum of cholera

The foregoing description is that of severe cholera which affects 10% of those infected with the El Tor biotype and rather more than this in those affected with the classical cholera biotype. As with any bacterial disease, there is a spectrum of infection. Many patients have moderate or mild diarrhoea not leading to significant dehydration and at the extreme end of the mild spectrum there are patients with entirely asymptomatic infections.

The diagnosis of cholera

The clinical picture of profuse watery diarrhoea, vomiting, severe dehydration and muscle cramps is very distinctive of cholera but is occasionally caused by other agents causing profuse small bowel diarrhoea.

Isolation of the vibrio

The laboratory gives confirmation of the clinical suspicion. Direct microscopy reveals, in severe cases, numerous comma-shaped bacilli with a characteristic spiral movement imparted by their flagella. Few other organisms have a similar appearance, and specific diagnosis is provided by the immediate immobilization of the organisms when a drop of anti-cholera serum is placed in the slide. In mild cases direct microscopy is less reliable because there are numerous other bowel organisms present in the preparation. Direct microscopy is useless in detecting asymptomatic infections. Fluorescence microscopy, in which a fluoroscein-conjugated specific anti-cholera serum is added to the slide, is more sensitive than dark field microscopy but much more complicated.

The most sensitive method of detecting the bacilli is isolation of the organisms on culture. The best media is TCBS (thiosulphate–citrate–bile salts–sucrose) agar. Small numbers of vibrios can be detected only using an enriched liquid medium such as akaline peptone water. The specimen is best taken by a rectal swab or by inserting a sterile rubber catheter into the anus. Specimens taken in the field can be transported to the laboratory in sealed plastic bags or after inoculation into a holding medium.

Indirect diagnosis

Following the patient's recovery from an attack of cholera, detectable antibodies to the organisms appear in the blood. Provided the patient has not received cholera vaccine recently these do allow a retrospective diagnosis to be made. This is of course of no clinical importance, but it may, in certain circumstances, be of epidemiological use.

Treatment of cholera

Initial rehydration

In a patient with severe cholera and circulatory collapse as described, the urgent immediate objective of the physician is to restore the circulating volume so that the kidneys are perfused. In severe cholera the total fluid deficit will be in the range of 10–15% and one-third of this amount can be given 'immediately', that is in the first 20–30 min. The outcome of severe cholera depends not so much on which fluid is given within certain limits, but of how much is given. In adults an isotonic fluid is needed. In children it is best to give hypotonic fluid after the initial restoration of blood volume.

A patient with severe cholera has collapsed veins, and the problem is how to get a good flow of rehydration fluid into the circulation. A cut down on the veins is not the answer. It is slow and when the veins are found they are invariably contracted and string-like, and even if a cannula can be placed in the lumen the flow is usually poor. To get a good initial flow of rehydration fluid, a large vein must be entered such as the femoral, subclavian or internal jugular. In the case of the femoral vein, which can usually be located without difficulty provided the femoral pulse is palpable, the position of the needle, being almost vertical to the skin, is unstable and the attending physician or other medical attendant must hold the needle in position until the initial fluid has run in. At the end of this period, the pulse will have returned, the circulation will have filled the peripheral veins, and the drip can be moved to a more stable and convenient site.

A safe rule for initial rehydration is to give one-third of the estimated total fluid in the first 20–30 min. Whether resuscitation has been adequate is judged by the return of the pulse. As soon as the systolic blood pressure rises above 90 mmHg renal perfusion is restored and the patient's kidneys are able to compensate for the acidosis.

The choice of rehydration fluid

The ideal rehydration fluid will be, in adults, isotonic and on the alkaline side. The single fluid that meets the needs of both adults and children is Ringer lactate solution BP, which contains sodium 131 mmol/l, potassium 5 mmol/l, calcium 2 mmol/l, lactate 37 mmol/l and chloride 111 mmol/l. It is suitable both for initial rehydration and maintenance therapy. The WHO intravenous diarrhoea treatment solution contains sodium 120 mmol/l, chloride 80 mmol/l, acetate 50 mmol/l and potassium 10 mmol/l, and is probably as good.

If isotonic sodium chloride solution 9 g/l is the only fluid available, it can be used with good results but will not correct the acidosis so quickly. It can be used successfully in combination with isotonic sodium bicarbonate, lactate or acetate if used in the ratio 2 volumes of saline to 1 volume of the other alkaline solutions. This is done not by mixing the solutions but by giving two bottles of one and one of the other in rotation.

It has been shown that chlorpromazine in small doses reduces the fluid loss to some extent, and a small dose such as 25 mg for an adult may also help to control vomiting. Vomiting normally ceases as soon as acidosis is corrected.

Maintenance hydration

After initial resuscitation, the remaining calculated deficit should be restored in the next 2 hours. The best way of nursing cholera patients is on a special 'cholera cot', a bed on a rigid frame covered with rubber which allows diarrhoeal fluid to drain away through a hole in the middle into a calibrated bucket under the bed. This enables fluid requirements in the next 4 h to be calculated, and greatly eases the managing of maintenance hydration. The fluid requirements are calculated on the basis of urine output plus stool output plus 500 ml added to allow for insensible losses.

The speed of recovery of a correctly managed patient with severe cholera is one of the most gratifying sights in medicine. The patient will stop vomiting and feel thirsty. Now is the time to introduce oral rehydration with a glucose/electrolyte solution. Oral rehydration with glucose/electrolyte solution can be used from the start in those with only moderate to minor dehydration. It depends on the fact that active absorption of glucose results in the active absorption of sodium from the lumen of the gut. The secret of successful oral rehydration is to give the fluid frequently but in small amounts. If this rule is not observed, the patient may merely vomit and nullify the benefit completely.

A widely used solution is made up as follows. In 1 l of sterile water: dextrose (glucose) 20 g; sodium chloride 3.5 g; sodium bicarbonate 2.5 g; potassium chloride 1.5 g. Its composition is as follows: sodium 90 mmol/l; potassium 20 mmol/l; chloride 80 mmol/l; bicarbonate 30 mmol/l.

There are a number of commercial preparations of a similar composition such as 'Dioralyte'. The patient drinks four times an hour, or the liquid is administered by nasogastric tube. In severe continuing diarrhoea the amount of fluid to aim at is 15 ml/kg per h. If that rate of administration cannot keep pace with fluid loss, and this corresponds to 20 l a day for an adult, parenteral fluid is needed. For mild to moderate diarrhoea the dose is 5–10 ml/kg per h.

The use of tetracycline in cholera

Tetracycline, chlortetracycline or oxytetracycline in a dose of 500 mg 6 hourly for 3 days, rapidly terminates the excretion of vibrios, renders the patient non-infectious, prevents the carrier state, and is cost effective as it considerably reduces the fluid requirements. Diarrhoea usually ceases within 3 days in contrast to 7 days in the untreated case. Furozolidone 400 mg daily for 3 days is equally effective.

AMOEBIC DYSENTERY

Most cases of amoebic dysentery do not present as a medical emergency; the natural history is for the disease to start gradually, increase in severity over a week or two, continue at a rate of moderate severity for a few further weeks then gradually to die away, only to relapse later. In the average case disability is usually small and because there is usually no fever or associated vomiting, dehydration is not a problem. The typical case of amoebic dysentery is 'ambulant dysentery' and the patient normally walks into the clinic. However exceptional cases can present as a grave emergency, with severe diarrhoea, extreme tenderness of the abdomen and, in the most fulminant cases, perforation of the colon. Such patients may present as a surgical emergency and the diagnosis of amoebic infection is then sometimes made only post-mortem.

If amoebic colitis is suspected, the salient diagnostic method is prompt examination of a freshly voided stool in which the haematophagous motile amoebae are normally found without difficulty.

The standard specific treatment for amoebic dysentery consists of metronidazole with or without supplemental diloxanide furoate (Furamide). In severe and fulminating cases it is useful to add emetine or dihydroemetine (DHE) to the regimen. A typical dose would be 60 mg of emetine or 100 mg of DHE subcutaneously or intramuscularly for a few days. It is usual to stop emetine as soon as symptoms improve. One of the older tetracyclines by mouth is also effective in amoebic dysentery, and in severe cases it is customary to add tetracycline itself to the regimen in a dose of 250–500 mg 4 hourly for 5 days. Even if given alone, tetracycline is usually effective in relieving the symptoms of amoebic dysentery but it cannot be relied on to achieve parasitological cure.

BACILLARY DYSENTERY

Bacillary dysentery seen in western Europe is most commonly due to *Shigella sonnei* and is usually mild. The severer forms of dysentery found in tropical and subtropical countries are usually caused by *Shigella dysenteriae* (known in the past as the Shiga bacillus) but this organism causes not only more damage to the colon but also a more severe generalized reaction and toxaemia. In severe cases of shigellosis, dysentery may be complicated by the haemolytic uraemic syndrome. Clinical illness identical with that caused by shigellosis can be caused by verotoxin-producing invasive strains of *Escherichia coli*.

Most bacillary dysentery patients respond to supportive and symptomatic treatment, but severe cases will require intravenous rather than oral rehydration.

Over the past two decades there has been an increasing amount of antibiotic resistance amongst strains of *Shigella*, the pattern of resistance reflecting that of antibiotic usage. Sulphonamide resistance was reported first, followed by resistance to the tetracyclines and chloramphenicol and nowadays many strains are isolated that are resistant to multiple antibotics. Antibiotic therapy in *Shigella* dysentery is normally confined to the most severe cases, and the clinician should choose an antibiotic to which the organism is almost certain to respond. Nowadays that would involve the use of one of the fluorinated quinolone antibiotics such as ciprofloxacin and its relatives. Enthusiasts for this group of antibiotics made claims to the effect that antibiotic resistance to them could never occur but this has proved not to be the case. However, resistance to ciprofloxacin amongst shigellae is at present very rare.

AMOEBIC LIVER ABSCESS

Amoebic liver abscess does not usually present as a medical emergency, but the fact that abscesses can rupture from time to time, with disastrous consequences, means that they have the potential for a medical emergency and must be treated without delay. The normal course of an amoebic liver abscess is for it to continue increasing in size until it ruptures. The complications of rupture depend on the anatomical site of the abscess: rupture through the chest wall will cause a fistula, right lobe abscesses rupture upwards and enter into bronchial tree and left lobe abscesses enter the pericardium. Inferior abscesses may drain into the lesser sac or peritoneal cavity.

The standard treatment of an abscess consists of metronidazole by mouth (400–500 mg 8 hourly for 5–10 days) supplemented by diloxanide furoate (Furamide) 500 mg 8 hourly for 10 days. The purpose of the Furamide is to ensure that no amoebae are left within the lumen of the colon and so eliminate the possibility of recurrence of the abscess due to reinfection of the liver from the gut.

Indications for drainage of an amoebic liver abscess are imminent rupture and failure of the abscess to respond to 72 h of effective medical treatment. Recognized indications for aspiration include very raised diaphragm and localized pointing. Some clinicians advocate aspiration of the abscess if ultrasonography or other imaging techniques indicate that it exceeds 100 ml in volume.

Aspiration should be with a wide-bore needle, under ultrasound control, using a three-way tap, and aspiration should be to dryness. If amoebae are being sought, the last few drops of the aspirate are most likely to contain them. In very large abscesses recurrence of symptoms may indicate the need to reaspirate. It seems very likely that reducing the pressure in the abscess by aspiration improves the penetration of metronidazole into the abscess wall and it may be that high pressure in an abscess cavity is responsible for those cases failing to respond to metronidazole initially.

The cavity in the liver left by an abscess when amoebae have been destroyed may take months to resolve and it serves no useful purpose carrying out repeated imaging examinations of the liver as this tends to make both the patient and the physician nervous.

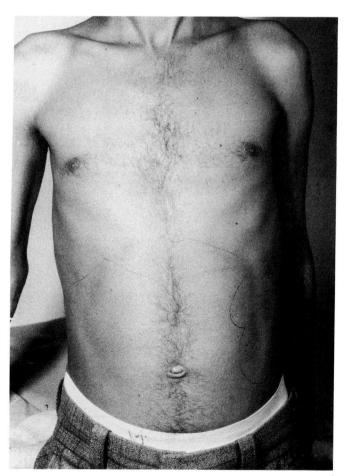

FIGURE I   A Yemeni patient with schistosomal fibrosis of the liver and portal hypertension due to *Schistosoma mansoni*. He had survived six previous episodes of haematemesis.

BLEEDING OESOPHAGEAL VARICES IN HEPATOSPLENIC SCHISTOSOMIASIS

The treatment of bleeding oesophageal varices due to portal hypertension secondary to hepatic fibrosis caused by schistosomiasis follows the same principles as the treatment of oesophageal varices caused by cirrhosis or any other pathology (Chapter 4). The main difference in the clinical picture is that in hepatosplenic schistosomiasis liver function is usually fairly well preserved and these patients tolerate their bleeds better than do for example those with cirrhosis, and hepatic encephalopathy is less common (Figures 1 and 2).

It used to be thought that the outlook in cases like this was hopeless in the long term and that there was, in consequence, little point in treating the underlying schistosomiasis. However 10 years ago a seminal paper from Egypt (Fareed et al, 1980) showed that using the drug oxamniquine, even advanced hepatosplenic

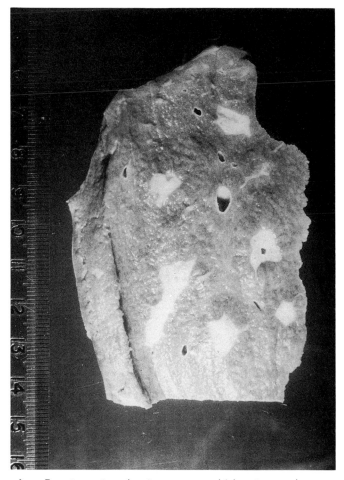

FIGURE 2 Liver from Egyptian patient showing pronounced 'clay pipe-stem' appearance in advanced schistosomal fibrosis.

schistosomiasis cases could show remarkable regression of the liver disease and a fall in portal pressure.

For this reason, nowadays it should be policy of the physician not only to treat the bleeding along conventional lines (endoscopic injection sclerotherapy being the preferred technique) but also to eradicate of the schistosome infection. There is little to choose between the drugs oxamniquine and praziquantel, but praziquantel has the advantage that sensitivity of strains of *Schistosoma mansoni* world-wide is more or less the same whereas different strains of *S. mansoni* show considerable differences in sensitivity to oxamniquine. Further, oxamniquine is without action against *S. japonicum* and praziquantel is effective against both species of parasites.

EMERGENCIES DUE TO *ASCARIS LUMBRICOIDES* (ROUNDWORM) INFECTION

The main abdominal emergency caused by *Ascaris* infection is intestinal obstruction, produced when a bolus of worms becomes impacted in the lumen of the small gut. Symptoms and signs of intestinal obstruction are often accompanied by a palpable mass in the abdomen, and if the mass moves it favours *Ascaris* rather than intussusception as the cause. When obstruction is intermittent, conservative treatment with intravenous fluids, nasogastric suction and an anthelmintic such as levamisole or piperazine may be successful. Where obstruction is persistent it will have to be relieved surgically.

Ascaris, in addition to causing obstruction due to a bolus, may also cause volvulus or intussusception. The worms have a tendency to penetrate suture lines in the gut, and if bowel surgery is carried out in a patient with *Ascaris*, the *Ascaris* are best removed from both above and below the incision manually. The chances of a worm penetrating the suture line can be further diminished by injecting a liquid preparation of piperazine into the gut lumen both above and below the suture line. *Ascaris* worms may also migrate up the common bile duct into the biliary tree where they may cause either an intrahepatic abscess or cholangitis (Figure 3). Worms that penetrate the pancreatic ducts may cause acute pancreatitis. In the past treatment of these complications has been by formal surgical removal. Nowadays, with modern endoscopic devices, per endoscopic removal is a possibility.

CONCLUSIONS AND THE WAY FORWARD

Acute diarrhoea from cholera or other bacterial infections, resulting in severe dehydration and hypovolaemia, remains the most serious common emergency of the gastrointestinal tract that the tropical physician is likely to face. Oral replacement solutions have been a major advance for mild to moderate cases but intravenous fluids, often in short supply, are essential for severely affected individuals. Real progress in prevention awaits improvements in hygiene and nutrition.

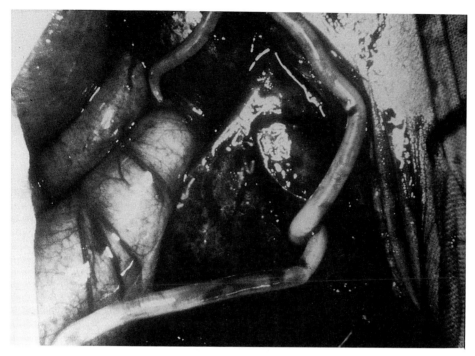

FIGURE 3   Peroperative photograph showing *Ascaris* being removed from bile ducts.

REFERENCES

Barua D & Burrows W (eds) (1974) *Cholera*. Philadelphia: W. B. Saunders.

Fareed Z et al (1980) Oxamniquine in advanced hepatosplenic *Schistosoma mansoni* infection. *Transactions of the Royal Society of Tropical Medicine* **74(3)**: 400–401.

Manson Bahr PEC & Bell DR (1987) Manson's *Tropical Diseases*, 19th edn, pp 259–274. London: Baillière Tindall.

18

SPONTANEOUS PERFORATION OF THE GASTROINTESTINAL TRACT

B. A. Taylor

INTRODUCTION

Perforation of any part of the gastrointestinal tract usually gives rise to a life-threatening emergency, which is most commonly managed by general surgeons. Furthermore, although the present incidences of both spontaneous rupture of the oesophagus and colonic perforation are relatively static, perforation of the stomach duodenum and small bowel is on the increase and likely to form a considerable proportion of our emergency workload for some years to come. An increasing proportion of elderly patients in western societies and the availability of powerful anti-inflammatory and analgesic medications combine to provide a fertile ground for upper gastrointestinal ulceration and its complications. This situation has been highlighted recently by a report which estimated a total of 24 million prescriptions for non-steroidal anti-inflammatory agents per year in the UK alone, and which also placed severe upper gastrointestinal side effects of non-steroidal anti-inflammatory drugs (NSAIDs) as the adverse reaction most commonly reported to the Committee on Safety of Medicines (Langman, 1987). The problem of unrecognized perforation of a viscus as a cause of death in the elderly has also recently been discussed in a report of 34 such deaths which were diagnosed only at post-mortem (Fulton et al, 1989). Advanced age, obesity, female sex, cardiovascular presentation and the absence of free gas on X-ray were all mentioned as possible confounding features, while the frequency of use of analgesics (26%), NSAIDs (44%) and steroids (21%) in this group serves as a reminder of the association between gastrointestinal tract ulceration and the ingestion of these agents.

This chapter consists of a discussion of the presentation and management of perforation of the gastrointestinal tract from the oesophagus to the colorectum, except for traumatic and iatrogenic perforation of the oesophagus and colorectum, both of which are covered elsewhere in this volume (see Chapter 14).

OESOPHAGUS

Non-instrumental perforation of the oesophagus is relatively uncommon and is often misdiagnosed unless a high index of suspicion is maintained. Such perforation may be truly spontaneous and related to an episode of vomiting (i.e. Boerhaave's syndrome), traumatic (e.g. gunshot wound) or related to a pre-existing pathological abnormality (such as Barrett's oesophagus), although this is excessively rare.

Presentation and initial assessment

The typical patient with Boerhaave's syndrome is an alcoholic who suffers a severe bout of vomiting following a 'binge', and immediately experiences marked lower chest and upper abdominal pain and prostration. The original description outlined the death in 1723 of a Dutch sea admiral, Baron van Wassener. The cause of his death was apparent at post-mortem when the Baron's previous meal of duck was found to be contaminating the mediastinum and pleural cavities. Herman Boerhaave carried out the post-mortem and his name has become eponymously attached to the condition (Williams, 1984). Forceable and prolonged vomiting against a closed cricopharnygeus muscle causes a dramatic rise in intra-oesophageal pressure which may give way at its weakest point—usually just above the diaphragm. The consequences tend to be more serious than those following instrumental perforation, since the condition almost always occurs on a full stomach, with gross chemical contamination of mediastinum and pleural spaces.

The possibility of a spontaneous oesophageal rupture must be borne in mind in any patient who has suffered a recent severe bout of vomiting, and who also then develops chest, back or abdominal pain or pain in the neck, associated with breathlessness. Obviously, this constellation of symptoms may lead the admitting physician towards more common diagnoses, and the condition is often mistaken for a cardiorespiratory problem such as myocardial infarction or pulmonary embolism, or for more common upper gastrointestinal emergencies such as pancreatitis or peptic ulceration. The condition is occasionally only suspected after a negative laparotomy, and it cannot be overemphasized that it will remain unrecognized until the outcome is inevitable unless it is considered in all potential cases.

The patient is usually in great pain, and may well be shocked, with hypotension and a tachycardia, cyanosis and breathlessness. It is apparent, therefore, how easily one might be misled into a suspicion of an underlying cardiorespiratory diagnosis. The physical sign which must be actively searched for, and the significance of which must not be overlooked, is that of subcutaneous crepitus of the skin of the neck, supraclavicular fossa and upper chest. This occurs most commonly with upper oesophageal perforations but air can track through the mediastinum from the lower oesophagus also. The presence of free mediastinal air may also be suggested by crepitus, audible on auscultation in time with the heartbeat. Further examination of the chest may reveal a pleural effusion with or without a pneumothorax, the extent of which will tend to influence the degree of respiratory embarrassment. In extreme cases there may be evidence of a tension pneumothorax with marked mediastinal shift. Examination of the abdomen is usually unremarkable, although guarding in the epigastrium may cause further diagnostic confusion.

Routine investigations will usually reveal a neutrophil leucocytosis with possible evidence of dehydration, such as a relative polycythaemia and uraemia. There is often arterial hypoxaemia depending on the extent of pre-existing and current respiratory embarrassment and the degree of arteriovenous shunting. However a chest X-ray (with both posterioanterior and lateral views) is the most important single investigation, and some care must be taken firstly that the film is of adequate quality, and secondly that the signs present, which may be quite subtle are not missed. Surgical emphysema (Figure 1) may be apparent either in the sub-cutaneous tissues of the neck or in the mediastinum and this may be most easily seen on a lateral film. There may be evidence of abnormal enlargement in the soft tissue space between the vertebral column and oesophagus in upper perforations, while mediastinal widening is occasionally all that is apparent on the initial chest film when the perforation is in the lower oesophagus. When the mediastinal pleura has been breached, signs of a hydropneumothorax may develop (more usually on the left side when the perforation affects the lower oesophagus), with possible progression to a tension pneumothorax. In doubtful cases, a contrast study using a water-soluble oral medium (e.g. gastrografin) will confirm the diagnosis and indicate the site and extent of the leak (Flynn et al, 1989; Yellin et al, 1989). A rare, intramural perforation (syn. intramural haematoma; submucosal dissection) may also be diagnosed by contrast radiology. The patient has a similar presentation to a patient with frank Boerhaave's syndrome although without the prostration, but the prognosis in general is good with conservative measures only (Williams, 1984).

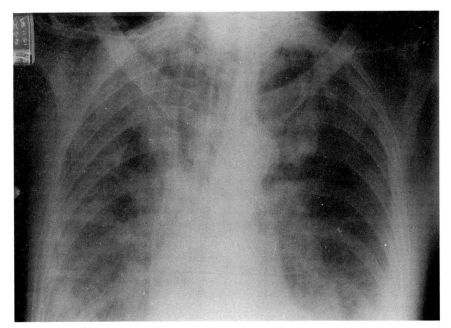

FIGURE I   Chest X-ray of patient with Boerhaave's syndrome, showing widespread pulmonary consolidation and extensive subcutaneous emphysema.

Perforation of the oesophagus is also very occasionally seen as a postoperative complication after prolonged vomiting (van Nooten et al, 1987), and also as a complication of pre-existing Barrett's oesophagus when peptic ulceration within the oesophagus gives rise to a transmural perforation, as it does more commonly in the stomach and duodenum (Cappell et al, 1989). Perforation of the oesophagus secondary to the ingestion of corrosives is an extremely difficult problem to deal with, and almost always requires multiple major procedures, initially to resect the damaged segment and later to restore intestinal continuity (Williams, 1984). Finally, iatrogenic injury to the cervical oesophagus has also recently been described as an uncommon complication of surgery to the cervical spine (most commonly after anterior spinal fusion, or Coward's procedure) (Newhouse et al, 1989). Management in this situation is conservative with a satisfactory outcome in most cases.

Treatment

A strategy for treatment may be considered in two phases; initial assessment and resuscitation, and definitive treatment. Between these two phases a decision must be made about the possibility of transfer to a specialist unit with facilities for thoracic and oesophageal surgery and for intensive care (Moghissi, 1988). A proportion of these patients will be most appropriately managed after transfer to a specialist unit, but the importance of adequate resuscitation before transfer must not be forgotten if outcome is not to be affected adversely. The definitive phase of management may be either operative or non-operative, depending on the delay in diagnosis, degree of constitutional disturbance, premorbid condition of the oesophagus and the site of injury.

Initial treatment

Oral intake is stopped and an intravenous infusion commenced. Broad spectrum antibiotics (e.g. metronidazole and cefuroxime) are administered parenterally. Adequacy of resuscitation is confirmed by a urinary catheter to monitor urine output and a central venous catheter to monitor right heart pressure. A central venous catheter specifically designated for parenteral feeding might also be positioned at this stage, since it will probably be required whether later definitive management is surgical or not. Where respiratory embarrassment is a significant feature and the chest film shows contamination of one or both pleural cavities, or perhaps even a tension penumothorax, intercostal tube drainage becomes a matter of some urgency and must be undertaken before consideration is given to transfer to a specialist unit. This will allow the lung to re-expand and will drain some of the material contaminating the pleural cavity.

Definitive treatment

The definitive form of treatment most appropriate to an individual case depends on the factors outlined earlier, and can range from a continuation of conservative measures (nil by mouth and broad spectrum antibiotics) to aggressive, radical surgery such as total oesophagectomy with delayed reconstruction. In general, perforations of the cervical oesophagus usually occur at the time of diagnostic or therapeutic endoscopy, can be diagnosed easily, do not cause major constitutional disturbances and can be managed very effectively by conservative measures (Brewer et al, 1986). Surgical intervention in such cases is likely to be confined to the establishment of a feeding gastrostomy (although long-term central venous feeding is an option) or the drainage of a cervical or superior mediastinal abscess in cases that present late.

Perforation of the thoracic oesophagus is more difficult to diagnose and therefore more commonly presents late. The consequences of uncontrolled sepsis and continuing leakage into the mediastinum and/or pleural cavity render this situation far more dangerous for the patient and are responsible for the much worse prognosis for patients with such injuries, compared to those whose injuries are located within the cervical oesophagus. Aggressive conservative measures, including balanced suction via multiple pleural and/or mediastinal drains together with a transnasal oesophagogastric drainage tube with holes cut above, below and opposite the site of the oesophageal injury are particularly indicated for those perforations presenting late, greater than 24 h after the initial injury. At this stage, operative repair is likely to be extremely difficult, if not impossible, because of the extent of the surrounding inflammation and oedema.

However, operative intervention is indicated in the majority of spontaneous thoracic oesophageal perforations presenting within 24 h of the initial injury. The left chest is opened to repair the lower oesophagus while a right thoracotomy gives more adequate access to the middle third. When contamination of the pleural cavity and mediastinum is minimal, and when operation is undertaken soon after injury, a direct primary repair of the tear is possible using interrupted non-absorbable sutures, combined with adequate debridement and drainage of both mediastinum and pleural cavities. The mucosal injury is often longer than that which is visible from the external aspect of the oesophagus, and the tear should be extended longitudinally so that all layers of the oesophagus can be repaired under direct vision. Various techniques have been described to buttress the repair, including using flaps of pleura, pericardium, intercostal muscle, diaphragm and omentum. When the injury is at or just above the cardia, direct repair of the perforation may be combined with a $360°$ Nissen-type fundoplication, in order to buttress the repair (Moghissi, 1988).

In cases of established Boerhaave's syndrome, mediastinal and pleural contamination is likely to be extensive, making direct primary repair of the injury impossible. In this situation, the only feasible option is to resect the damaged and partly necrotic oesophagus. Whether or not gastrointestinal continuity is restored at the same initial procedure depends largely on the physical condition of the patient and the extent of intrathoracic contamination. In the elderly, unstable patient with extensive contamination, the simplest, quickest and safest procedure would be the removal of the oesophagus and closure of the gastro-oesophageal junction, construction of a cervical oesophagostomy, and a feeding jejunostomy. At the second stage, some 3 or 4 months later, continuity is restored either by mobilizing the stomach to the cervical oesophagus or by bridging the gap between the two using transverse colon. However continuity is achieved, it is likely to be a difficult procedure for the surgeon and a dangerous procedure for the patient. The alternative is to undertake a restorative procedure at the first operation, which can be undertaken only when the patient is reasonably fit, since it is likely to involve a protracted general anaesthetic as the final anastomosis ought to be on the neck away from the contaminated thoracic cavity. Orringer and Stirling (1990) recently described a series of 24 patients who underwent immediate resection for oesophageal perforation secondary to a variety of conditions. Thirteen of this series also had a cervical oesophagogastric anastomosis performed at the same procedure with good results. These authors do not advocate conservative measures or surgical approaches less radical than resection in the management of thoracic oesophageal perforation, and although their results in general were good, the life-threatening severity of the situation cannot be overemphasized.

STOMACH AND DUODENUM

The great majority of perforations of the stomach or duodenum are complications of peptic ulceration. Such patients make up a considerable part of the emergency workload of the average general surgeon. The demography of this condition has been changing over the past several decades with the result that it is no longer relatively fit young males who make up the majority of such patients, but frail elderly patients, most of whom are female and many of whom are suffering from significant intercurrent disease (Coggon et al, 1981). Non-steroidal anti-inflammatory agents are implicated very frequently in this situation. The question of the best form of surgical management is one which has been addressed by numerous authors, and opinions tend to be divided between simple and definitive approaches. Various patient-related factors have been suggested as important in this decision-making process, and these will be discussed below. Another condition posing problems of management is spontaneous perforation of gastric malignancy.

Perforation of a peptic ulcer in a hiatus hernia is thankfully rare, since it may be extremely difficult both to diagnose and to treat. Usually an attempt can be made to close the perforation directly, assuming the hiatus hernia can be mobilized into the abdomen. Perforation of a stomal ulcer can be managed by an omental patch/oversew although if the stoma has been fashioned during the course of a previous operation for peptic ulcer, the addition of a manoeuvre designed to reduce acid output still further might be appropriate (gastrectomy after previous gastroenterostomy; vagotomy after previous gastrectomy). Finally, there are occasional reports of gastroduodenal perforations secondary to Crohn's disease and tuberculosis, while a very recent report has suggested an association between gastroduodenal perforation and the abuse of cocaine, although the possible mechanism remains obscure (Lee HS et al, 1990).

Perforated peptic ulcer

There is unfortunately no longer any such thing as the 'typical patient' with a perforated peptic ulcer. The young, male smoker with a dyspeptic history and a sudden onset of severe epigastric pain followed by prostration is still seen occasionally, but the condition is not confined to specific demographic groups and indeed the clinical picture can vary from that described above to that in which symptoms are entirely absent. Often there is a sudden onset of epigastric pain with pre-existing dyspepsia, but a more common antecedent history is one of NSAID ingestion. No attempt may be made to differentiate gastric from duodenal ulcer perforation on the basis of the clinical picture since the two are indistinguishable. Most recent series suggest that perforated gastric ulcers make up approximately 20% of all perforated peptic ulcers (Brown et al, 1976), and there seem to be at least two distinct subgroups—those elderly, usually female patients (often on NSAIDs) with a fundic gastric perforation, and young male patients with prepyloric perforation (Lanng et al, 1988). This latter group probably has more in common with patients with typical duodenal ulcer perforation than with gastric perforation.

The patient is usually in severe pain which is exacerbated by movement, hence the development of involuntary epigastric guarding. However, it should not be forgotten that leakage of gastric contents from an acutely perforated ulcer into the right paracolic gutter may simulate acute appendicitis, with relatively few upper abdominal signs. Shoulder tip pain may also be a feature, thought to be related to irritation of the lower surface of the diaphragm. The degree of constitutional disturbance will depend on the extent and duration of leakage of gastric contents into the peritoneal cavity and will vary from none at all to severe prostration. There may be clinical evidence of dehydration, with oliguria and hypotension, and bowel sounds may be scanty or absent.

Investigation may reveal a neutrophil leucocytosis, marginally elevated serum amylase and evidence of dehydration. Abdominal X-rays may be remarkably normal, but a well-penetrated erect chest X-ray will confirm perforation of a viscus by demonstrating free gas under the diaphragm in approximately 60% of cases. Otherwise, free intraperitoneal gas may be demonstrated on a lateral film, or perhaps even by using ultrasound, which is said to be sensitive to the presence of intraperitoneal gas (Lee DH et al, 1990). Occasionally, when the clinical suspicion of a perforation is high but confirmation is lacking, a water-soluble contrast study may provide useful information (Bell et al, 1987), while abdominal CT scanning may help in the difficult situation of a perforation arising in a duodenal diverticulum. Rarely, a gastroduodenal perforation is diagnosed at the time of upper gastrointestinal endoscopy.

Management

The initial management includes adequate resuscitation and the provision of oxygen, antibiotics and analgesia, in the same way as was outlined for oesophageal perforation. Care should be taken, however, since many of these patients will be elderly and frail, with relatively poor cardiorespiratory reserve. Resuscitation will almost certainly involve the placement of a central venous line and a urinary catheter with regular monitoring of urine output, right heart pressure and arterial blood gases. An indwelling arterial cannula and a Swan–Ganz catheter may be needed in those patients whose intercurrent illness and degree of cardiorespiratory compromise are most severe.

Although there are many series in the literature that describe good results from the conservative (non-operative) management of perforated peptic ulcers (Taylor, 1957), the place for this form of treatment nowadays is strictly limited. It has a role in those patients who refuse consent to operation, in those who are so severely unwell that intervention of any kind would be extremely dangerous, and in those who are very well and whose perforation can be demonstrated to be relatively localized, using contrast studies. However, any sign of deterioration in this last group should precipitate operative intervention. Operative intervention has the advantages that an alternative diagnosis (such as colonic perforation) will not be missed, that peritoneal lavage can be undertaken and a definitive ulcer operation performed if this is considered appropriate.

There does seem to be general agreement that those patients at greatest risk of operation should receive the simplest possible procedure of oversewing the perforation. However, the definition of a high risk group is the subject of some debate (Schein et al, 1990). Advanced age, major medical illness, perforation of long duration and the presence of preoperative shock have been highlighted as significant operative risk factors, in the absence of which definitive surgery may be undertaken safely (Boey et al, 1982b). Other authors have attempted more sophisticated scoring systems that can stratify patients into negligible, moderate and excessive risk groups (e.g. the Apache II Score; Schein et al, 1990). However, subsequent attempts to use such a score prospectively in order to decide between definitive and minimal surgical approaches failed to reduce mortality, albeit in a small number of patients. With the current availability of powerful antisecretory agents, many surgeons are opting for a conservative surgical approach to the majority of perforations, followed by long-term H_2 receptor blockade or omeprazole. However, the decision regarding the extent of surgery is usually made not only in the light of the associated morbidity and mortality but also after consideration of ulcer recurrence and reoperation rates and long-term clinical outcome.

Perforated gastric ulcer

Although considerably less common than perforated duodenal ulcer, perforated gastric ulcer remains a far more dangerous condition, with a mortality of approximately 25–30% (Steinheber, 1985). In general these patients are older than those with perforated duodenal ulcers, with more significant intercurrent illness and higher prevalence of smoking and NSAID ingestion (Wilson-MacDonald et al, 1985). There is commonly no antecedent dyspeptic history, and delayed presentation, possibly with a perigastric or lesser sac abscess, is common. A proportion of these ulcers (up to 10%) will also be malignant (Peel and Raimes, 1988).

The elective operation of choice for benign gastric ulcer is a Billroth I gastrectomy with gastroduodenal anastomosis. In the emergency setting, when malignant perforation cannot be excluded confidently, a more radical procedure such as a Billroth II resection might seem more appropriate although usually the patient is too unstable to undergo such a procedure. Gratifying results, with possibly improved mortality, may be achieved with lesser operations such as truncal vagotomy and drainage with excision of the ulcer and primary closure of the defect, or at least four quadrant biopsy of the ulcer followed by oversew (Collier and Pain, 1985). The plethora of antisecretory agents currently available means that aggressive medical management can be instituted at the same time as surgical intervention, and healing of the ulcer, together with confirmation of its benign nature, can be obtained in the postoperative period. Indeed, in a recent survey of

297 patients operated upon in Denmark between 1975 and 1984 for perforated gastric ulcer, 83% had biopsy and simple closure alone, without vagotomy (Lanng et al, 1988). The postoperative mortality of the whole group was only 21% while the incidence of both early and late reperforation, long considered to be the major danger of simple closure of perforated gastric ulcer, was only 2.4% It would appear therefore that the surgical approach to perforated gastric ulcer has become more conservative over the past decade.

Perforated duodenal ulcer

There are several factors to consider in deciding on the type of surgery required for a perforated duodenal ulcer. Firstly, the relative safety of the planned procedure must be assessed, and in this regard there will be both operation-related and patient-related factors to consider. Secondly, the need for a definitive procedure must be assessed on the basis of the patient's antecedent history and in the knowledge of the likely rate of ulcer recurrence and reoperation following simple closure of the perforation. Finally, some consideration should be given to the likely long-term side effects of definitive surgery (Blackett, 1990). With this background the present availability of a variety of antisecretory drugs must also be borne in mind since their effectiveness in healing ulcers is beyond doubt, and their side effects few.

Morbidity and mortality

Morbidity and mortality following operation for perforated duodenal ulcer vary with the constitutional disturbance, the adequacy of preoperative preparation and the experience of both surgeon and anaesthetist. There is no good evidence that the type of procedure *per se* influences results but such adequately controlled data would necessarily be difficult to acquire. Mortality is, however, directly related to the age of the patient, with those over 80 years of age having a mortality of approximately 80% (Blackett, 1990). Overall, mortality for simple closure varies between 0 and 16%, but similar figures have also been reported for definitive procedures such as highly selective vagotomy or vagotomy and pyloroplasty (Peel and Raimes, 1988). Definitive surgery undoubtedly takes longer (43 min for simple closure; 82 min for truncal vagotomy and drainage; 127 min for proximal gastric vagotomy; Boey et al, 1982a), while an emergency operation carries a higher mortality than the same operation undertaken electively (Clark et al, 1985). However, in very high risk patients it should be remembered that any operative procedure carries a very high mortality which may be as high as 41% in high risk patients treated even by simple closure (Jordan, 1982). Most deaths in this situation are primarily related to cardiorespiratory complications, but reperforation and bleeding after simple closure also carry a very high mortality of their own. They may be reduced by the concurrent administration of antisecretory drugs.

Need for a definitive procedure

The frequency with which perforated duodenal ulcers recur and cause symptoms following oversewing is related to the antecedent history, with 70% of patients with chronic duodenal ulcers experiencing recurrent ulcer symptoms compared to 20–30% of patients with acute ulcers. However, it is not always easy to differentiate the two either clinically or at the time of surgery. Many recurrent ulcers will be manageable medically but most series report reoperation rates of about 50–60% for chronic ulcers treated by simple closure, compared to about 20% for acute ulcers treated by the same technique (Gillen et al, 1986). More importantly, although most of these patients will undergo reoperation because of failed medical management, a small proportion will suffer a further life-threatening emergency such as reperforation, bleeding or gastric outlet obstruction. There is a case to be made for definitive operation in this group of patients, assuming the absence of adverse risk factors, not only to reduce the requirement for subsequent elective surgery but also to reduce the incidence of later emergency procedures. There is also, of course, an occasional requirement for further surgery for recurrent ulceration following definitive emergency surgery but this is mostly of the order of 5% or less.

Those prospective studies which have been undertaken support the role for definitive surgery in perforated duodenal ulcers. In 101 fit patients with perforated chronic duodenal ulcers randomized to simple closure or definitive treatment in Hong Kong, 63.3% of ulcers recurred endoscopically after simple closure, compared to 11.8% after vagotomy and drainage and 3.8% after proximal gastric vagotomy (Boey et al, 1982a). However, it cannot be overemphasized that the operation must be tailored to the patient's needs, and not to the ability of the operating surgeon. If a definitive procedure is considered to be indicated, then a suitably experienced surgeon must be involved.

Long-term clinical outcome

If one accepts that there is a case for a definitive procedure in some patients with perforated chronic duodenal ulcers, and there are some authors who do not (Raimes and Devlin, 1987), the two procedures which probably have a place are truncal vagotomy with drainage and highly selective vagotomy. There are, however, no definitive procedures for duodenal ulcer without significant long-term side effects, and the more extensive the initial procedure the more common are its side effects. Highly selective vagotomy probably comes closest to the ideal operation and can be carried out as an emergency procedure without increased morbidity and with acceptably low frequency of long-term side effects (Jordan, 1982). The unfortunate corollary is that rates of ulcer recurrence following highly selective vagotomy can be very high, varying between 1% and 40%, with a median of approximately 10% that continues to increase with time (Johnston, 1986). However, the vast majority of these recurrences following highly selective vagotomy can be managed by continuous or intermittent antisecretory agents. It is apparent that those authors reporting acceptable results and low ulcer recurrence rates using highly selective vagotomy for perforated duodenal ulcers are enthusiasts, and if such an approach is to be adopted, the experience of the individual surgeon is paramount. Truncal vagotomy and drainage is perhaps still a more conventional definitive procedure in perforated duodenal ulcer but approximately 15% of these patients will ultimately achieve a poor result (Visick grades III and IV), either because of intractable symptoms such as postvagotomy diarrhoea, or because they develop a symptomatic recurrent ulcer (Clark et al, 1985). It should also be remembered, however, that 60–70% of patients will achieve poor long-term clinical results (Visick grades III and IV) after simple closure of a duodenal ulcer, which reinforces the argument in favour of a definitive procedure at the time of perforation. In an attempt to predict those patients suffering a 'severe ulcer diathesis', there are some authors who would advocate a definitive procedure only if an ulcer perforates while the patient is on H_2 antagonists or if the patient has suffered a previous ulcer-related complication (Raimes and Devlin, 1987).

H_2 receptor antagonists

Theoretically, one might expect the introduction of H_2 receptor antagonists to have affected the demographic patterns of patients presenting with perforated duodenal ulcers and to some extent this is true. A small proportion of patients with duodenal ulcer suffer perforation while taking H_2 receptor blocking agents (both full and maintenance doses) (Gillen et al, 1986). Furthermore, while the frequency of elective ulcer operations has decreased dramatically over the past years, the number of patients having emergency operation is unchanged, although there is a suggestion that the majority of these patients now have acute rather than chronic ulceration (Watkins et al, 1984), and that NSAIDs play an important role. Whether or not H_2 receptor blocking agents can affect reoperation rates in patients who have had a perforated duodenal ulcer treated by simple closure remains unclear, but what data are available (and these data are not perfect) suggest that they do not (Gillen et al, 1986). There is need for a large, prospective trial with at least 6 months therapy and routine endoscopy to assess healing.

In conclusion, there is a good case to be made for a definitive, ulcer-curing operation in selected cases of perforated duodenal ulcer. However, the exact procedure undertaken will be dictated largely by the clinical situation, in the knowledge that highly selective vagotomy plus closure provides a means of minimizing the possible long-term complication rate. A blanket policy of simple closure for all peptic duodenal perforations cannot be justified if the only reason is inexperience of a junior surgeon.

Perforated gastric neoplasms

The prognosis for gastric neoplasia in the United Kingdom is relatively very poor, and perforation implies free access of tumour cells to the peritoneal cavity and an accordingly worsened prognosis. This is a relatively uncommon presentation for gastric neoplasia. In general, a laparotomy and resection will be undertaken, although perforation of an unresectable carcinoma is a difficult situation since local drainage will inevitably be followed by a malignant fistula. In those elderly, unfit patients in whom a perforated but unresectable tumour is suspected, it may be prudent to adopt a conservative approach in the knowledge that many of these patients will not survive longer than a few days.

SMALL INTESTINE

Perforation of the small intestine is relatively uncommon in westernized societies, except in regions where typhoid fever (Gibney, 1989), tuberculosis (Kakar et al, 1983) and parasitic infestations are endemic (Archampong, 1985). In Europe and North America the potential underlying abnormalities are extremely varied and include local conditions affecting isolated areas of the small intestine such as foreign bodies, enteric ulceration and blunt abdominal trauma, or generalized conditions such as Crohn's disease, intestinal lymphoma and the various vasculitides. In some instances there is no obvious abnormality of the bowel whatsoever, perforation having taken place through apparently normal bowel. The clinical picture tends to be rather non-specific early in the disease and patients sometimes undergo extensive investigation for occult gastrointestinal bleeding or for vague abdominal pain before presentation with frank peritonitis. However, the mortality within a series of 35 patients with small bowel perforation not related to trauma was 31%, and was thought to be directly related to delayed diagnosis and the presence of sepsis (Mischinger et al, 1989). Earlier diagnosis and surgical intervention might be expected to improve these figures.

Aetiology (see Table I)

In a recently collected series of 273 cases from nine centres (Mischinger et al, 1989), foreign bodies proved to be the most common cause, with fish and chicken bones, toothpicks and the clips used to secure plastic bags being particularly common. Although not strictly foreign bodies, gallstones occasionally cause perforation at or just above the site of impaction in the ileum, although obstruction is the more usual presentation. In the same series of 273 cases, idiopathic or non-specific ulceration causing perforation was even more common than perforation secondary to foreign bodies, although in this group the underlying abnormality is obscure (Thomas and Williamson, 1985). Some of these cases were undoubtedly related to the ingestion of drugs such as enteric-coated potassium supplements (Campbell and Knapp, 1966), although other agents such as NSAIDs, steroids and some chemotherapeutic agents have also been implicated.

Duodenal and small bowel diverticula are usually acquired lesions which are mostly entirely asymptomatic but which can cause bleeding, malabsorption, peridiverticulitis and perforation (Thomas, 1990). When situated in the duodenum, the inflammatory process causes a phlegmon around the pancreatic head, and possibly also a retroperitoneal abscess. Drainage of the abscess and resection of the diverticulum are usually required. Perforation of a jejunal diverticulum necessitates a simple small bowel resection. Perforation of such a diverticulum is occasionally related to a foreign body, the presence of an enterolith or even to air insufflation at the time of upper gastrointestinal endoscopy (Brown et al, 1986). Meckel's diverticulum is a congenital variety of small bowel diverticulum which may cause perforation by any of the mechanisms described above, but also as a complication of peptic ulceration, assuming the presence of ectopic gastric mucosa.

TABLE I
Aetiology of small bowel perforation

Mechanical	Strangulating obstruction
	Foreign body
	Trauma (blunt/perforating)
Idiopathic	'Non-specific' ulcers
Drug related	Potassium supplements
	NSAIDs
	Steroids
	Chemotherapeutic agents
Inflammatory	Jejunoileal diverticula
	Meckel's diverticulum
	Crohn's disease
	Zollinger–Ellison syndrome
	Coeliac disease
Neoplastic	Primary/secondary carcinomas
	Lymphoma
	Leukaemia
Infective	Typhoid
	Tuberculosis
Parasitic	Ascariasis
Vascular	Mesenteric infarction
Connective tissue	Polyarteritis nodosa
	Systemic lupus erythematosus
	Wegener's granulomatosis
	Scleroderma
Metabolic	Amyloid
Iatrogenic	Operative injury
	Radiation enteritis

The list of alternative underlying diagnoses in patients with small bowel perforation is very long indeed, but other broad areas that ought to be mentioned briefly include acute radiation injury following radiotherapy, malignant processes such as primary and secondary epithelial neoplasms, lymphomas and leukaemic infiltration, and connective tissue disorders such as polyarteritis nodosa, systemic lupus erythematosus and Wegener's granulomatosis. The prognosis in the majority of such cases will depend on that of the underlying condition. Finally, spontaneous intraperitoneal perforation of a small bowel adenocarcinoma complicating previously bypassed Crohn's disease has been recently described (Greenstein et al, 1987).

Presentation and management

In a recent series of 53 patients from a centre in Austria, presenting between 1974 and 1988 with small bowel perforation, 18 were secondary to trauma while the remainder were related to a variety of underlying conditions (Mischinger et al. 1989). This work load represented 0.4% of all surgical admissions with acute abdominal complaints, with an incidence of 0.3 cases per 100 000 population per year. The majority of these patients had generalized abdominal tenderness and a leucocytosis, although in only 18% was a pneumoperitoneum detectable on abdominal and/or chest X-rays. Thirty-nine per cent of perforations had occurred in the terminal ileum, the remainder being distributed relatively evenly throughout the length of the small bowel.

The operative procedure is largely governed by the likely underlying abnormality. When the perforation has occurred during blunt or penetrating abdominal trauma, the bowel wall itself is normal and the degree of peritoneal contamination slight. In this situation a direct repair can usually be undertaken without intestinal resection, although the extent of damage to adjacent structures, such as the small bowel mesentery, will obviously also be important (Chapter 14).

When the small bowel abnormality is more diffuse, as in Crohn's disease, or when multiple perforations are relatively close together in the same segment, intestinal resection and reanastomosis are indicated. The extent of resection will obviously depend on a clinical assessment of the extent of the disease process at the time of operation. If there is any question of vascular compromise, a resection must be sufficiently extensive to ensure viability of the ends used to fashion the anastomosis. However, in the case of a perforation occurring in Crohn's disease, it should be remembered that the current surgical approach tends to be relatively conservative, with preservation of as much bowel as possible. There is no evidence that anastomoses fashioned in bowel affected by Crohn's disease heal any less well than those in normal bowel, and in patients with diffuse jejunoileal involvement the superimposition of a short-bowel syndrome on widespread Crohn's disease may render the subsequent clinical situation extremely precarious.

The management of certain well-defined conditions affecting the small intestine, such as acute mesenteric infarction, perforated Crohn's disease and strangulated hernia, are covered in other areas within this text (see Chapters 8, 10 and 11, respectively), but there is still room within this chapter to stress one or two practical points. The first is that in perforated Crohn's disease, where there may be a large inflammatory mass with extensive sepsis and possible involvement of other organs, there is still a definite place for the fashioning of a temporary stoma, both to defunction the bowel beyond and to avoid the potential problems of intestinal anastomosis in malnourished and septic patients. Although this necessarily commits the patient to a further laparotomy, this course of action is often the safest in an otherwise difficult situation. It can also be useful to fashion a stoma in a case in which the small bowel is of doubtful viability following a limited resection for intestinal ischaemia. A 'second-look' laparotomy (approximately 48 h after the first operation) is occasionally beneficial in a patient who has had patchy ischaemic changes from whatever cause. It may be that a further resection can be undertaken before frank necrosis and reperforation occur.

LARGE INTESTINE

Perforation of the large intestine represents a major surgical challenge to the clinician, not simply because the technical aspects of the operation may be difficult, but more importantly because the situation is rapidly lethal in the type of compromised patients in whom the condition usually presents. In westernized societies there are only two common diagnoses, diverticular disease and colonic carcinoma, whereas in developing countries infective conditions, such as amoebiasis, are important (Luvuno, 1990). Other less common causes include volvulus and mesenteric vascular abnormalities. The underlying cause influences the type of operation more than in the small intestine. Furthermore, the type of operation is also influenced by the relationship between the site of perforation and the site of any other pathological process (such as an obstructing carcinoma). If perforation occurs remote from an obstructing sigmoid carcinoma, management is likely to be significantly different to that used in a stercoral perforation immediately adjacent to an obstructing tumour, or indeed at the site of the tumour.

Perforation of the large intestine is a rapidly fatal condition, death being caused by sepsis from peritoneal contamination with various enteric pathogens, both aerobic and anaerobic. The main aims of treatment are to control established sepsis, to minimize contamination and to treat the underlying cause of the condition. Before addressing specific causes of large bowel perforation, there are certain common features of management which are fundamental if morbidity and mortality are to be reduced to an acceptable level.

Presentation, assessment and initial management

Patients presenting with large bowel perforation unrelated to trauma may give little history to enable the clinician to reach a correct preoperative diagnosis. Indeed, many of these patients will ultimately undergo a laparotomy on the basis of established peritonitis from a presumed perforation of an unknown viscus. There are some features in the clinical presentation that might point towards large bowel disease, such as a previous history of acute diverticulitis or current investigation of anaemia or altered bowel habit, but in general large bowel perforation will be suspected because of the age of the patient and an absence of features suggesting a gastroduodenal perforation (e.g. NSAID ingestion). Patients whose diverticular perforation is initially localized often present with a rather vague history of lower abdominal pain, possibly with a mass on examination. A sudden exacerbation of symptoms and deterioration in the general condition of the patient must alert the clinician to the possibility that a localized paracolic abscess has perforated.

On examination, the patient will usually be markedly unwell and may in fact be septicaemic. There is usually obvious guarding or rigidity with quiet or absent bowel sounds. Digital examination of the rectum should not be forgotten and will occasionally demonstrate an unsuspected rectal carcinoma or suggest a carcinoma lying within the pelvis, although it may be impossible to differentiate this situation from one in which a large diverticular mass prolapses into the pelvis.

The investigation, as in the patient with suspected gastroduodenal perforation, is directed towards establishing fitness to withstand a major operation. Blood tests must include a full blood count, urea and electrolytes and a cross-match. An erect chest X-ray is essential as a preoperative measure in an ill patient about to undergo abdominal surgery, and because it may demonstrate free intraperitoneal gas. An ECG is essential in elderly patients. A plain abdominal film may show evidence of fluid between bowel loops, or abnormal collections of gas in extraperitoneal tissues or in the bowel wall itself. If obstruction is also a feature, an erect abdominal X-ray is usually obtained in order to confirm the diagnosis. The size of the dilated colon in this situation might indicate an impending large bowel perforation, the caecum being the usual site of such an event.

In those cases that are clear cut and in which a laparotomy is indicated urgently, contrast radiology has no place. However, when the clinical picture is rather more vague, for example in a localized perforation of the sigmoid colon secondary to diverticular disease, contrast radiology, possibly followed by endoscopic assessment and biopsy, has a definite role, although it should be remembered that invasive procedures undertaken early in the course of the illness have the capacity to make the clinical situation considerably worse.

The initial management of these patients involves more aggressive resuscitation than is required in gastroduodenal perforations. Faecal peritonitis from large bowel perforation represents a very significant challenge to the patient, and profound endotoxaemia and septic shock may be the result. Adequacy of fluid replacement may again be monitored using the usual parameters such as blood pressure, pulse and urine output, while the placement of right heart and pulmonary artery catheters will be influenced by the degree of haemodynamic disturbance and the presence of pre-existing cardiorespiratory diseases. Pre- and postoperative pharmacological support using suitable vasopressor agents such as dopamine, both to maintain urine output and systolic blood pressure, are frequently required. Broad spectrum antibiotics are administered early, as soon as gastrointestinal perforation is suspected. A combination of an aminoglycoside or a cephalosporin plus metronidazole is usual, and should probably be continued for a week in established peritonitis. Copious intra-operative irrigation of the peritoneal cavity with warm saline to remove all particulate faecal matter and frank pus is also important, although topical tetracycline lavage (1 g tetracycline in 1 l normal saline) is probably more beneficial to the patient, since at the concentrations achieved in the peritoneal cavity tetracycline is bacteriocidal to most enteric organisms (Krukowski et al, 1987). In general, drains should be reserved for specific purposes such as draining established abscesses or potential spaces such as that in front of the sacrum following rectal mobilization. If contamination is extensive, the superficial layers of the abdominal wound can be left open and allowed to heal by secondary intention, although primary wound healing can be achieved in 95% of all 'dirty' abdominal wounds, assuming adequate peritoneal lavage and protecting of wound edges (Krukowski and Matheson, 1988). Little is lost, however, by opening the wound at a later date if and when a wound infection becomes apparent, although the hospital stay may be prolonged by a few days. Most of these patients will develop a significant postoperative ileus, which may be prolonged for several days or weeks if continued sepsis is a problem, and nasogastric intubation or perhaps gastrostomy may avoid some of the associated problems.

Surgical management of specific types of perforation

Large bowel perforation secondary to ischaemia, inflammatory bowel disease and iatrogenic or instrumental causes have been covered elsewhere (Chapters 8, 10 and 14 respectively).

Perforation secondary to diverticular disease

Perforated diverticular disease can give rise to a spectrum of clinical situations, from a small pericolic abscess when the process is relatively contained and contamination minimal, to frank faecal peritonitis with its associated marked systemic disturbance. Between these two extremes, localized perforation, abscess formation and adherence to adjacent structures can give rise to fistulae into hollow organs such as the bladder, or into soft tissues such as the retroperitoneum, and thence to the back, buttocks and thighs. Perforated diverticular disease is one of the few causes of psoas abscess, along with perforated colonic carcinoma and Crohn's disease. Diverticula of the caecum are seen either in very extensive diverticulosis elsewhere, or as an isolated, probably congenital abnormality. The congenital variety occasionally perforates, usually giving rise to a localized abscess, but the clinical situation is indistinguishable from that seen in acute appendicitis. A local resection is adequate treatment for the condition, but a right colectomy is undertaken more commonly, either because of the associated inflammatory mass or because the situation is difficult to differentiate at operation from a perforated caecal carcinoma (Kovalcik and Sustarsic, 1981).

Those patients presenting acutely with an inflammatory paracolic mass usually can be managed conservatively, with bowel rest and broad spectrum antibiotics, to be investigated later by ultrasound, contrast radiology and/or endoscopy to confirm the benign nature of the process. In general, once the acute process has settled, the decision to resect the involved segment electively can be made on the basis of the patient's general medical condition, the presence of symptoms (which may be few even in the presence of grossly involved bowel) and on the likelihood of further complications. In the elective situation, a straightforward sigmoid colectomy with primary anastomosis is the usual surgical option. However in extensive disease some care must be taken to construct an anastomosis between proximal colon and normal rectum, since there is a risk of recurrent attacks of acute diverticulitis in approximately 11% of cases, probably when an involved segment is left below the anastomosis (Wolff et al, 1984). Complicated diverticular disease in which fistulae exist either into adjacent organs or into nearby soft tissues is usually managed by primary resection and immediate anastomosis (Hackford et al, 1985), although an assessment of associated sepsis will have to be made at the time of surgery in the knowledge that anastomosis occasionally will be deemed inadvisable or indeed impossible.

If at operation an inflammatory mass surrounding the sigmoid colon is detected, with or without an associated paracolic abscess but without free perforation of the bowel, there is a case to be made for conservative measures using peritoneal lavage and drainage only (Killingback, 1983), since a significant proportion of such patients will have few symptoms subsequently and will not have been committed to a further major surgical procedure. Approximately 20% will, however, develop a colocutaneous fistula indicating that a perforation was presumably present but undetected at the time of operation. Most of these will heal spontaneously. A more aggressive approach in this situation is to resect the involved segment and undertake an immediate anastomosis, such as is advocated by clinicians at the Lahey clinic (Schoetz, 1990), with a transverse loop colostomy if the septic focus is 'extensive'. My own personal preference would be to divert the faecal stream using a loop ileostomy and to undertake antegrade lavage in order to empty the proximal colon prior to primary anastomosis (Radcliffe and Dudley, 1983).

The management of the case in which there is a free perforation of the large bowel with purulent or faecal peritonitis presents more of a problem, and current surgical options revolve around immediate resection of the involved segment, usually without a primary anastomosis. Although a staged approach obviously has a significant role, the operation of transverse loop ('decompressive') colostomy and drainage of the associated pelvic sepsis as the initial procedure (Smithwick, 1942), has now been largely abandoned. The results of this approach are very poor, with the mortality approaching 30% and failure to proceed to the second or third stage in a significant proportion of patients (Wara et al, 1981). However, there are still some authors who question primary resection rather than drainage in the management of severe complications of diverticular disease, based on mortality figures from small groups of patients with peritonitis and abscesses compared to historical controls (Peoples et al, 1990). The majority of authors do, however, support the concept of primary resection of the diseased segment as the manoeuvre most likely to reduce mortality and morbidity (Auguste and Wise, 1981; Underwood and Marks, 1984; Nagorney et al, 1985). Although the fashioning of a mucus fistula of the rectosigmoid colon, usually through the lower end of the abdominal incision, undoubtedly facilitates the second stage simply because the distal segment is easier to find, my own preference is for a Hartmann's procedure with stapled or hand-sewn closure of the upper rectum. In any case, it is often impossible to bring the rectosigmoid to the surface in an obese patient whose colon is foreshortened because of diverticular disease, while the reversal of a Hartmann's resection has been greatly facilitated by the introduction of end-to-side stapling techniques (Ramirez et al, 1983). As a point of operative technique, mobilization of the rectum away from the sacrum at the first operation can only make subsequent procedures more difficult, and should be avoided if at all possible. Some authors also advocate leaving non-absorbable marker sutures on the closed rectal stump to facilitate its subsequent mobilization (Madure and Fiore, 1983).

Perforated colonic neoplasms

Colonic carcinomas may cause either local perforation or, more commonly, perforation secondary to closed loop obstruction. As a presenting feature perforation is relatively uncommon, accounting for somewhat less than 10% of all cases of colonic carcinoma (Badia et al, 1987), and in general is associated with decreased survival (Sugarbaker, 1981). Free intraperitoneal perforation of a carcinoma itself might be expected to liberate viable tumour cells, but why obstruction and higher perforation should be associated with decreased survival is unknown.

A colonic carcinoma that has perforated either locally to form an abscess or more generally into the peritoneal cavity should be resected if at all possible. The operation may involve the in-continuity resection of adjacent, involved structures such as small bowel or parietal peritoneum, and may also involve leaving unresectable tumour within the abdomen. Other operative considerations, such as the liberal use of tetracycline lavage, apply in this situation as they do in perforated diverticular disease, and the decision to undertake a primary anastomosis is based on the same criteria as were detailed in the previous section. In general, perforated carcinomas of the right colon can be resected with immediate anastomosis in almost all cases, while for lesions in the sigmoid colon and rectum Hartmann's procedure is more suitable when contamination is extensive. Data relating to anastomotic healing in the presence of sepsis and/or faecal contamination are conflicting (Matheson, 1989), although there is no doubt that the risks to the patient's life following anastomotic dehiscence are very significant (Schrock et al, 1973). Most authors would therefore favour resection without anastomosis in a low colonic perforation with significant contamination, although there is probably a place for the procedure described in the previous section—that is, primary resection of the involved segment, on-table antegrade lavage to empty the colon above, immediate anastomosis and loop ileostomy. However, when obvious macroscopic tumour has been left within the pelvis following the palliative excision of a perforated low carcinoma, I favour Hartmann's procedure since local recurrence is very predictable in this situation. The potential large bowel obstruction which results may be very difficult to deal with and will almost certainly necessitate a further laparotomy.

When a carcinoma has caused a large bowel perforation above, the only feasible surgical option is a subtotal colectomy to excise both the primary lesion and the perforated colon. Many of these patients are relatively elderly, with obstructing lesions in the sigmoid colon and the potential for extensive contamination of the whole peritoneal cavity following caecal rupture. An end ileostomy with oversewing of the distal rectum is really the only option in such a case, since elderly patients with ileorectal anastomoses tend to have rather poor functional results, with faecal incontinence being a significant problem. If contamination is not excessive and the obstructing lesion is in the upper sigmoid or descending colon, an immediate anastomosis is a suitable alternative, with more acceptable functional results.

Other mechanical problems

Volvulus, either sigmoid or caecal, is a condition which is uncommonly associated with large bowel perforation. It more usually presents with large or small bowel obstruction, often recurrent, and usually can be diagnosed on plain abdominal films. The diagnosis may be confirmed by contrast radiology, and it almost always requires intestinal resection although various temporizing measures such as the passage of a flatus tube and colonoscopic decompression have been described. If the volvulus is sufficiently advanced to compromise the vascular supply within the mesenteric attachment of the segment involved, ischaemic necrosis will be followed by perforation and peritonitis. In this situation, resection of the involved segment is mandatory, although the decision to undertake an immediate anastomosis must depend on local conditions at the time of operation.

Pseudo-obstruction (syn. Ogilvie's syndrome) is a relatively common condition characterized by massive colonic distension without mechanical obstruction. It presents typically in elderly patients who usually have a variety of other non-surgical conditions, but can be associated with massive caecal distension and perforation in up to 21% of patients (Soreide et al, 1977). Having confirmed the diagnosis by contrast radiology, conservative measures, such as the use of therapeutic decompressive colonoscopy or of prokinetic agents such as ceruletide and cisapride, are indicated in an attempt to prevent perforation. Lack of resolution remains one of the few indications for tube caecostomy. Once free perforation has taken place, the right colon will almost certainly have to be resected, and possibly also the colon beyond if viability is doubtful. Immediate anastomosis in such a situation would be extremely hazardous, since continuing large bowel inertia would almost certainly lead to anastomotic leakage.

Stercoral perforation occurs as a result of impaction of inspissated faeces, which leads to ulceration of mucosa and pressure necrosis of otherwise normal colonic wall. The degree of contamination of the peritoneal cavity tends to be slight, since faeces are usually scybalous and can be removed very easily. A limited resection can be undertaken to remove the perforated segment, followed by antegrade lavage and primary anastomosis or temporary colostomy, again depending on the extent of contamination.

CONCLUSIONS AND THE WAY FORWARD

This chapter covers a significant part of the emergency workload of the average general surgeon and the principles of management of cases such as these are therefore of considerable importance. Refinements in the operative procedures themselves are unlikely to have a major impact on morbidity and mortality. Preoperative, perioperative and postoperative management are, however, of paramount importance and it is by attention to these complementary areas that improvements in outcome are still possible. Early diagnosis is certainly an aim worth striving for, and to this end, the maintenance of a high degree of suspicion in at-risk patients and contrast radiology where there is doubt will improve diagnostic accuracy. Operative intervention in patients who are adequately prepared is likely to improve outcome, and vigorous resuscitation and inotropic support when necessary, will ensure that in this group of high risk patients a satisfactory result will be achieved. Confirmation that resuscitative measures are effective must be sought by monitoring routine physiological parameters and, where necessary, by using invasive techniques such as right heart catheterization, peripheral arterial cannulation and the placement of pulmonary artery catheters. Facilities for postoperative intensive care including ventilatory support and the availability of haemofiltration and dialysis are also likely to improve outcome. Sepsis and contamination of body cavities are the major reasons for failure in these cases, and such complications will be minimized by the use of broad spectrum, systemic antibiotics, together with antibiotic lavage of peritoneal and pleural cavities and the raising of defunctioning stomas and placement of drains where necessary.

For the future, the current explosion of interest in laparoscopic abdominal surgery will no doubt bring about a laparoscopic approach to diagnosis in some of these cases and also to the treatment of, for example, acute perforation of anterior duodenal ulcers. Indeed, this has already been carried out in some centres, although it is perhaps more difficult to see what role it will have to play in the management of perforation of other regions of the gastrointestinal tract. It is also possible that the prophylactic use of cytoprotective prostaglandin El analogues in selected patients on NSAIDs (for example, those who become symptomatic during treatment with NSAIDs or who have a previous history of peptic ulceration) might influence the current increase in perforations of the upper gastrointestinal tract related to the ingestion of NSAIDs. However, the indiscriminate use of prostaglandin El analogues in all patients on NSAIDs would have very major financial implications for the NHS and cannot be justified on currently available evidence. Patients with non-instrumental perforation of the gastrointestinal tract will continue to provide major diagnostic and management challenges well into the future and may constitute an increasing proportion of the emergency workload of most general surgeons.

REFERENCES

Archampong EQ (1985) Tropical diseases of the small bowel. *World Journal of Surgery* **9**: 887–896.

Auguste LJ & Wise L (1981) Surgical management of perforated diverticulitis. *American Journal of Surgery* **141**: 122–127.

Badia JM, Sitges-Serra A, Pla J, Rague JM, Roqueta F & Sitges-Creus A (1987) Perforation of colonic neoplasms: a review of 36 cases. *International Journal of Colorectal Disease* **2**: 187–189.

Bell KE, McKinstry CS & Mills JOM (1987) Iopamidol in the diagnosis of suspected upper gastro-intestinal perforation. *Clinical Radiology* **38**: 165–168.

Blackett RL (1990) Perforated duodenal ulcer and benign gastric outlet obstruction. *Surgery* **1(81)**: 1924–1927.

Boey J, Lee NW, Koo J, Lam PHM, Wong J & Ong GB (1982a) Immediate definitive surgery for perforated duodenal ulcer. *Annals of Surgery* **196**: 338–344.

Boey J, Wong J & Ong GB (1982b), A prospective study of operative risk factors in perforated duodenal ulcers. *Annals of Surgery* **195**: 265–269.

Brewer LA, Carter R, Mulder GA & Stiles QR (1986) Options in the management of perforations of the esophagus. *American Journal of Surgery* **152**: 62–69.

Brown MW, Brown RC & Orr G (1986) Pneumoperitoneum complicating endoscopy in a patient with duodenal and jejunal diverticula. *Gastrointestinal Endoscopy* **32**: 120–121.

Brown RC, Langman MJS & Lambert PM (1976) Hospital admissions for peptic ulcer during 1958–1972. *British Medical Journal* **i**: 35–37.

Campbell JR & Knapp RW (1966) Small bowel ulceration associated with thiazide and potassium therapy: review of 13 cases. *Annals of Surgery* **163**: 291–296.

Cappell MS, Sciales C & Biempica L (1989) Esophageal perforation at a Barrett's ulcer. *Journal of Clinical Gastroenterology* **11**: 663–666.

Clark CG, Fresini A, Araujo JGC, Moore F & Boulos P (1985) Truncal vagotomy and drainage: a comparison of elective and emergency operations. *British Journal of Surgery* **72**: 149–151.

Coggon D, Lambert P & Langman MJS (1981) Twenty years of hospital admission for peptic ulcer in England and Wales. *Lancet* **i**: 1302–1304.

Collier DStJ & Pain JA (1985) Perforated gastric ulcer. A reappraisal of the role of biopsy and oversewing. *Journal of the Royal College of Surgeons of Edinburgh* **30**: 26–29.

Flynn AE, Verrier ED, Way LW, Thomas AN & Pellegrini CA (1989) Esophageal perforation. *Archives of Surgery* **124**: 1211–1215.

Fulton DJ, Peebles SE, Smith GD & Davie JW (1989) Unrecognised viscus perforation in the elderly. *Age and Ageing* **18**: 403–406.

Gibney EJ (1989) Typhoid perforation. *British Journal of Surgery* **76**: 887–889.

Gillen P, Ryan W, Peel ALG & Devlin HB (1986) Duodenal ulcer perforation: the effect of H₂ antagonists? *Annals of the Royal College of Surgeons of England* **68**: 240–242.

Greenstein AJ, Gennuso R, Sachar DB & Aufses AH Jr (1987) Free perforation due to cancer in Crohn's disease. *International Journal of Colorectal Disease* **2**: 201–202.

Hackford AW, Schoetz DJ Jr, Coller JA & Veidenheimer MC (1985) Surgical management of complicated diverticulitis: the Lahey Clinic experience, 1967–1982. *Diseases of the Colon and Rectum* **28**: 317–321.

Johnston D (1986) Duodenal ulcer. *Surgery* **1(39)**: 930–935.

Jordan PH (1982) Proximal gastric vagotomy without drainage for treatment of perforated duodenal ulcer. *Gastroenterology* **83**: 179–183.

Kakar A, Aranya RC & Nair SK (1983) Acute perforation of the small intestine due to tuberculosis. *Australian and New Zealand Journal of Surgery* **53**: 381–383.

Killingback M (1983) Management of perforative diverticulitis. *Surgical Clinics of North America* **63**: 97–115.

Kovalcik PJ & Sustarsic DL (1981) Cecal diverticulitis. *American Surgeon* **47**: 72–73.

Krukowski ZH & Matheson NA (1988) Ten year computerised audit of infection after abdominal surgery. *British Journal of Surgery* **75**: 857–861.

Krukowski ZH, Al-Sayer HM, Reid TMS & Matheson NA (1987) Effect of topical and systemic antibiotics on bacterial growth kinesis in generalised peritonitis in man. *British Journal of Surgery* **74**: 303–306.

Langman MJ (1987) The changing face of peptic ulceration. *Scandanavian Journal of Gastroenterology Supplement* **136**: 37–40.

Lanng C, Palnaes Hansen C, Christensen A, Thagaard CS, Lassen M, Klaerke A, Jonnesen H & Ostgaard SE (1988) Perforated gastric ulcer. *British Journal of Surgery* **75**: 758–759.

Lee DH, Lim JH, Ko TY & Yoon Y (1990) Sonographic detection of pneumoperitoneum in patients with acute abdomen. *American Journal of Roentgenology* **154**: 107–109.

Lee HS, Lamaute HR, Pizzi WF, Picard DL & Luks FI (1990) Acute gastroduodenal perforations associated with use of crack. *Annals of Surgery* **211**: 15–17.

Luvuno FM (1990) Role of intra-operative prograde colonic lavage and a decompressive loop ileostomy in the management of transmural amoebic colitis. *British Journal of Surgery* **77**: 156–159.

Madure JA & Fiore AC (1983) Reanastomosis of a Hartmann rectal pouch. *American Journal of Surgery* **145**: 279–280.

Matheson NA (1989) Management of obstructed and perforated large bowel carcinoma. *Balliere's Clinical Gastroenterology* **3**: 671–697.

Mischinger HJ, Bergen A, Kronberger L & Fellbaum C (1989) Spontaneous small bowel perforation: a rare cause of acute abdomen. *Acta Chirurgica Scandinavica* **155**: 593–599.

Moghissi K (1988) Instrumental perforations of the oesophagus. *British Journal of Hospital Medicine* **39**: 231–236.

Nagorney DM, Adson MA & Pemberton JH (1985) Sigmoid diverticulitis with perforation and generalized peritonitis. *Diseases of the Colon and Rectum* **28**: 71–75.

Newhouse KE, Lindsey RW, Clark CR, Lieponis J & Murphy MJ (1989) Esophageal perforation following anterior cervical spine surgery. *Spine* **14**: 1051–1053.

Orringer MB & Stirling MC (1990) Esophagectomy for esophageal disruption. *Annals of Thoracic Surgery* **49**: 35–42.

Peel ALG & Raimes SA (1988) Perforation of the stomach. In RCG Russell (ed.), *Recent Advances in Surgery*, vol. 13. Edinburgh: Churchill Livingstone.

Peoples JB, Vilk DR, Maguire JP & Elliott DW (1990) Reassessment of primary resection of the perforated segment for severe colonic diverticulitis. *American Journal of Surgery* **159**: 291–293.

Radcliffe AG & Dudley HAF (1983) Intraoperative antegrade irrigation of the large intestine. *Surgery, Gynecology and Obstetrics* **156**: 721–723.

Raimes SA & Devlin HB (1987) Perforated duodenal ulcer. *British Journal of Surgery* **74**: 81–82.

Ramirez OM, Hernandez-Pombo J & Marupundi SR (1983) New technique for anastomosis of the intestine after the Hartmann's procedure with the end-to-end anastomosis stapler. *Surgery, Gynecology and Obstetrics* **156**: 366–368.

Schein M, Gecelter G, Freinkel Z & Gerding H (1990) Apache II in emergency operations for perforated ulcers. *American Journal of Surgery* **159**: 309–313.

Schoetz DJ Jr (1990) Colonic perforation. In Williamson RCN & Cooper MJ (eds), *Emergency Abdominal Surgery. Clinical Surgery International*, vol. 17. Edinburgh: Churchill Livingstone.

Schrock TR, Deveney CW & Dunphy JE (1973) Factors contributing to leakage of colonic anastomoses. *Annals of Surgery* **177**: 513–518.

Smithwick RH (1942) Experiences with surgical management of diverticulitis of the sigmoid. *Annals of Surgery* **115**: 969–985.

Soreide O, Bjerkeset T & Fossdal JE (1977) Pseudo-obstruction of the colon (Ogilvie's Syndrome): a genuine clinical condition? *Diseases of the Colon and Rectum* **20**: 487–491.

Steinheber FU (1985) Ageing and the stomach. *Clinics in Gastroenterology* **14**: 657–688.

Sugarbaker PH (1981) Carcinoma of the colon: prognosis and operative choice. *Current Problems in Surgery* **18**: 753–826.

Taylor H (1957) The non-surgical treatment of perforated peptic ulcer. *Gastroenterology* **33**: 353–368.

Thomas WEG (1990) Complications of small bowel diverticula. In Williamson RCN & Cooper MJ (eds), *Emergency Abdominal Surgery. Clinical Surgery International*, vol. 17. Edinburgh: Churchill Livingstone.

Thomas WEG & Williamson RCN (1985) Enteric ulceration and its complications. *World Journal of Surgery* **9**: 876–886.

Underwood JW & Marks CG (1984) The septic complications of sigmoid diverticular disease. *British Journal of Surgery* **71**: 209–211.

Van Nooten G, Azagra JS, Alle JL, Deuvaert FE, de Paepe J, Jacobs D, Osmani A & Primo G (1987) Spontaneous rupture of the esophagus after coronary artery bypass. *Acta Chirurgica Belgica* **87**: 367–370.

Wara P, Sorensen K, Berg V & Amdrup E (1981) The outcome of staged management of complicated diverticular disease of the sigmoid colon. *Acta Chirurgica Scandinavica* **147**: 209–214.

Watkins RM, Dennison AR & Collin J (1984) What has happened to perforated peptic ulcer? *British Journal of Surgery* **71**: 774–776.

Williams TG (1984) Oesophageal rupture. *Surgery* **1(14)**; 320–322.

Wilson-MacDonald J, Mortensen NJMcC & Williamson RCN (1985) Perforated gastric ulcer. *Postgraduate Medical Journal* **61**: 217–220.

Wolff BG, Ready RL, McCarty RL, Dozois RR & Beart RW Jr (1984) Influence of sigmoid resection on progression of diverticular disease of the colon. *Diseases of the Colon and Rectum* **27**: 645–647.

Yellin A, Schachter P & Lieberman Y (1989) Spontaneous transmural rupture of the esophagus—Boerhaave's Syndrome. *Acta Chirurgica Scandinavica* **155**: 337–340.

INDEX